Oxford Medical Publications

Cognition in schizophrenia

Cognition in schizophrenia

Impairments, importance, and treatment strategies

Edited by

Tonmoy Sharma

Department of Psychological Medicine, Institute of Psychiatry, London, UK

And

Philip Harvey

Professor of Psychiatry and Chief Psychologist, Mt Sinai Hospital, New York, USA

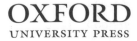

List of Contributors

Abi-Saab, W. Department of Psychiatry, Yale University School of Medicine, New Haven, CT, USA

Addington, J. Department of Psychiatry, University of Calgary, Calgary, Alberta, Canada.

Anand, A. Department of Psychiatry, Yale University School of Medicine, New Haven, CT, USA

Belger, A. Department of Psychiatry, Yale University School of Medicine, New Haven, CT, USA

Blyler, C.R. Maryland Psychiatric Research Center, Department of Psychiatry, University of Maryland School of Medicine, P.O. Box 21247, Baltimore, MD 21228, USA

Braff, D.L. Department of Psychiatry, University of California, San Diego, 9500 Gilman Drive, La Jolla, CA 92093-0804, USA

Cadenhead, K.S. Department of Psychiatry, University of California, San Diego, 9500 Gilman Drive, La Jolla, CA 92093-0804, USA

Charney, D.S. Department of Psychiatry, Yale University School of Medicine, New Haven, CT, USA

Chou, J.C.-Y. Nathan Kline Institute for Psychiatric Research, Department of Psychiatry, New York University School of Medicine, New York, USA

David, A.S. Institute of Psychiatry and GKT School of Medicine, London SE5 8AF, UK

D'Souza, C. Department of Psychiatry, Yale University School of Medicine, New Haven, CT, USA

Friedman, J.I. Department of Psychiatry, Mount Sinai School of Medicine, Box 1230, One Gustave Levy Place, New York, NY 10029, USA

Gold, J.M. Maryland Psychiatric Research Center, Department of Psychiatry, University of Maryland School of Medicine, P.O. Box 21247, Baltimore, MD 21228, USA

Goldberg, T.E. Clinical Brain Disorders Branch, NIMH/NIH, Bethesda, MD 20892, USA

Green M.F. UCLA Department of Psychiatry and Biobehavioral Sciences, Department of Veterans Affairs, VISN 22 Mental Illness Research, Education, and Clinical Center, Los Angeles, CA 90024-1759, USA

Gur, R.C. University of Pennsylvania Medical Center, Neuropsychiatry Section, Department of Psychiatry, Philadelphia, PA 19104-4283, USA

Harvey, P.D. Department of Psychiatry, Box 1229, Mt. Sinai School of Medicine, New York, NY 10029, USA

Heaton, R.K. Department of Psychiatry, University of California, San Diego, CA, USA

Kee, K.S. UCLA Department of Psychiatry and Biobehavioral Sciences, Department of

Veterans Affairs, VISN 22 Mental Illness Research, Education, and Clinical Center, Los Angeles, CA 90024-1759, USA

Keefe, R.S.E.   Box 3270, Duke University Medical Center, Durham, NC 27710, USA

Kern, R.S.   UCLA Department of Psychiatry and Biobehavioral Sciences, Department of Veterans Affairs, VISN 22 Mental Illness Research, Education, and Clinical Center, Los Angeles, CA 90024-1759, USA

Krystal, J.H.   Department of Psychiatry, Yale University School of Medicine, New Haven, CT, USA

Madonick, S.   Department of Psychiatry, Yale University School of Medicine, New Haven, CT, USA

McGurk, S.R.   Department of Psychiatry, The Mount Sinai School of Medicine, New York, NY 10029, USA

Moelter, S.T.   Neuropsychology Program, Drexel University, Philadelphia, PA 19104-4283, USA

Moghaddam,B.   Department of Psychiatry, Yale University School of Medicine, New Haven, CT, USA

Mueser, K.T.   Departments of Psychiatry, and Community and Family Medicine, New Hampshire-Dartmouth Psychiatric Research Center, 105 Pleasant Street, Concord, NH 03301, USA

Palmer, B.W.   Department of Psychiatry, University of California, San Diego, CA, USA

Phillips, M.L.   Institute of Psychiatry and GKT School of Medicine, London SE5 8AF, UK

Powchik, P.   CNS Pharmaceuticals, Sepracor, Inc., Marlborough, MA 01752, USA

Ragland, J.D.   University of Pennsylvania Medical Center, Neuropsychiatry Section, Department of Psychiatry, Philadelphia, PA 19104-4283, USA

Robertson, M.J.   UCLA Department of Psychiatry and Biobehavioral Sciences, Department of Veterans Affairs, VISN 22 Mental Illness Research, Education, and Clinical Center, Los Angeles, CA 90024-1759, USA

Sergi, M.J.   UCLA Department of Psychiatry and Biobehavioral Sciences, Department of Veterans Affairs, VISN 22 Mental Illness Research, Education, and Clinical Center, Los Angeles, CA 90024-1759, USA

Serper, M.R.   Department of Psychology, Hofstra University, and Department of Psychiatry, New York University School of Medicine, New York, 10016, USA

Sharma, T.   Section of Cognitive Psychopharmacology, Institute of Psychiatry, DeCrespigny Park, Denmark Hill, London SE5 8AF, UK

Weickert, T.W.   Clinical Brain Disorders Branch, NIMH/NIH, Bethesda, MD 20892, USA

Wykes, T.   Institute of Psychiatry, King's College, London, SE5 8AF, UK

1 The course of cognitive impairment in patients with schizophrenia

Thomas W. Weickert and Terry E. Goldberg

Introduction

Although a vast literature pertaining to neuropsychological deficits in schizophrenia has amassed over the past 45 years, the exact timing and course of the neuropsychological deficits remains obscure. Some authors have provided evidence for a decline of intellect from premorbid levels subsequent to the onset of schizophrenia, while others have failed to obtain evidence for such a decline of intellect. Finally, some studies have suggested that patients with schizophrenia suffer severe cognitive and intellectual damage early in their development, while other studies would, by inference, imply that there is no basis for such severe cognitive deficits early in the development of patients with schizophrenia. The focus of this chapter will be to review the literature pertaining to the nature and extent of cognitive deficits in schizophrenia including studies pertaining to the presence or absence of intellectual decline in an effort to synthesize these disparate findings into a unified description of the course of cognitive impairment in schizophrenia.

General intellectual decline

Numerous investigators have described a decline in the intellectual abilities of patients with schizophrenia subsequent to the onset of disease. In a small sample of 10 hospitalized patients with schizophrenia, Rappaport and Webb (1950) obtained an average deficit of 33 points between pre- and postmorbid measures of Intelligence Quotient (IQ). In a group of US Armed Forces inductees who went on to develop schizophrenia, Lubin *et al.* (1962) observed declines from premorbid cognitive levels ranging between 0.17 and 0.3 standard deviation units. In a group of Canadian armed forces servicemen who went on to develop schizophrenia subsequent to their initial testing, Schwartzman and Douglas (1962) demonstrated a 15.2 point decline between pre- and postmorbid intellectual levels.

In a group of 63 hospitalized patients with schizophrenia, Nelson *et al.* (1990) observed significant differences between present and premorbid estimates of IQ. Premorbid estimates of IQ have been used routinely as a means of comparing current cognitive deficits with prior intellectual ability or potential before the onset of illness. These premorbid estimates are based upon the traditional belief that certain neuropsychological tests are sensitive to brain damage (the so-called 'no hold' tests) while others remain insensitive (the so-called 'hold' tests, for example the ability to read and pronounce words which is usually acquired at an early age). Several studies have demonstrated the validity of using reading and pronunciation tests as estimates of premorbid intellectual ability in patients with schizophrenia. Dalby and Williams (1986) demonstrated that although there were high correlations between reading and intelligence in normal controls, average reading ability was contrasted with lower intellectual levels in patients with schizophrenia. Nelson *et al.* (1990) also obtained premorbid intellect estimates in patients with schizophrenia that were significantly below the average for normal. Additionally, the findings of Kremen *et al.* (1996) further supported the construct of 'hold' versus 'no hold' tests in patients with schizophrenia by showing similarities between spelling and reading scores while current IQ and arithmetic scores represented relative deficits from spelling and reading.

In a group of 57 hospitalized patients with schizophrenia, Goldberg *et al.* (1993a) obtained differences between a premorbid measure of IQ (reading words) and current 'postmorbid' IQ levels. In monozygotic twin pairs discordant for schizophrenia, Goldberg *et al.* (1995) have demonstrated an IQ discrepancy in which the unaffected twin scored on average 10 points higher than the affected twin. This finding suggests that the genetic potential of the twin with schizophrenia would be 10 points above their current IQ score. Additionally, in a group of first-episode psychotic adolescent inpatients, Goldberg *et al.* (1988a) also observed a significant difference between performance IQ scores and reading relative to a control group of non-psychotic adolescents.

Although the finding of intellectual decline after the onset of disease is common in studies of schizophrenia, it is by no means exclusive. In a group of patients with schizophrenia, Albee *et al.* (1963) were unable to obtain evidence of a deficit between pre- and postmorbid measures of IQ. More recently, based on a sample of 34 patients with schizophrenia displaying low pre- and postmorbid IQ scores, Russell *et al.* (1997) suggested that any deficit in the intellectual function of patients with schizophrenia is due to an early decline which pre-dates the onset of disease.

The results of Albee *et al.* (1963) and Russell *et al.* (1997) may be interpreted alternatively as reflecting a sampling bias since only low functioning individuals were studied, which may have influenced the outcome. The Albee *et al.* sample was drawn from inner city students, while patients in the Russell *et al.* study were drawn from a population of children who had received treatment at a child psychiatry clinic due to behavior and learning problems, of which a substantial minority were already psychotic. These limitations, however, do not obviate the fact that some patients with schizophrenia manifest obvious cognitive limitations from early in development (Torrey *et al.*, 1994).

Evidence for severe early developmental cognitive impairment

Numerous reports document low premorbid IQ scores in children who later developed schizophrenia (Lane and Albee, 1964, 1965; Offord and Cross, 1971; Offord, 1974; Jones and Offord, 1975; Nelson *et al.*, 1990). This would suggest that early developmental anomalies might be responsible for the cognitive impairment observed in schizophrenia. In a meta-analysis of the research pertaining to the premorbid intelligence of patients with schizophrenia, Aylward *et al.* (1984) determined that the premorbid intelligence of children with schizophrenia is below that observed in normal children that do not go on to develop schizophrenia. In a birth cohort study in which 4746 people born in Great Britain during one week of 1946 were followed up to 16 years of age, Jones *et al.* (1994) have shown that those participants that went on to develop schizophrenia displayed low premorbid levels of educational achievement, retardation in the attainment of neuromotor developmental milestones and premorbid speech abnormalities. Effect sizes ranged between 0.37 and 0.51 for mathematics, 0.26 and 0.60 for non-verbal abilities and between 0.33 and 0.60 for verbal abilities. In another birth cohort study, a small but significant diminution in the intellect of patients with schizophrenia was observed prior to onset of psychotic symptoms (Crow *et al.*, 1995). In a large population-based cohort of Swedish army conscripts, David *et al.* (1997) reported that a higher frequency of patients that went on to develop schizophrenia displayed low premorbid IQ scores (<96) relative to non-psychotic individuals.

Additionally, other studies (Taylor and Abrams, 1984; Braff *et al.*, 1991; Goldstein and Shemansky, 1995) make a strong case that there are groups or clusters of patients with schizophrenia who display rather severe and diffuse cognitive impairments in adulthood which, at least in some patients, may have existed before the emergence of diagnostic symptoms. On the basis of a cluster analysis, Goldstein and Shemansky (1995) identified a group of severely cognitively impaired patients with schizophrenia whose cognitive performance was indistinguishable from the performance of dementia patients. Braff *et al.* (1991) provided evidence that patients with schizophrenia displayed diffuse neuropsychological deficits encompassing multiple cognitive domains. Finally, Taylor and Abrams (1984) obtained marked to severe cognitive impairment that encompassed all cortical regions with the exception of the non-dominant temporal cortex in a group of patients with schizophrenia.

Evidence for minimal cognitive impairment

In stark contrast to studies that report severe and extensive cognitive deficits in patients with schizophrenia, several studies have characterized groups of relatively high functioning patients with schizophrenia. On a circumscribed battery of neuropsychological tests, Schwartz (1967) obtained similar performances in college-educated patients with schizophrenia and normal controls. Thirty one percent of the 54 patients with schizophrenia who were administered the Wechsler Adult Intelligence Scale (WAIS) in the Dudek (1969) study had a Full-Scale IQ (FSIQ) in the range of 120–140. More recently, on the basis of a cluster analysis of the neuropsychological data obtained from 186 patients with schizophrenia, Goldstein and Shemansky (1995) were able to identify a high functioning group of patients. Finally, Palmer *et al.* (1997) reported a subgroup of 27% from a study of 171 patients with schizophrenia whose neuropsychological performance, inclusive of IQ, was indistinguishable from the performance of a normal control group. Results from these studies clearly suggest that there is also a subgroup of patients with schizophrenia who do not experience intellectual decline or severe cognitive impairment before or after the onset of illness.

Variation of cognitive abilities in schizophrenia

The inconsistencies present in the literature may be due to the inclusion of non-representative samples and a focus on specific neuropsychological variables pertinent to the specific hypotheses being tested. In a recent study (Weickert *et al.*, in press), we assessed a sample of 117 chronic, hospitalized patients with schizophrenia who were admitted consecutively to a tertiary care research facility. Furthermore, these patients were characterized on the basis of preserved or compromised intellectual abilities in an attempt to clarify the nature and extent of cognitive deficits manifest in schizophrenia. Thus, we assessed premorbid intellect in addition to measuring neuropsychological function in a variety of cognitive domains, such as memory, attention, working memory and perception. All participants were administered a four-subtest version of the Wechsler Adult Intelligence Scale-Revised (WAIS-R), consisting of the Arithmetic, Digit Symbol Substitution Test (DSST), Picture Completion and Similarities subtests, in order to obtain an estimate of their current FSIQ as described by Missar *et al.* (1994) and Kaufman (1990). Additionally, all participants received the Reading subtest of the Wide Range Achievement Test-Revised (WRAT-R) in order to obtain an estimate of premorbid intellectual levels. As noted above, the Reading subtest of the WRAT-R is thought to reflect preserved abilities since it is a test of decoding skills which are acquired routinely prior to the onset of disease and appear to remain unaffected by the disease process in analogous fashion to the 'hold' subtests of the WAIS-R (Dalby and Williams, 1986; Nelson *et al.*, 1990; Kremen *et al.*, 1996). We specifically sought to answer the following questions: (i) is there a pattern of intellectual change from before to after illness onset that is characteristic of schizophrenia; and (ii) what are the nature and extent of cognitive deficits in patients with schizophrenia?

Based on previous findings, an attempt was made to divide the sample of patients with schizophrenia into two groups as follows.

(i) To define a group of patients that undergo *intellectual deterioration* from premorbid levels as defined by a drop of at least 10 points from the premorbid IQ estimate. We used 10 points as a cut-off because it was about one standard deviation from the mean difference score in our control sample.

(ii) Identify a group of patients that do not undergo *intellectual deterioration* from premorbid levels as defined by a drop of <10 points, no change or a slight increase from premorbid IQ estimate. The non-declining group was subdivided further based on previous findings and our own clinical observation as follows:

    (a) Specify a group of *premorbidly compromised* patients defined as exhibiting premorbid IQs below 90 and no decline in current IQ from the premorbid level.

    (b) Describe a *cognitively preserved* group defined as exhibiting premorbid IQs above 90 and no decline in current IQ from the premorbid level.

At first glance, this scheme may appear arbitrary, as it would necessarily be inclusive. However, there was no *a priori* reason to suggest that the proportions of patients that met criteria for these three subgroups would differ by chance.

The results of our study demonstrate a decline of intellectual abilities occurring with psychotic symptoms in half of the chronic inpatients sampled. Therefore, this intellectually

Diagnostic subtype, symptoms and age of onset

With respect to relationships between clinical symptoms and intellectual stability, those individuals classified as disorganized on the basis of clinical interview were somewhat more likely to experience a decline in intellect from premorbid levels. While we did not find differences between our groups with respect to negative symptoms displayed during the entire course of the disease, we recognize that our measure was related to the presence or absence of symptoms and not to severity of symptoms. A select positive symptom, auditory hallucinations, was found to occur at the highest frequency in the premorbidly compromised group. Additionally, patients experiencing later manifestation of cognitive deficits, the intellectually deteriorated group, displayed an increased frequency of delusional thinking.

Furthermore, we found a lack of a differential age of onset between the groups, especially with respect to the premorbidly compromised group. This would suggest that even though the disease may manifest itself non-specifically as cognitive deficits relatively early in development, the psychotic features are not triggered until later, usually in early adulthood. Thus, the organization and activational changes that initiate the cognitive deficits may not always be related directly to the initiation of the psychotic features of the disease. Alternatively, because all of our patients were chronic and to some degree treatment refractory, we may have been unable to detect differences in age of onset because of cohort effects.

IQ and schizophrenia

Although the decline in IQ of the intellectually deteriorated group involved to some degree the four subtests of the WAIS-R, the measures that are thought to demand more working memory, DSST and Arithmetic, appear to be more severely affected. Interestingly, with respect to WAIS-R measures, in our study even the cognitively preserved patient group differed from the normal control group only on the basis of their Age Scaled Scores on the WAIS-R DSST (though FSIQ did not differ). The DSST is thought to be an indicator of working memory integrity in so far as it involves self-monitoring, the brief maintenance of information including that of locations, and oculo-motor scanning (Wilson *et al.*, 1993). Thus, IQ does not reflect simply a unitary function, but, as has been demonstrated repeatedly, is comprised of multiple factors. In particular, IQ does not decline *en masse*, but rather the freedom from distractibility or working memory factor appears to be most susceptible to the core neurobiological disturbance underlying schizophrenia.

Overall, we believe that these results may be interpreted from at least two broad perspectives. First, they could be viewed as reflecting a severity dimension in which the premorbidly compromised group is most impaired with widespread cortical involvement (as evidenced by deficits in most cognitive domains), and the intellectually preserved group is least impaired with specific and circumscribed alteration in frontal system function (evidenced by working memory and attention deficits). On the other hand, it is possible that the groups are genetically and/or environmentally distinct, involving different neural trajectories that manifest themselves via different cognitive courses. They thus would represent valid subtypes of illness. These alternatives cannot be resolved with the available data.

Synthesis of the findings

Results from the current study suggest that the cognitive deficits associated with schizophrenia may emerge along three developmental trajectories based on the degree and timing of impairment of general intellect. One course suggests that the disease process manifests itself as cognitive impairment that may be relatively profound and widespread at an early stage of development and is present subsequent to the onset of psychotic symptoms. These premorbidly compromised patients may have experienced early developmental stressors and/or a genetic predisposition leading to the observed cognitive deficits. A second course suggests that the cognitive deficits may become manifest concurrently with the onset of psychotic symptoms, resulting in a more circumscribed pattern of deficits that encompasses the cognitive domains of executive function, attention and long-term memory. This process is, however, self-limiting, as patients do not go on to a full-blown dementia (for discussions, see Goldstein and Zubin, 1990; Heaton *et al.*, 1994; Hyde *et al.*, 1994; Mockler *et al.*, 1997). This occurs in the presence of intellectual decline. Finally, the third course suggests that while cognitive impairment may be concurrent with symptom onset, the debilitating cognitive deficits associated with the disease process may be relatively subtle, being restricted to the domains of executive function/working memory and attention. It is unclear whether the deficits in this group precede symptoms or emerge concurrently.

Furthermore, based on these findings, it would appear that deficits associated with the function of the prefrontal cortex, i.e. deficits of executive function/working memory and attention, constitute a necessary and perhaps sufficient type of cognitive impairment in schizophrenia. With the exception of the DSST of the WAIS-R, the number of categories attained on the WCST and correct responding on the CPT were the only cognitive measures that provided significant differences between the cognitively preserved group of patients and the normal control group. As such, these deficits can be considered to be 'core' cognitive deficits in schizophrenia.

References

Albee, G.W., Lane, E.A., Corcoran, C. and Werneke, A. (1963) Childhood and intercurrent intellectual performance of adult schizophrenics. *Journal of Consulting Psychology*, **27**, 364–366.

Aylward, E., Walker, E. and Bettes, B. (1984) Intelligence in schizophrenia: meta analysis of the research. *Schizophrenia Bulletin*, **10**, 430–459.

Braff, D.L., Heaton, R., Kuck, J. *et al.* (1991) The generalized pattern of neuropsychological deficits in outpatients with chronic schizophrenia with heterogenous Wisconsin Card Sorting Test results. *Archives of General Psychiatry*, **48**, 891–898.

Buchanan, R.W., Strauss, M.E., Kirkpatrick, B., Holstein, C., Breier, A. and Carpenter. W.T., Jr (1994) Neuropsychological impairments in deficit vs nondeficit forms of schizophrenia. *Archives of General Psychiatry*, **51**, 804–811.

Buchanan, R.W., Strauss, M.E., Breier, A., Kirkpatrick, B. and Carpenter, W.T., Jr (1997) Attentional impairments in deficit and nondeficit forms of schizophrenia. *American Journal of Psychiatry*, **154**, 363–370.

Crow, T.J., Done, D.J. and Sacker, A. (1995) Childhood precursors of psychosis as clues to its evolutionary origins. *European Archives of Psychiatry and Clinical Neuroscience*, **245**, 61–69.

Dalby, J.T. and Williams R. (1986) Preserved reading and spelling ability in psychotic disorders. *Psychological Medicine*, **16**, 171–175.

David, A.S., Malmberg, A., Brandt, L., Allebeck, P. and Lewsi, G. (1997) IQ and risk for schizophrenia: a population based cohort study. *Psychological Medicine*, **27**, 1311–1323.

DeWolfe, A.S., Barrell, R.P., Becker, B.C. and Spaner, F.E. (1971) Intellectual deficit in chronic schizophrenia and brain damage. *Journal of Consulting and Clinical Psychology*, **36**, 197–204.

Donnelly, E.F. (1984) Neuropsychological impairment and associated intellectual functions in schizophrenic and other psychiatric patients. *Biological Psychiatry*, **19**, 815–824.

Dudek, S.Z. (1969) Intelligence, psychopathology, and primary thinking disorder in early schizophrenia. *Journal of Nervous and Mental Disease*, **148**, 515–527.

Elliott, R., McKenna, P.J., Robbins, T.W. and Sahakian, B.J. (1995) Neuropsychological evidence for frontostriatal dysfunction in schizophrenia. *Psychological Medicine*, **25**, 619–630.

Evans, J.J., Chua, S.E., McKenna, P.J. and Wilson, B.A. (1997) Assessment of dysexecutive syndrome in schizophrenia. *Psychological Medicine*, **27**, 635–646.

Fey, E.T. (1951) The performance of young schizophrenics and young normals on the Wisconsin Card Sorting Test. *Journal of Consulting Psychology*, **15**, 311–319.

Frith, C. (1996) Neuropsychology of schizophrenia: what are the implications of intellectual and experiential abnormalities for the neurobiology of schizophrenia? *British Medical Bulletin*, **52**, 618–626.

Gold, J.M., Hermann, B.P., Randolph, C., Wyler, A.R., Goldberg, T.E. and Weinberger, D.R. (1994) Schizophrenia and temporal lobe epilepsy: a neuropsychological analysis. *Archives of General Psychiatry*, **51**, 265–272.

Goldberg, T.E., Karson, C.N., Leleszi, J.P. and Weinberger, D.R. (1988a) Intellectual impairment in adolescent psychosis: a controlled psychometric study. *Schizophrenia Research*, **1**, 261–266.

Goldberg, T.E., Kelsoe, J.R., Weinberger, D.R., Pliskin, N.H., Kirwin, P.D. and Berman, K.F. (1988b) Performance of schizophrenic patients on putative neuropsychological tests of frontal lobe function. *International Journal of Neuroscience*, **42**, 51–58.

Goldberg, T.E., Gold, J.M., Greenberg, R. *et al.* (1993a) Contrasts between patients with affective disorders and patients with schizophrenia on a neuropsychological test battery. *American Journal of Psychiatry*, **150**, 1355–1362.

Goldberg,, T.E., Torrey, E.F., Gold, J.M., Ragland, J.D., Bigelow, L.B. and Weinberger, D.R. (1993b) Learning and memory in monozygotic twins discordant for schizophrenia. *Psychological Medicine*, **23**, 71–85.

Goldberg, T.E., Torrey, E.F., Gold, J.M. *et al.* (1995) Genetic risk of neuropsychological impairment in schizophrenia: a study of monozygotic twins discordant and concordant for the disorder. *Schizophrenia Research*, **17**, 77–84.

Goldstein, G. and Shemansky, W.J. (1995) Influences on cognitive heterogeneity in schizophrenia. *Schizophrenia Research*, **18**, 59–69.

Goldstein, G. and Zubin, J. (1990) Neuropsychological differences between young and old schizophrenics with and without associated neurological dysfunction. *Schizophrenia Research*, **3**, 117–126.

Heaton, R., Paulsen, J.S., McAdams, L.A. *et al.* (1994) Neuropsychological deficits in schizophrenics: relationship to age, chronicity and dementia. *Archives of General Psychiatry*, **51**, 469–476.

Hyde, T.M., Nawroz, S., Goldberg, T.E. *et al.* (1994) Is there cognitive decline in schizophrenia? A cross-sectional study. *British Journal of Psychiatry*, **164**, 494–500.

Jones, M.B. and Offord, D.R. (1975) Independent transmission of IQ and schizophrenia. *British Journal of Psychiatry*, **126**, 185–190.

Jones, P., Rodgers, B., Murray, R. and Marmot, M. (1994) Child developmental risk factors for adult schizophrenia in the British 1946 birth cohort. *Lancet*, **344**, 1398–1402.

Kaufman, A.S. (1990) *Assessing Adolescent and Adult Intelligence*. Allyn and Bacon, Needham, MA.

Kremen, W.S., Seidman, L.J., Faraone, S.V., Pepple, J.R., Lyons, M.J. and Tsuang, M.T. (1996) The '3 R's' and neuropsychological function in schizophrenia: an empirical test of the matching fallacy. *Neuropsychology*, **10**, 22–31.

Lane, E.A. and Albee, G.W. (1964) Early childhood intellectual differences between schizophrenic adults and their siblings. *Journal of Abnormal and Social Psychology*, **68**, 193–195.

Lane, E.A. and Albee, G.W. (1965) Childhood intellectual differences between schizophrenic adults and their siblings. *American Journal of Orthopsychiatry*, **35**, 747—753.

Lubin, A., Gieseking, C.F. and Williams, H.L. (1962) Direct measurement of cognitive deficit in schizophrenia. *Journal of Consulting Psychology*, **26**, 139–143.

Mirsky, A.F., Lochhead, S.J., Jones, B.P., Kugelmass, S., Walsh, D. and Kemdler, K.S. (1992) On familial factors in the attentional deficit in schizophrenia: a review and report of two new subject samples. *Journal of Psychiatric Research*, **26**, 383–403.

Missar, C.D., Gold, J.M. and Goldberg, T.E. (1994) WAIS-R short forms in chronic schizophrenia. *Schizophrenia Research*, **12**, 247–250.

Mockler, D., Riordan, J. and Sharma, T. (1997) Memory and intellectual deficits do not decline with age in schizophrenia. *Schizophrenia Research*, **26**, 1–7.

Nelson, H.E., Pantelis, C., Carruthers, K., Speller, J., Baxendale, S. and Barnes, T.R. (1990) Cognitive functioning and symptomatology in chronic schizophrenia. *Psychological Medicine*, **20**, 357–365.

Offord, D.R. (1974) School performance of adult schizophrenics, their siblings and age mates. *British Journal of Psychiatry*, **125**, 12–19.

Offord, D.R. and Cross, L.A. (1971) Adult schizophrenia with scholastic failure or low IQ in childhood. *Archives of General Psychiatry*, **24**, 431–436.

Palmer, B.W., Heaton, R.K., Paulsen, J.S. *et al.* (1997) Is it possible to be schizophrenic yet neuropsychologically normal? *Neuropsychology*, **11**, 437–446.

Paulsen, J.S., Heaton, R.K., Sadek, J.R. and Perry, W. (1995) The nature of learning and memory impairments in schizophrenia. *Journal of the International Neuropsychological Society*, **1**, 88–99.

Rappaport, S. and Webb, W. (1950) An attempt to study intellectual deterioration by premorbid and psychotic testing. *Journal of Consulting Psychology*, **14**, 95–98.

Russell, A.J., Munro, J.C., Jones, P.B., Hemsley, D.R. and Murray, R.M. (1997) Schizophrenia and the myth of intellectual decline. *American Journal of Psychiatry*, **154**, 635–639.

Schwartz, S. (1967) Cognitive deficit among remitted schizophrenics: the role of a life-history variable. *Journal of Abnormal Psychology*, **72**, 54–58.

Schwartzman, A.E. and Douglas, V.I. (1962) Intellectual loss in schizophrenia: part I. *Canadian Journal of Psychology*, **16**, 1–10.

Servan-Schreiber, D., Cohen, J.D. and Steingard, S. (1996) Schizophrenic deficits in the processing of context: a test of a theoretical model. *Archives of General Psychiatry*, **53**, 1105–1112.

Sullivan, E.V., Shear, P.K., Zipursky, R.B., Sagar, H.J. and Pfefferbaum, A. (1994) A deficit profile of executive, memory, and motor functions in schizophrenia. *Biological Psychiatry*, **36**, 641–653.

Taylor, M.A. and Abrams, R. (1984) Cognitive impairment in schizophrenia. *American Journal of Psychiatry*, **141**, 196–201.

Torrey, E.F., Bowler, A.E., Taylor, E.H. and Gottesman, I.I. (1964) *Schizophrenia and Manic–Depressive Disorder*. Harper Collins, NY.

Vrtunski, P.B., Simpson, D.M., Weiss, K.M. and Davis, G.C. (1986) Abnormalities of fine motor control in schizophrenia. *Psychiatry Research*, **18**, 275–284.

Watson, C.G. (1965) WAIS profile patterns of hospitalized brain-damaged and schizophrenic patients. *Journal of Clinical Psychology*, **21**, 294–295.

Weickert, T.W., Goldberg, T.E., Gold, J.M., Bigelow, L.B., Egan, M.F. and Weinberger, D.R. in press. Differential patterns of cognitive impairment in patients with schizophrenia displaying perserved and compromised intellect. *Archives of General Psychiatry*.

Weinberger, D.R. (1987) Implications of normal brain development for the pathogenesis of schizophrenia. *Archives of General Psychiatry*, **44**, 660–669.

Wilson, F.A.W., Scalaidhe, S.P.O. and Goldman-Rakic, P.S. (1993) Dissociation of object and spatial processing domains in primate prefrontal cortex. *Science*, **260**, 1955–1958.

happened a few seconds before, and are therefore no longer physically present. Although there were numerous models of memory developed in the 1960s, the prototypic model was the modal model (Atkinson and Shiffrin, 1968), which assumed that long-term learning depends on holding information in a temporary short-term storage system until it is transferred to a long-term storage system. The term 'working memory' may have been used first by Atkinson and Shiffrin (1968), referring to the notion that this type of memory storage system was necessary for the performance of many other cognitive tasks, such as long-term memory and learning, and was thus active and working. However, these early models generally were refuted by data suggesting that long-term learning was possible without short-term learning.

In 1972, Craik and Lockhart suggested that the durability of a memory trace depended on the manner in which the stimulus was coded. The deeper the encoding, the more durable the memory. At about the same time, Baddeley and Hitch (1974) developed the notion underlying the currently accepted definition of working memory. They noticed that subjects were able to perform digit-span tasks at their full capacity while performing other tasks. Although performance declined slightly, the degree of disruption was far less than expected. They thus suggested that the idea of a single unitary short-term memory was inadequate, and proposed a system of working memory that serves temporarily to hold and manipulate information during the performance of a range of cognitive tasks such as comprehension, learning and reasoning.

According to the Baddeley model, general working memory (WMG) refers to the temporary storage of information that is being processed in any of a range of cognitive tasks. WMG is differentiated from specific working memory (WMS), which describes a model of the structures and processes involved in performing the tasks requiring WMG. In the model, a number of subsystems are controlled by a limited capacity executive system. The supervisory controlling system is referred to as the central executive. This system, which Baddeley later revised to incorporate Norman and Shallice's (1980) supervisory attentional system, is aided by two 'slave' systems, one which is specialized for processing language material (*the articulatory loop*) and the other which is concerned with visuospatial memory (*the visuospatial sketchpad*). The central executive is viewed as having attentional capacities, and is capable of selecting and operating control processes. The Baddeley model was limited to visual and auditory stimuli, and did not include systems for maintaining stimuli from tactile, olfactory and gustatory sensory systems. Very little work has been completed on these systems.

While Baddeley and Hitch's original notion has been pursued in thousands of studies since its conception, controversies remain. Baddeley (1986) assumed that the concept of a working memory implies a common system that operates across a wide range of tasks. Others disagreed. Allport (1980) and Barnard (1985) assumed the presence of a series of interacting yet relatively independent subsystems, and argue against the notion of a unitary working memory. As detailed below, this controversy has been pursued by researchers attempting to determine the specific aspects of working memory dysfunction in schizophrenia.

The notion of a single limited-capacity working memory would need to be supported by data suggesting that: (i) the capacity of the system is indeed limited, and (ii) absorbing a substantial amount of the available processing capacity should have broadly comparable effects across a range of different cognitive tasks. The WMG model predicts that performance will deteriorate substantially if a substantial amount of capacity is used by a supplementary task. One of the key characteristics of a working memory task may be the assessment of performance on a primary task such as problem solving, while simultaneously performing a secondary task such as recalling words or digits (Daneman and Carpenter, 1980). The cognitive process of maintaining the information from the primary task 'in mind' while conducting the secondary task is the core of working memory functioning. If the secondary task disrupts the primary one, this is attributable to the limitations of the working memory system.

The components of the working memory system

The phonological loop

There is substantial evidence for the presence of a temporary phonological storage system that relies on a fading trace which can be maintained by subvocal rehearsal (Baddeley *et al.*, 1975; Vallar and Baddeley, 1982). There are two components of the phonological loop (Baddeley and Lewis, 1981; Baddeley, 1992a): a phonological store that can hold acoustic or speech-based information for 1–2 s, and an articulatory control process, described by Baddeley (1992a) as analogous to inner speech in that it involves some form of acoustic image that is independent of articulation. Baddeley's studies of deaf and mute subjects suggest that the ability to speak is not essential for phonological encoding or subvocal rehearsal.

The presence and characteristics of the phonological loop subsystem can be determined by four well-established effects (Baddeley, 1992a; Baddeley, 1992b; Salame *et al.*, 1998). The first is that visually presented phonemes that sound similar to one another will be recalled more poorly than phonemically different items (Conrad, 1964). For example, subjects will be able to recall different-sounding words such a 'pit, day, cow, pen' better than similar-sounding words, such as 'man, cap, can, map'. Thus, verbal information presented visually is coded into a speech-based phonemic form. The second effect is that immediate memory span is correlated directly with the length of time taken to rehearse the items to be remembered. Long words are recalled less well than short ones because they need more time to be rehearsed (Baddeley *et al.*, 1975). The third effect is referred to as 'articulatory suppression' (Baddeley, 1986). Repeatedly uttering a redundant word such as 'the' prevents the to-be-remembered items from being rehearsed, and significantly reduces the length of the material that can be recalled (Levy, 1971). Lastly, simple listening to speech-based material impairs the immediate recall of visually presented items (Salame and Baddeley, 1982). This effect is assumed to occur because speech-based and visual to-be-remembered material compete for space in the phonological store (Salame and Baddeley, 1989). The phonological loop is thus a speech-based system, and is assumed to be called upon for tasks requiring the temporary manipulation and limited storage of a finite number of items (Salame *et al.*, 1995).

The visuospatial sketchpad

Baddeley described the visuospatial sketchpad as a temporary storage system for generating and manipulating visuospatial images. The term 'sketchpad' is used to imply that the system is used in much the same way as a pad of paper might be used by someone attempting to work out a geometric puzzle. Baddeley's original interest in this aspect of working memory derived from an experience he had attempting to listen to an American football game while driving along a California highway. He found that as the visual images of the game intensified, his steering became more erratic and he felt the need to switch to a less hazardous music radio station. Baddeley's misfortune of being unable to process these tasks simultaneously (listening to football games is not one of the leading causes of road accidents in the US) was science's fortune. He applied his highway experience to a laboratory experiment that required subjects to complete a pursuit rotor tracking task (keeping a stylus on a certain circular path along a turntable) while they maintained the shapes of upper case letters in mind so that they could describe aspects of the letters' shape. The spatial letter processing task disrupted tracking performance, while a verbal task had minimal effect (Baddeley and Hitch, 1974). Tracking performance could also be impaired by requiring subjects to keep spatial words (e.g. above, below, left and right) maintained in working memory during the task. Non-spatial words (e.g. good, bad, slow and quick) had no effect on tracking performance. Further work suggested that the spatial working memory system is not modality specific, in that a non-visual tracking test (blindfolded subjects follow a beeping pendulum with a flashlight) will disrupt a visuospatial working memory test more than will a simple visual task (Baddeley and Lieberman, 1980). Other work (e.g. Byrne, 1974; Carpenter and Just, 1977) similarly has suggested that the spatial components of a task such as reading verbal material have a greater impact on simultaneously performed spatial tasks than the visual components of the task have on simultaneous visual tasks. However, a heavy spatial component is not an essential feature of the operation of the visuospatial working memory system (Logie, 1986).

More recent conceptualizations of visuospatial working memory have included two components: a passive visual temporary store (a visual cache) responsible for temporary retention of visual properties of objects and scenes, and an active spatially based rehearsal mechanism (an inner scribe) responsible for planning and controlling movement (Reisberg and Logie, 1993; Logie, 1995). It has been suggested that generation of action is dependent upon visuospatial working memory functions as well as more general executive functions (Salway and Logie, 1995).

Perhaps the most important development in the relevance of working memory functions to schizophrenia has been the clarification of the neural systems that mediate working memory in humans and non-human primates. In a series of elegant studies of non-human primates, Goldman-Rakic and her colleagues have traced the neural networks that mediate various working memory functions, including visuospatial (e.g. Goldman-Rakic, 1987), visual object working memory (Wilson et al., 1993) and auditory–spatial working memory. While these different working memory functions have been found to be mediated by slightly different neural circuits, all of them in some way involve the operations of the prefrontal cortex. Initial functional imaging studies of working memory functions in humans have suggested that the circuitry that mediates working memory is homologous in human and non-human primates (McCarthy et al., 1994; McCarthy, 1995). Human brain activation during working memory tasks is widespread and varies depending upon the stimuli that are being held in mind. Similarly to non-human primates, consistent activation of the dorsolateral prefrontal cortex

(DLPFC) is found independently of the content of the stimuli (summarized in Frith and Dolan, 1996).

Many studies of working memory in humans have followed the methodology originally developed by Goldman-Rakic in her series of studies on non-human primates. In the visuo-spatial version of these working memory tests, a monkey is trained to fixate on a stimulus in the middle of a computer screen. A very brief visual stimulus is presented to peripheral vision. In the sensory-guided condition, the monkey immediately looks to where the stimulus was, indicating its ability to identify its location in space. In the memory-guided condition, the monkey is trained not to move his eyes to the stimulus, but rather to look to where the stimulus had been presented following a delay period, thus expressing his ability to keep the peripheral visual stimulus in mind. The delay period used varies across studies, but is usually between 3 and 10 s.

There are at least two subcomponents of the sketchpad: pattern- or object-based and spatial. In her early review of the data, Farah (1988) concluded that spatial and visual working memory functions may be functionally and anatomically separable. More recent anatomical studies support different dimensions of the sketchpad, possibly composed of object-based and spatial components (Wilson *et al.*, 1993). These two working memory systems appear to correspond anatomically to the dorsal and ventral 'streams' of neural connections originating at posterior regions (occipital and temporal regions for object perception and occipital and parietal regions for spatial stimuli) and feeding forward to the prefrontal cortex. The spatial working memory functions in non-human primates are mediated by regions of the DLPFC different from those mediating object working memory functions (Wilson *et al.*, 1993). Early human imaging studies also support these divisions (McCarthy, 1995).

The central executive or supervisory attentional system (SAS)

The supervisory attentional system (SAS) regulates the allocation of resources toward the phonological loop and the visuospatial sketchpad in addition to any other cognitive system that is involved in processing information 'on-line'. The SAS is assumed to have a limited capacity. It is called upon in a variety of circumstances, including the following: (i) tasks that involve planning or decision making; (ii) situations in which the automatic processes appear to be running into difficulties, necessitating troubleshooting of some sort; (iii) tasks that involve novel or poorly learned sequences; (iv) situations that are judged to be dangerous or technically difficult; and (v) situations in which a strong habitual response or temptation is involved or needs to be avoided (Baddeley, 1986).

Many complex tasks require SAS functioning. The series of 'Tower' tasks, which differ more in terms of the city from which they are said to derive than their methodology, are in many ways classic tests of the SAS. The Tower tasks, such as the Tower of London, require subjects to move disks on pegs from one arrangement to another in the smallest number of steps. Thus, Tower tasks require subjects to keep in mind the goal arrangement while initiating the steps along the way and deciding whether those movements are proceeding toward the goal arrangement in the expected manner.

Many 'dual tasks' also require the functioning of the SAS. In a classic dual task, subjects are required to perform two tasks simultaneously, such as repeating aloud lists of words while performing a visual Continuous Performance Test (Serper *et al.*, 1990;Granholm *et al.*, 1991). The Wisconsin Card Sorting Test (WCST) certainly requires some of the functions that fall under the umbrella of 'supervisory attention', as it demands that the subject change his strategy in response to feedback, make decisions and resist strategies that are attractive yet ineffective. However, the WCST also requires a variety of other functions that are not considered to be in the domain of working memory (Keefe, 1995).

Working memory deficits in schizophrenia

A large number of studies have demonstrated that working memory functions are impaired in patients with schizophrenia. These impairments are not attributable to treatment with antipsychotic medication (reviewed below) or anticholinergic treatment of extrapyramidal symptoms (Granholm *et al.*, 1997; Pantelis *et al.*, 1997; Salame *et al.*, 1998). Studies of working memory in schizophrenic patients have often varied considerably in the tasks used to assess working memory functions. Thus, the description of the working memory tasks will be detailed. Only those studies that have used a definition of working memory consistent with the literature reviewed above will be included.

Phonological loop impairment in patients with schizophrenia

One of the first methods for assessing the phonological loop, which has also been referred to as 'verbal working memory' is the Brown–Peterson paradigm. In these tasks, subjects are presented with verbal stimuli and then engage in a distraction task for brief periods of time until they are given a signal to recall the original verbal stimuli. The verbal stimuli are subject to decay (Brown, 1958) unless updated by the workings of the phonological loop, including vocal maintenance rehearsal (Morris, 1986).

Patients with schizophrenia perform less well than controls on Brown–Peterson tasks. In a study using a design that required subjects to recall consonant trigrams after delays of 0, 3, 9 and 18 s, schizophrenic patients performed less well than normal or psychiatric controls (Stuss *et al.*, 1982). Interestingly, schizophrenic patients without frontal leukotomy performed less well than patients who had received leukotomy. In a study using a Brown–Peterson paradigm in which words were recalled following a 12 s interval filled with various levels of distraction, schizophrenic patients were found to recall fewer words than normals following complex distraction such as counting and repeating serial 3s, but not following finger tapping (Fleming *et al.*, 1995). Thus, the degree of demand on the capacity of the phonological loop had a direct impact on the extent of the impairment in the patients with schizophrenia.

The phonological loop has also been assessed with the Letter–Number Test, originally devised by Gold *et al.* (1997), and incorporated into the most recent versions of both the Wechsler Adult Intelligence Scale (WAISIII) and the Wechsler Memory Scale (WMS-3). In this test, subjects listen to series of letter–number combinations of increasing length, beginning with one letter and one number, and increasing to four letters and four numbers. Subjects are required to recite the letter–number sequences in the following order: the numbers first, lowest to highest, followed by the letters in alphabetical order. Thus, the stimulus 8G2U would require a response of '28GU'. Schizophrenic patients perform significantly less well than normal controls on this test. One of the drawbacks of using this measure to assess the phonological loop specifically is that it may involve the visuospatial sketchpad as well. Performance on this task may be improved if subjects rearrange the stimuli for this task by using visuospatial images.

In the Item Recognition Test (Sullivan *et al.*, 1997; originally developed from Sagar *et al.*, 1988), subjects are required to read from 233 index cards presented serially with a noun printed on each card. At random times throughout the series, patients are asked whether they have seen a word before. Recognition of words presented two cards prior to the question is considered an index of working memory functioning. One of the advantageous features of this test is that an analogous visual task has been designed using colored wallpaper swatches consisting primarily of geometric shapes. In this task, recognition of items presented 3–50 cards earlier was considered to be a measure of longer term memory. Schizophrenic patients perform far less well on the working memory components of this test than on the long-term memory measures (Sullivan *et al.*, 1997).

The Sentence Span Test (Leahy, 1987), developed for clinical populations based on the Reading Span Test (Daneman and Carpenter, 1980), measures memory for the final words in serial sentences that are presented in sets of gradually increasing size (two sets of two sentences each; two sets of three sentences; three sets of four; three sets of five; three sets of six; three sets of seven; one set of eight). An individual's sentence span is the largest set size for which all final words are recalled correctly. Subjects are advised that they will hear a series of sentences after which they will be asked to recall the final word of each sentence in each set. Performance on this test has been found to be impaired in patients with schizophrenia (Condray *et al.*, 1996).

The relative dysfunction of schizophrenic patients on verbal and non-verbal auditory working memory tests was determined by Wexler *et al.* (1998). The verbal working memory test was the Word Serial Position Test. Subjects heard four words spoken by the experimenter. Following delays of 1, 5 or 9 s, the subject was presented with one of the words, and asked to indicate the word's serial position. The non-verbal auditory working memory test was similar except that three different tones were presented. Following the same delay periods, subjects were presented with one of the tones, and were required to indicate its serial position. Patients performed significantly less well on the verbal working memory task. Patients who could perform at normal levels at discriminating the tones did not perform significantly less well than controls on the non-verbal working memory test. These results argue for the dissociation of verbal and non-verbal auditory working memory systems, and suggest that only the verbal auditory working memory system is impaired in schizophrenia.

Visuospatial sketchpad impairment in patients with schizophrenia

Several studies have been completed demonstrating impairment of visuospatial working memory in patients with schizophrenia (Park and Holzman, 1992; Keefe *et al.*, 1995), although normal performance has been reported (Kolb and Whishaw, 1983).

Much of the work investigating impairment in the visuospatial sketchpad in patients with schizophrenia has followed some form of the delayed response task. Human analogs of

Goldman-Rakic's methodology have been used to demonstrate that patients with schizophrenia have severely impaired visuospatial working memory. Park and Holzman (1992) used an oculomotor working memory test that required human subjects either to look immediately to a black circle presented on a computer monitor or to wait after a 5 or 30 s delay period to look to the location where the stimulus had been presented. During the delay period, to prevent verbal rehearsal of the location of the stimuli (i.e. preventing the functioning of the articulatory loop), subjects performed word categorization or digit subtraction tests. The location of eye position was measured to determine the subject's ability to recall the position of the stimuli. The performance of the schizophrenic patients during the delayed recall conditions was worse than that of normal controls and patients with bipolar illness. A haptic version of the task, requiring subjects to recall the physical location of where they had placed their finger behind a curtain, also revealed spatial working memory deficits in the patients with schizophrenia, suggesting that the spatial working memory impairment in schizophrenia is not limited to the visual modality. In later work, Park and McTigue (1997) assessed working memory using a computerized task requiring subjects to point with a finger to where on the screen a black dot had been presented. The working memory impairment in schizophrenia persisted using this methodology. The consistency of working memory impairment independent of the response methodology is consistent with the non-human primate literature suggesting that dorsolateral prefrontal cortex lesions induce working memory deficits whether the tasks require oculomotor (Funahashi *et al.*, 1993) or manual (Goldman and Rosvold, 1970) responses.

Various other computerized tests of working memory functions have been developed. The following method has been developed by Carter *et al.* (1996) to measure visuospatial working memory: subjects sit before a computer monitor, fixated on a central cross. A small 'probe' stimulus appears for 150 ms at one of 12 locations along a radius 9° eccentric to fixation. The screen is then blank and, after either 0 or 8000 ms, an array of 18 letters appears, one of which marks the location of the probe. Subjects are required to respond by identifying the letter that marks the location at which the probe appeared. Two blocks of 24 trials are completed, with 12 trials in each block at each delay period. Schizophrenic patients demonstrated a greater increase in errors during the delayed trials, indicating a visuospatial working memory deficit.

Work from our laboratory has suggested that the working memory impairment in patients with schizophrenia can be observed with simple pen-and-paper tests such as the 'Dot Test' (Keefe *et al.*, 1995, 1997). For the no-delay trials of this task, subjects were presented with a solid black dot, 0.5 cm in diameter, on a piece of standard white paper. Simultaneously, they were given an entirely blank sheet of paper and were instructed to copy the dot on the blank paper in the same location as the dot they saw on the stimulus page. No-delay performance for each trial was calculated by measuring the distance between the actual dot and the subject's mark. The performance over the 14 copying trials was averaged to determine an overall no-delay score. For the delayed recall trials, the procedure described above was repeated with the following exceptions: following the 5 s presentation of the dot, subjects were presented with a list of words to read aloud in order to inhibit verbal mediation of stimulus location memory during the delay period; after the delay period, subjects were asked to make a mark where they remembered the dot to have been. Over two separate studies, delay periods of 10, 20 and 30 s were used. Schizophrenic patients were able to perform at normal levels for the no-delay copying trials, but performed significantly less well than normals in each of the delay conditions. Thus, marking a piece of paper is as sensitive as an oculomotor assessment task in identifying working memory deficits in schizophrenia. In a separate study comparing the pen-and-paper method of the Dot Test with oculomotor measurement, we found that many of the patients with schizophrenia were unable to complete the computerized oculomotor task (Keefe *et al.*, 1996). In those patients who were able to complete both the eye movement and pen-and-paper versions of the paradigm, performance on each of the tests was significantly correlated.

Visuospatial working memory was assessed by Salame *et al.* (1998) with a pattern span task. In this task, subjects were presented with increasingly complex patterns of black and white squares. After each presentation, subjects were required to reproduce the pattern on a blank card. Schizophrenic patients had significantly reduced pattern span compared with normal controls (7.05 ± 0.23 versus 5.55 ± 0.32; $F1,38 = 14.29$; $P < 0.0006$).

The sketchpad was assessed by Stratta *et al.* (1997) by placing two sets of 12 identical cards from the WCST (1–4 red triangles, 1–4 green stars, 1–4 blue circles) face down in a random sequence in a 4 by 6 matrix. Subjects turned two cards at a time in order to find the location of each card and its identical 'match'. Compared with normal controls, schizophrenic patients required significantly more trials and more time to form the 12 matches.

The methods of Spindler *et al.* (1997) combined computerized and pen-and-paper components, requiring subjects to fixate on a cross in the center of a computer screen while a sequence of black dots was presented on the screen for 250 ms per dot. The number of dots presented sequentially on the screen increased incrementally from two to seven. Following the dot sequence presentation and a 3 s delay, subjects were given a sheet of paper on which they indicated at which of the eight locations the dots had been presented. Subjects received two trials of each stimulus length, and the test was stopped when subjects failed both trials of any given length. Two analogous tests were used to assess object working memory. In the color condition, dots of different colors were presented in the same manner as in the spatial condition, and subjects pointed to the colors of the dots following the delay period. In the shapes condition, irregular shapes were presented instead of colors. In a dual task condition, the presentation of the dots in different locations was followed immediately by the presentation of two of the irregular shapes in the center of the screen. The subject was required to indicate on a piece of paper the location of the dots and the shapes of the figures. Schizophrenic patients performed less well than controls on each of the single presentation working memory tasks, but not on the dual task condition. These results are considered further below in the section on supervisory attentional system deficits in schizophrenia.

This section has served to review the various methods used to assess visuospatial sketchpad functioning in patients with schizophrenia. Although the methods have varied considerably between studies, visuospatial working memory impairment in patients with schizophrenia has been remarkably consistent.

Impairment in the central executive or SAS in schizophrenia

The literature on cognitive deficits in schizophrenia is rich with studies assessing the SAS. Tower tasks such as the Tower of London have been found to be severely impaired in patients with schizophrenia (Pantelis *et al.*, 1997). Although the extent to which the WCST can be seen as utilizing the SAS is controversial, significant and widespread impairment on the WCST in schizophrenic patients is unambiguous (Goldberg *et al.*, 1987; see review by Van der Does and Van den Bosh, 1992). In fact, Kraepelin's notion of a frontal cortex dysfunction in schizophrenia received much of is momentum in the 1980s based upon the poor performance and hypoactivation of the prefrontal cortex in schizophrenic patients during the WCST (Weinberger, 1987).

More recent work on SAS impairment in patients with schizophrenia has targeted more specific functions of resource allocation as outlined by Baddeley (1986, 1992a) and Norman and Shallice (1980). These studies have yielded important data regarding the relative dysfunction in schizophrenia of the SAS and 'slave' systems.

The functioning of the central executive in patients with schizophrenia was assessed by Bressi *et al.* (1996) with the use of a dual task paradigm. The primary task was a tracking task in which subjects followed a square on a computer monitor with a light pen. The difficulty level of the tracking test was calibrated based upon each subject's ability. During tracking, subjects were exposed to a series of increasingly interfering secondary tasks: articulatory suppression, foot-press reaction time to tones; and digit span. Schizophrenic patients performed progressively less well than normals with increasing interference. Thus, schizophrenic patients appear to manifest increasingly poor motor performance as processing demands are placed on the SAS.

The relative dysfunction of the visual working memory system and the SAS in schizophrenia was assessed with tests of visuospatial working memory, working memory for shapes, working memory for colors and dual-task versions of the shapes and location tests (Spindler *et al.*, 1997). Patients performed less well than controls in all conditions, yet their performance in the dual-task conditions was not significantly worse than in each of the single working memory conditions. Although patients performed significantly better than chance on the dual tasks, their performance was very poor (mean = 0.571 out of a possible 12 correct responses), and did not worsen in the dual-task condition, suggesting that either the dual-task condition did not provide an additional processing load to test the supervisory attentional system, or that floor effects were present in that the schizophrenic patients could not reasonably do less well than they had in the single-task working memory conditions. Thus, the impairment of the SAS relative to the visuospatial sketchpad was not measured adequately.

The relationship of the phonological loop and the SAS in schizophrenic patients was assessed by Tracy *et al.* (1998) by relating performance on the Auditory Consonant Trigrams Test to performance on tests of time estimation. One test measured time interval production (i.e. 'tell me when 15 s has elapsed'). The other test measured time interval estimation (i.e. after a specific time period is demarcated for the subject, he is asked 'how much time elapsed?'). The tasks were completed either in isolation or in combination with reading aloud during the intervals. The performance of schizophrenic patients on the time interval production test declined more than that of normals when the reading task was added, suggesting impairment of the SAS. Furthermore, dual task performance deficits in schizophrenic patients were significantly correlated with Auditory Consonant Trigrams Test performance, suggesting that deficiencies of the phonological loop may contribute to impaired SAS functioning. In other words, a limited working memory capacity for verbal stimuli may place a greater demand on the SAS, leading to errors in cognitive functions such as time estimation, which require the utilization of the SAS as well as the phonological loop. However, a more parsimonious explanation of the results from this study may be that time estimation tests also place demands on the phonological loop.

All three components of Baddeley's working memory system were assessed in a study of patients with schizophrenia and age- and education-matched controls (Salame *et al.*, 1998). To assess the SAS, a dual task was conducted requiring subjects to perform an oral digit-span task while completing a crossing task consisting of placing crosses into boxes joined along an erratic path on a sheet of paper. The Corsi block task was used to assess visuospatial working memory. This task requires subjects to touch a series of blocks in the same sequence as the experimenter following a brief delay. The phonological loop was assessed through an articulatory suppression test. Subjects were required to recall digits presented visually at the length of their individual span under conditions of: quiet; while listening to reading in Arabic; while listening to noise with intensity variations mirroring the Arabic speech; and while repeating the word 'bla' continuously at an average of 3–4 times per second (articulatory suppression). Performance did not differ significantly between patients and control in the dual task or digit span. Patients performed significantly less well on the Corsi block test, and on all conditions of the serial recall test. The patients were not affected differentially by articulatory suppression, suggesting that patients were equally as effective as normals in ignoring irrelevant information. This study suggested more severe impairments in the visuospatial and phonological slave systems compared with the SAS. While the authors conclude that their pattern of results suggests that working memory impairment in schizophrenia is associated with reduced processing speed, an alternative interpretation may be that schizophrenic patients performed poorly on tests that required a greater time period between the encoding of stimuli and their recall. As has been reported frequently elsewhere (Park and Holzman, 1992), patients had normal digit-span capabilities; however, serial recall tasks that require ongoing processing for several seconds are more vulnerable to impairment. Thus, an inability to maintain information 'on-line' during delay periods may be the hallmark of the working memory deficit in schizophrenia.

In the second experiment of this study, the SAS was assessed with a random letter-generation task. Visuospatial working memory was assessed with a pattern span task. In this task, subjects were presented with increasingly complex patterns of black and white squares. After each presentation, subjects were required to reproduce the pattern on a blank card. The phonological loop was measured by reading rate. Schizophrenic patients systematically deviated from randomness more than controls in the random letter-generation task. They also performed significantly less well than controls on the visuospatial pattern span task and the reading rate task. These results indicated impairments in all aspects of the working memory system. Re-analyses of the first experiment were performed on all tasks after dividing the schizophrenic group into those with a normal reading rate ($n = 14$) and those with a slow reading rate ($n = 6$). In the slow reading patients, all tests of the phonological loop were impaired, including serial recall and digit span, while the normal reading patients performed similarly to the controls. Visuospatial working memory functions were impaired in the slow and fast reading subjects alike. Regarding the SAS, dual task performance was significantly worse in the slow reading patients only. The results from the random generation task were only slightly affected, with slow readers performing less well than fast readers only when letters were generated at 1/s. The authors concluded that reading rate may underlie performance on phonological loop and SAS tests; however, it is very important to note that these results may reflect the differential impact of neuroleptic medications on different patients. Although reported as a non-significant difference, extrapyramidal symptoms, as measured by the Simpson–Angus Scale, differed between groups by two standard deviations (SDs). Thus, the slowness factor may have been mediated more by medication differences than by inherent cognitive difficulties of the six slow readers.

In summary, the few studies to date comparing the relative dysfunction of the visuospatial sketchpad, phonological loop and SAS have yielded conflicting data. The results of these studies have differed substantially due to the differences in the tests chosen to measure the different aspects of the working memory system. While it is likely that all three components of the working memory system are impaired in schizophrenia, the relative impairment of each to the others is uncertain.

Working memory deficits in relatives of schizophrenic patients and individuals with schizotypal symptoms

Deficits on tests of working memory are not limited to patients with full-blown schizophrenia psychosis. The non-psychotic relatives of patients with schizophrenia as well as individuals with schizotypal personality also appear to demonstrate working memory deficits, although normally in a milder form. Interestingly, patients with bipolar disorder (Park and Holzman, 1992) and patients with personality disorders outside of the 'odd cluster' (Lees Roitman et al., 2000) do not demonstrate significant impairment compared with normal controls.

When assessed on Park and Holzman's (1992) oculomotor apparatus, college students who scored high on the Chapmans' inventory – aimed to assess experiences of perceptual aberration – make significantly more visuospatial working memory errors than those college students who had very few or no signs of schizotypy (Park et al., 1995a). However, only ~25% of the students were considered to be in the 'impaired' range. Visuospatial working memory was assessed in 89 undergraduate students using a computerized task requiring subjects to point with a finger to where on the screen a black dot had been presented (Park and McTigue, 1997). Total scores on the Schizotypal Personality Questionnaire (SPQ) (Raine, 1991) were only slightly correlated with working memory performance ($r = 0.14$, $P < 0.10$). Of nine subscales of the SPQ, only one, 'no close friends', was significantly correlated with working memory score ($r = 0.29$, $P < 0.01$)

Individuals with Schizotypal Personality Disorder as defined by the Diagnostic and Statistical Manual for Psychiatric Disorders also demonstrate poorer performance than normal controls and patients with non-odd cluster personality disorder diagnoses on the Dot Test of visuospatial working memory (Lees Roitman et al., 2000). These deficits were not as severe as those found in patients with schizophrenia.

Working memory impairment may even extend beyond the spectrum of schizophrenia-related disorders. The relatives of schizophrenic patients have been found to be impaired on visuospatial working memory tasks (Park et al., 1995b) whether the mode of response is with eye movements or with a manual response. However, these relatives were not assessed for schizotypal personality symptoms, which have also been found to be elevated in the relatives of patients with schizophrenia (Kendler *et al.*, 1981). Thus, the presence of working memory deficits as an expression of the schizophrenia phenotype independent of schizotypal psychopathology has not been established.

Relevance of working memory deficits to schizophrenia

While it is clear that working memory is impaired in schizophrenia, it is not clear to what extent working memory impairment is associated with other aspects of the illness, including the symptoms of the disorder and the wide range of cognitive impairments that are found in most patients with schizophrenia. The recent literature assessing these associations will now be reviewed.

Association with other cognitive deficits

Thus far, clear relationships between 'working memory' as a singular construct and other cognitive deficits in patients with schizophrenia have been elusive. The absence of consistent findings may be due to the absence of a consistent method to measure working memory functions. While measures of the phonological loop and the visuospatial sketchpad both involve the manipulation of information held 'in mind' for brief periods, the differences between these domains may outweigh their similarities. For instance, verbal working memory, as assessed by the Paced Auditory Serial Attention Test, and visuospatial working memory, as measured by the Dot Test, were found to have correlations close to zero in schizophrenic patients and in normal controls (Gold, 1998). Conversely, unpublished data on a small number of schizophrenic subjects in our laboratoy suggest that correlations between the Dot Test and the letter–number span test were high ($r = 0.73$, df $= 7$, $P = 0.027$). These data suggest that the performance of schizophrenic patients on working memory tests may depend upon factors unrelated to pure working memory functions. Even within the visuospatial domain, for instance, it is unlikely that the delayed response deficit can be accounted for by any single cognitive impairment. In a comparison of visuospatial working memory deficits and eye tracking deficits in patients with schizophrenia, response errors that were never corrected were associated with eye tracking abnormalities, while errors attributable to interference from other stimuli were independent of eye tracking deficits (Park and O'Driscoll, 1996).

Association with Wisconsin Card Sorting Test performance

No neurocognitive test has received more attention in schizophrenia research than the WCST. In general, working memory tasks have been found to be correlated with performance on the WCST. Some authors have even referred to this test as a 'working memory test', but there are numerous other cognitive functions measured by the WCST (Keefe, 1995).

Visuospatial working memory has been found to be correlated with various WCST measures. In a sample of 14 schizophrenic patients, Park (1997) reported correlations between oculomotor working memory performance and WCST categories achieved ($r = -0.61$, $P<.05$), number of errors ($r = -0.78$, $P <0.001$) and the number of perseverative errors ($r = -0.58$, $P <0.05$). Similar results were reported by Keefe *et al.* (1995). In this study of 34 patients with schizophrenia, performance on the Dot Test was found not to be correlated with a broad range of neuropsychological measures, yet was significantly correlated with WCST perseverative errors ($r = -0.41$, $P = 0.01$). In contrast, Stratta *et al.* (1997) found no significant correlation between WCST performance and a visuospatial working memory test involving the memory of the location of face-down WCST cards in a 4 by 6 card matrix. This test may have differed from traditional measures of the visuospatial sketchpad in that subjects needed to maintain visuospatial information in mind for minutes at a time. These results suggest that visuospatial working memory deficits in patients with schizophrenia may underlie some performance deficits on the WCST, but that other cognitive factors are also important.

The relationship between the phonological loop and WCST performance was assessed by Gold *et al.* (1997) using the letter–number span test. Although letter–number test performance in schizophrenic patients was associated with several other domains of cognitive functioning, including full-scale IQ, trailmaking, memory, attention and verbal fluency, the correlation with WCST categories was particularly high ($r = 0.74$, $P <0.01$), and was significantly higher than in normal controls. These results suggest that the role of working memory impairment in WCST performance in schizophrenia is not limited to the visuospatial domain. Rather, it suggests that either impairments in both 'slave' systems help to account for WCST deficits, or that general working memory impairment underlies some WCST deficits. Multiple regression techniques used in this study suggested that the letter–number span test accounted for more variance in WCST categories than any other cognitive measure. In fact, the differences between schizophrenic patients and controls on the WCST categories was non-significant when the contribution of the letter–number span test was statistically controlled. However, the obverse was not true; group differences in the letter–number span test remained after the contribution of WCST performance was statistically controlled. Thus, verbal working memory appears to be a significant component of WCST performance, and may account for a major component of the cognitive impairment that accounts for WCST performance in patients with schizophrenia.

Association with planning

Since planning involves complex cognitive operations requiring a number of subprocesses (Luria, 1965), it could be expected that the ability to keep planned operations in mind via working memory functions would underlie performance on tests of planning such as the Tower of London test (Frith and Dolan, 1996). Tower tests require subjects to rearrange, in the minimum number of moves, a set of three colored balls arranged on pegs to attain a final configuration that matches a pre-specified goal (Shallice, 1982).

The relationship between working memory and planning has been investigated in a series of elegant studies using the Cambridge Neuropsychological Test Automated Battery (CANTAB) (Pantelis *et al.*, 1997). The CANTAB includes a computerized working memory test in which subjects are required to search through a number of boxes for hidden tokens. Trials differ in difficulty according to the number of boxes (three, four, six and eight). On each trial, only one box contains a token. The key instruction is that once a token has been found, that box will not be used to hide a token again. Two types of errors are measured: a between-search error occurs when a subject returns to open a box in which a token has already been found; a within-search error occurs when a subject returns to a box already opened in the same sequence. Between-search errors represent shorter term working memory failures; within-search errors are likely to be longer term memory failures. An efficient strategy for performing this task greatly enhances performance (Hutton *et al.*, 1998), suggesting that central executive functions are also being measured with this test.

When performing the tests of the CANTAB, patients with schizophrenia were found to have worse working memory functions than patients with neurological disorders matched for age, sex and National Adult Reading Test (NART) score (Pantelis *et al.*, 1997). The performance of the schizophrenic patients on tests of visuospatial working memory and executive functions (as measured by a 'Tower of London' test) was even worse than that of patients with frontal lobe lesions, and far worse than that of patients with focal temporal lobe lesions. It is noteworthy that the strategies of schizophrenic patients in performing the spatial working memory test were severely impaired, suggesting that executive functions may in some cases underlie the poor working memory performance of patients with schizophrenia. In contrast, working memory performance was not correlated with performance on the Tower of London test, suggesting that the impairments in planning found in the schizophrenic group were not caused by impaired working memory. The results of this study need to be tempered by the fact that the schizophrenic patients were receiving very high doses of typical neuroleptic medication (1401.1 ± 218.6 mg in chlorpromazine equivalents).

The CANTAB was administered to 30 schizophrenic or schizophreniform patients presenting for the first time for psychiatric treatment (22 patients were tested within 8 weeks of starting medication and six within 6 months) and 30 healthy controls matched for NART IQ score. Patients made significantly more between-search errors than controls on the spatial working memory test, which depends upon strategy utilization (>1.5 SDs below the normal mean), and significantly worse on a spatial span test, a computerized Corsi block-type test (~0.75 SD below the normal mean). Spatial memory span was significantly correlated with between-search errors in the patient group only ($r = -0.44$, $P < 0.05$). Interestingly, there was no significant between-group difference in errors on this test if scores were covaried using a score of strategy utilization; conversely, between-group differences remained even after scores were covaried for spatial span. Thus, the impaired visuospatial working memory performance of the patients in this study can be accounted for by the differences between the two groups in their use of a search strategy rather than in their short-term memory capacity as measured by spatial span. These results may derive from the fact that this study used a working memory test for which performance depends heavily upon strategy utilization rather than the pure ability to keep visuospatial information in mind for brief periods of time. Along these same lines, spatial span was found not to underlie performance on a Tower of London test requiring patients to keep in mind a series of moves while carrying them out. These data suggest the primacy of the SAS in other aspects of working memory dysfunction in schizophrenia.

Somewhat inconsistent with these cognitive data are the neuroimaging data reported in a series of studies by Chris Frith and his colleagues at the Institute of Neurology in London, summarized by Frith and Dolan (1996). In these studies, spatial working memory tasks and a Tower of London test activated very similar neural networks. The only difference between the activation patterns was an activation of the rostrolateral frontal cortex during the planning component of the Tower tests. This series of cognitive and neuroimaging studies suggests that the rostrolateral frontal cortex may be an area of particular interest in the investigation of the neuroanatomical dysfunction of schizophrenia.

Relationship to other memory functions

While it would seem that shorter term memory functions such as working memory are fundamental cognitive 'stepping stones' to longer term memory retrieval, a clear relationship between working memory and delayed recall has not been demonstrated. Memory tests can be classified as strategic versus non-strategic in that strategic tests require subjects to develop a strategy for retrieving or manipulating information. Non-strategic tests, such as recognition tests, require explicit retrieval from long-term memory but have little additional reasoning or working memory demands. Tests of free recall require strategic memory in that the subject must develop a plan for arranging the information in order to facilitate retrieval. Stone *et al.* (1998) assessed working memory using a task developed by Salthouse and Babcock (1991). Subjects heard a series of sentences aloud, then immediately were required to answer a simple question about each sentence. At the end of the series of sentences, subjects were asked to recall the last word in a series of sentences. The number of sentences presented on each trial increased successively from one to seven, with three trials presented at each series length. A subject's working memory span was determined by the largest number of sentences with correctly answered questions and correctly recalled last words on at least two of the three trials. A computational analog using one-digit addition and subtraction problems was also used. Schizophrenic patients performed less well than controls on these working memory tests as well as on tests of long-term verbal memory. In analyses of covariance, group differences in working memory capacity could not be accounted for by digit span performance. Between-group differences on all three tests of strategic long-term memory (free recall, memory for temporal order and self-ordered pointing) could be accounted for by working memory capacity. Non-strategic memory, as measured by recognition performance, could not be accounted for by working memory capacity. It is important to note that the task demands of the working memory tests and the strategic memory tests were similar in that they both required the development of strategies for rehearsal and retrieval of information. However, these data suggest that some aspect of working memory functions may underlie long-term memory functions that require strategic recall.

It is possible that the modalities of the stimuli to be recalled are important determinants of the relationship between working memory and delayed recall. Verbal working memory, as measured by the letter–number span, has been found to be related to general memory functions (Gold *et al.*, 1997), yet visuospatial working memory is not related to delayed recall of verbal material (Keefe *et al.*, 1995).

Sullivan *et al.* (1997) demonstrated that when scores were controlled for age and IQ estimated from the NART, the working memory deficits of schizophrenic patients were far more severe than their deficits in longer term memory functions. This finding was remarkably consistent across verbal and visual stimuli, as well as for working memory for the temporal order of the stimuli. In fact, schizophrenic patients performed >4 SDs below the normal mean on a test of working memory for the order of verbal stimuli; their performance on longer term recognition of order was <1 SD below the normal mean. In summary, the relationship between working memory and longer term memory functions is complex and may depend upon the modality of the stimuli and the strategies employed by subjects to encode and retrieve stored information.

Relationship to processing capacity

The relative impact of distractibility and processing capacity on verbal working memory was assessed by Goldberg *et al.* (1998) by administering serial span tasks of either three or six digits to schizophrenic patients and healthy controls. Controls attained 100% accuracy on the three-digits forward test, and nearly 90% accuracy on the six-digits forward tests. Schizophrenic patients attained accuracy rates of 98 and 60% respectively, suggesting that verbal working memory span deficits are more likely to be attributable to processing capacity limitations than attentional deficiencies. In a second experiment, a Brown–Peterson task was used with variable numbers of words (two, four or six) per presentation and variable delay intervals (5, 10 or 15 s). On half of the trials, the experimenter indicated to the subject that he should engage in a color naming task during the delay period. The patients' performances were affected by the interference task to a greater degree than those of the controls, suggesting that schizophrenic patients may rely more heavily than normal controls on covert articulatory rehearsal strategies. When these strategies are disrupted by simple word reading, performance worsened further, suggesting that schizophrenic patients may not be as adept at developing alternative mechanisms to facilitate short-term recall. As the size of the word set increased from two to six, the performance of schizophrenic patients compared with controls worsened at a greater rate, supporting the notion that schizophrenic patients may have limitations in their processing capacity. Taken together, these two experiments suggest that schizophrenic patients do not perform poorly on verbal working memory tests due to a lack of verbal rehearsal; rather, the fundamental deficit may lie in processing capacity limitations or possibly the ability to generate alternative processing strategies. Thus, in Baddeleyian terms, the so-called phonological loop may be relatively intact compared with the dysfunction of the central executive.

Relationship to processing speed

Correlations were demonstrated in schizophrenic patients between working memory as measured by backwards digit span and several different memory measures, including free recall, recognition and encoding (Brebrion *et al.*, 1998). Backwards digit span was also correlated significantly with digit–symbol substitution test performance. However, the relationships between working memory and other memory functions were not significant if they were covaried for processing speed as measured by the digit–symbol substitution test. The relationships between digit–symbol and the memory measures remained significant after they were covaried for digits backwards performance. A significant correlation between a visuospatial working memory task (remembering the location of WCST cards in a 6 by 4 matrix) and digit–symbol performance has also been reported (Stratta *et al.*, 1997). These data suggest that processing speed may be an important factor underlying working memory deficits in schizophrenia.

Relationship to language comprehension

A significant correlation between performance on the Sentence Span Test and language comprehension in patients with schizophrenia was reported by Condray *et al.* (1996). However, only the patient group was analyzed separately in this study; it is likely that this relationship also exists in the general population, and may not be specific to schizophrenia.

Relationship to eye tracking

Within a group of 18 schizophrenic patients, a significant bi-serial correlation has been reported between the quality of eye tracking performance (rated as 'good' or 'impaired') and the accuracy of oculomotor working memory performance ($r = 0.51$, df = 16, $P < 0.05$) (Park and Holzman, 1993).

In summary, poor performance on a variety of tests of working memory has been found to be related to other cognitive deficits in patients with schizophrenia. It is difficult to discern a clear pattern among these correlations; however, tests sensitive to frontal dysfunction appear to be correlated most strongly with working memory functions. This may be due in part to the greater number of studies investigating these particular constructs. In addition, many different cognitive tests require subjects to hold information of some sort (if only the directions for the test procedures) 'on-line' for brief periods of time. The extent to which tests demand information to be maintained in awareness and manipulated may correlate directly with the strength of the correlation with purer tests of working memory.

Association with negative symptoms

Working memory deficits may have a clear clinical impact on negative symptoms in patients with schizophrenia. Patients with working memory deficits may be far more distractable than patients with normal working memory functions. Since they lose awareness of important stimuli, they may attend to irrelevant stimuli with greater frequency. This has an obvious interpersonal impact, as patients who are unable to pay attention to the flow of conversation are more susceptible to social withdrawal. On a larger scale, patients with these types of cognitive deficits will have greater difficulty maintaining social relationships, keeping jobs and functioning independently (Green, 1996).

In a study of 18 schizophrenic patients who had been withdrawn from oral antipsychotic medication for at least 10 days, a significant correlation ($r = 0.50$, df = 16, $P < 0.05$) was reported between visuospatial working memory performance and negative symptoms as measured by either the Negative Symptoms Assessment or the Schedule for the Assessment of Negative Symptoms (Carter *et al.*, 1996).

It is often assumed that cognitive deficits such as working memory deficits are mediated by negative symptoms such as amotivation. I have argued elsewhere that it is likely that the arrow of causality should be pointed in the opposite direction: working memory deficits and other aspects of cognitive dysfunction are likely to be the underlying features of many negative symptoms (Keefe, in press). An example of this relationship is demonstrated by a series of studies conducted by Eric Granholm on pupillary response in patients with schizophrenia.

An index of pupillary response has been used as an indication of whether an individual is engaged sufficiently in working memory tasks (Granholm *et al.*, 1996). Increases in pupil size are associated with increased cognitive processing demands; pupil size begins to decline when the demands of the task exceed the processing resources available. Thus, pupillary responses can be used to determine if an individual is engaged sufficiently in a task to perform adequately. If the working memory deficits of schizophrenic patients were due to lack of interest or motivation, we could expect that their pupillary responses would be low throughout the period of cognitive assessment. However, patients with schizophrenia demonstrate normal pupillary responses during the low processing conditions of a working memory task, namely the recall of four-digit sequences following a 2 s delay period (Granholm *et al.*, 1997). It is only during high processing conditions (recall of 10-digit sequences) that patients with schizophrenia have reduced pupillary responses. These results suggest that schizophrenic patients put in a normal amount of effort during tests of working memory, yet their decreased processing capacity leads them to be unable to engage in difficult tasks.

The working memory deficits of schizophrenia thus do not appear to be accounted for by patients' reduced motivation. It seems likely that the causal relationship between these two factors is in the opposite direction. Patients who have working memory deficits may be less likely to be motivated to have goals and pursue them. Those patients with severe working memory deficits are likely to be met with failure if they attempt to pursue employment, social and even recreational avenues that require cognitive skill. These repeated failures are likely to cause discouragement and reduced motivation even in people without mental illness.

One caveat to the notion that working memory deficits underlie some aspects of negative symptoms is the fact that patients with severe negative symptoms may take longer to perform working memory tests, which will extend the delay period, thus increasing the difficulty of the test for those patients only.

Association with formal thought disorder

By the time a schizophrenic patient with working memory deficits finishes a complicated sentence, it is likely that he will have lost awareness of his original intention. Thus, the speech of patients with working memory deficits will be filled with loose associations and derailments. This notion, described by Rochester (1978) and enriched by Hoffman *et al.* (1986), has been supported recently by empirical data. A correlation of 0.51 between ratings of formal thought disorder and performance on a visuospatial working memory test was reported by Spitzer (1993). Unpublished data from our laboratory support this correlation. We found that formal thought disorder, as rated by the Thought, Language and Communication Scale (Andreasen, 1982), was significantly correlated ($r = 0.65$, df = 21, $P < 0.05$) with visuospatial working memory functions. The fact that this correlation crosses the modality dichotomy between visual and verbal functions supports the notion that in some patients with schizophrenia there is a general system of working memory that fails.

Association with positive symptoms

The relationships between cognitive deficits and positive, or psychotic, symptoms are poorly understood. While the lower reliability of positive symptom assessment is a crucial factor (Strauss, 1993), it has been believed generally that performance on standard neuropsychological tests is not strongly correlated with severity of psychotic symptoms in patients with schizophrenia (Addington *et al.*, 1991; Perlick *et al.*, 1992; Gold and Harvey, 1993; Goldberg *et al.*, 1993; Strauss, 1993). These studies generally have used tests designed to measure cognitive functions in individuals with brain injury following normal premorbid histories; these tests may not be appropriate for the study of the specific cognitive deficits associated with specific psychotic symptoms in schizophrenia (Frith and Done, 1988; Gray *et al.*, 1991; Strauss, 1993).

Several of the psychotic symptoms of schizophrenia suggest that patients with this disorder are unable to monitor the initiation of certain types of self-generated thought (Frith and Done, 1989; Frith, 1992). These symptoms include some of those described by Schneider (1959): thought insertion; passivity experiences such as made actions, made impulses and made feelings; delusions of control; and many hallucinatory experiences. Patients with these symptoms may share a common underlying cognitive deficit, possibly a working memory deficit, in monitoring the generation of their own thoughts, which then results in their conclusion that these self-generated thoughts came from an external source. This deficit has been referred to as autonoetic agnosia, which literally means 'the inability to identify self-generated mental events' (Keefe, 1998).

Autonoetic agnosia has been measured with various experimental cognitive tests, including tests of source monitoring (Hashtroudi *et al.*, 1989), reality monitoring (Johnson and Raye, 1981) and 'generation-effect' paradigms (Slamecka and Graf, 1978; Hirshman and Bjork, 1988). Source monitoring refers to the ability to remember the source of information obtained. In a standard source monitoring paradigm, subjects are asked to discriminate among items of information that either have been presented previously by one of several sources or are new (i.e. have not been presented before). Reality monitoring is a specific kind of source monitoring in which individuals have to remember if information originated from an external source or was self-generated (internal source). For example, some reality monitoring tasks assess an individual's ability to remember whether an event actually occurred or whether it was only imagined (Johnson *et al.*, 1993). The generation-effect refers to the tendency of normal individuals to remember self-generated information better than information that comes from external sources. These paradigms have been used to suggest that autonoetic agnosia is present in patients with schizophrenia, and that it may be associated with specific symptoms. All of these paradigms require that subjects keep this source information 'on-line' for brief periods of time; thus, it is likely that working memory deficits may underlie autonoetic agnosia in schizophrenia.

The relationship between autonoetic agnosia and the specific type of working memory deficit may depend upon the modality of the stimuli being kept in working memory. Deficits in the phonological loop, especially deficits in monitoring stimuli in 'inner speech' described by Baddeley (1992a), may be identified inaccurately as originating from an outside source in the form of a hallucination. Symptoms of thought insertion may originate from deficits in the visuospatial sketchpad or the phonological loop, depending upon the nature of the thought that the patient experiences as 'inserted.' Symptoms such as delusions of passive control reveal the limitations of Baddeley's working memory model. Intentions to initiate movement also require processing, yet are not clearly represented in either of the visuospatial or phonological slave systems. In disagreement with this notion, Salway and Logie (1995) have argued that the intention to produce motor movement is a part of the visuospatial working memory system.

Although the relationship between working memory functions and autonoetic agnosia has not been directly investigated empirically, there is some evidence to suggest that, unlike cognitive deficits in general, working memory functions may be associated with some types of delusions and hallucinations in patients with schizophrenia. A modest correlation has been reported between visuospatial working memory functions and Brief Psychiatric Rating Scale (BPRS)-positive symptoms ($r = 0.46$, $P < 0.08$) (Carter et al., 1996). Similarly, a significant positive correlation between deficits on a test of central executive working memory functions as measured by dual task performance and the severity of positive symptoms has been found ($r = 0.58$, $P < 0.001$) (Bressi et al., 1996). Patients may experience positive symptoms because they are unable to monitor two or more competing events. Thus, when monitoring one event, unmonitored automatic thoughts and physiological changes may seem to arise spontaneously and may be interpreted as coming from an external source in the form of experiences such as hallucinations and thought insertion (Frith and Done, 1988; Keefe, 1998).

In a recent study from our laboratory (Keefe et al., in review), we assessed autonoetic agnosia using a source-monitoring paradigm in 29 patients with schizophrenia and 19 controls. Patients with schizophrenia demonstrated deficits in monitoring the source of self-generated information, yet performed similarly to controls in monitoring the source of information that derived from visual and auditory sources. Schizophrenic patients with specific 'target' symptoms such as auditory hallucinations and thought insertion had greater deficits than patients without these symptoms in recognizing self-generated information. The data from this study support the notion that patients with schizophrenia manifest autonoetic agnosia, and that the relationship between positive symptoms and working memory deficits may depend upon the source of the stimuli being monitored and processed with the working memory system.

The relationship between phonological loop deficits and psychotic symptoms was investigated (Leudar et al., 1992) using the Reporter Test, originally devised by Renzi and Vignolo (1962). This test requires the subject to watch an experimenter carry out a series of operations with colored shapes, and then 'report' verbally what the experimenter is doing. For instance, as the experimenter moves a large red square onto a small white circle, the subject must describe the experimenter's actions accurately, including color, shape, relative size and position of the objects being moved. Patients with schizophrenia have been found to perform less well than normal controls on this test in that they issued more incorrect instructions and more incomplete instructions about the actions of the experimenter (Leudar et al., 1992). Increasing numbers of incorrect and incomplete instructions were associated with poorer performance on backward digit span, but the differences between controls and patients remained even after variance accounted for by the backward digit-span scores was removed.

In the Leudar study, there was no difference between controls and schizophrenia patients without hallucinations in the adequacy of the repair of wrong instructions; the frequency of inadequate repair, however, increased with increasing verbal hallucinations. This result supports Hoffman's (1986) notion that verbal hallucinations are related to discourse disturbances in schizophrenic patients. It is possible, however (consistent with the Baddeley model), that patients experiencing hallucinations during testing may have performed less well because their hallucinations produced a greater processing load (e.g. an additional stress on the articulatory loop). Their discourse error may thus have resulted from their attention to their hallucinations. It is important to note that this type of assessment measures the monitoring of observable behavior, not the monitoring of self-generated thought. As such, it is not directly relevant to the notion of working memory deficits and autonoetic agnosia underlying psychotic symptoms in patients with schizophrenia.

In summary, a few studies have demonstrated correlations between working memory impairment and positive symptoms, in contrast to the absence of such a relationship between positive symptoms and other cognitive deficits. Furthermore, specific cognitive tests aimed at measuring the inability of patients with schizophrenia to monitor self-generated mental events suggests that to the extent that working memory is involved in self-monitoring, it is correlated with the presence of psychotic symptoms.

Imaging studies of working memory in schizophrenia

A large body of literature suggests that prefrontal functions are impaired in patients with schizophrenia. Brain imaging studies using a variety of different tasks sensitive to frontal dysfunction have demonstrated that patients with schizophrenia have reduced activation of the prefrontal cortex (reviewed by Weinberger and Berman, 1996). One of the drawbacks of these studies has been that they have often used standard neuropsychological tests such as the WCST to activate the frontal cortex. For many of these tasks, there are a large number of different cognitive domains active throughout the course of the test (Keefe, 1995). One of the advantages in using working memory tasks to assess frontal dysfunction in schizophrenia is that unlike with the standard neuropsychological tests used previously, working memory tasks involve relatively few disparate cognitive operations. Furthermore, as reviewed by McCarthy (1995), many of these studies have concluded that, similarly to the single-neuron activation studies completed on non-human primates, the prefrontal cortex is very important in mediating working memory functions. Thus, tests of working memory functions are natural tools to determine the nature of prefrontal dysfunction in patients with schizophrenia (Keefe, 1995).

In the few studies completed to date, patients with schizophrenia performing working memory tasks demonstrate reduced activation of the prefrontal cortex. An 'N-back' task was used in a positron emission tomography (PET) study of eight schizophrenic patients and eight controls matched for age, sex and parental education (Carter et al., 1998). During an easy working memory task (zero-back), for which subjects were required to press one of four buttons labeled 1–4 corresponding to the number presented, patients and controls performed similarly. Despite similar performance, patients had less activation of the right DLPFC than the controls. When the working memory load increased to a two-back task, for which subjects were required to press the button corresponding to the numeral that had been presented two numerals prior to the current one, patients' performance worsened more than that of the controls. The increase in activation of the right DLPFC and the posterior parietal cortex associated with greater working memory load was significantly less in the patients than in the controls.

Using a refined functional magnetic resonance imaging (fMRI) methodology, regional activation was assessed by Callicott *et al.* (1998a) in six schizophrenic patients compared with six controls, also using an 'N-back' task. Subjects were matched on the extent of regional activation of motor areas during the cognitive task. Compared with this 'internal activation standard', the patients with schizophrenia had less relative activation of the DLPFC than control subjects. The most recent data from this laboratory, however, suggest that when schizophrenic patients perform at near-normal levels during an N-back task, they have increased frontal activity (Callicott *et al.*, 1998b).

Recent neuroimaging data suggest that the circuitry that mediates verbal working memory tasks may be particularly impaired in patients with schizophrenia. First, normal controls demonstrate increases in DLPFC activation with increases in verbal working memory load, yet patients with schizophrenia demonstrate reductions in DLPFC activation at the higher levels of verbal working memory load (Fletcher *et al.*, 1998). Further, tests of verbal auditory working memory may reveal greater differences than non-verbal auditory working memory tasks in the functioning of the prefrontal cortex in schizophrenic patients (Stevens *et al.*, 1998). The Word Serial Position Task (described above) was used in this study to reveal differences between patients and controls in the inferior frontal gyrus (Brodmann areas 6 and 44). These differences were significantly greater than those produced using the Tone Serial Position Task. These data may suggest that patients with schizophrenia are more likely to have impairment in the neural circuitry that mediates verbal working memory than that for non-verbal auditory working memory tasks.

An investigation of the neural circuitry impairment underlying SAS deficits in schizophrenia was conducted by Andreasen *et al.* (1992). Three different samples were assessed: (i) 13 neuroleptic-naive schizophrenic patients; (ii) 23 non-naive schizophrenic patients who had been relatively chronically ill but were medication free for at least 3 weeks; and (iii) 15 healthy normal volunteers. Regional cerebral blood flow was measured using single-photon emission computed tomography (SPECT) with xenon 133 as the tracer. The control condition consisted of looking at undulating colored shapes on a video monitor, while the experimental task was the Tower of London. The Tower of London activated the left mesial frontal cortex (possibly including parts of the cingulate gyrus) and the right parietal cortex in healthy normal volunteers. Both the neuroleptic-naive and the non-naive patients lacked these areas of activation. Decreased activation occurred only in the patients with high scores for negative symptoms.

In summary, working memory tests have served to support and refine theories of prefrontal dysfunction in schizophrenia. The short duration of working memory trials is ideal for current functional imaging methods. The most recent data from patients with schizophrenia suggest that the relationship between prefrontal activation and performance on working memory tasks is complex. While schizophrenic patients demonstrate reduced prefrontal activation compared with normals at higher levels of working memory load, at reduced loads their activation is normal or even higher than normal. This pattern of results is consistent with the notion that patients with schizophrenia demonstrate a reduced capacity or inefficient strategy for processing information in working memory stores. Thus, the neural circuitry impairments associated with working memory deficits could be attributable to dysfunction of the SAS or the component 'slave' systems. Further work is needed to disentangle the various neural impairments in schizophrenia and how they underlie the different working memory deficits.

Treatment of working memory dysfunction in schizophrenia

If, as has been argued in this chapter, working memory deficits are central to various aspects of the schizophrenia syndrome, then treatment of these deficits would be of utmost importance. Conventional antipsychotics block dopamine receptors in the prefrontal cortex, which has been found to impair working memory functions in non-human primates under normal conditions (Sawaguchi and Goldman-Rakic, 1994). Furthermore, dopamine agonism with bromocriptine improves visuospatial working memory in normal subjects (Luciana *et al.*, 1992). It could thus be expected that conventional antipsychotics would impair working memory functions in patients with schizophrenia. However, an extensive literature has suggested that this is not the case. Conventional antipsychotic medications such as haloperidol do not impair or improve working memory functions in patients with schizophrenia (see reviews by Medalia *et al.*, 1988; Cassens *et al.*, 1990; Goldberg and Weinberger, 1996). However, following conditions of intense auditory stress, intended to mimic human psychopathology, haloperidol serves to protect monkeys from suffering stress-related impairments in visuospatial working memory functions (Arnsten and Goldman-Rakic, 1998). This effect was found with a low dose of haloperidol (0.005 mg/kg), but not with a higher dose (0.01–0.03 mg/kg). Thus, in patients suffering from psychosis, who may have an altered system of dopaminergic transmission (Davis *et al.*, 1991), working memory functions may be relatively unaffected by dopaminergic blockade. Very low doses of dopamine receptor antagonists may be useful in treating working memory impairment in psychotic patients. Higher doses of neuroleptics may be ineffective owing to excessive blockade of dopamine receptors in the prefrontal cortex or impaired striatal function producing response deficits (Arnsten and Goldman-Rakic, 1998).

While there is evidence to suggest that cognitive deficits in general are improved by novel antipsychotic medication, including clozapine, the evidence to support clozapine-related enhancement of working memory functions is weak. In non-human primates, clozapine has been found to reverse spatial working memory deficits induced by excessive dopamine stimulation in the prefrontal cortex (Murphy *et al.*, 1997). However, clozapine reverses FG7142-induced spatial working memory deficits only at lower doses (1–3 mg/kg p.o.); doses in the clinical range (e.g. 6 mg/kg, p.o.) do not improve cognitive function in most animals. These results from non-human primates suggest that the clozapine doses commonly used to treat schizophrenia may not be optimal for treating working memory deficits in these patients.

Clinical data from studies of patients with schizophrenia have supported this prediction.

While one study reported improvement in all cognitive tests, including auditory consonant trigrams, with clozapine treatment (Galletly *et al.*, 1997), other work suggests that treatment with clozapine does not improve verbal working memory as assessed by auditory consonant trigrams (Hagger *et al.*, 1993; Lee *et al.*, 1994) or digits backward (Grace *et al.*, 1996).

Risperidone may improve all three aspects of working memory functions. Risperidone treatment had a greater beneficial effect than haloperidol treatment on verbal working memory as assessed by a digit-span distraction test (Green *et al.*, 1997). The treatment effect remained significant after the effects of adjunctive benztropine treatment, change in psychotic symptoms and change in negative symptoms were controlled. A small but statistically significant risperidone-related improvement has also been reported in schizophrenic patients performing digits backwards (Rossi *et al.*, 1997). Meltzer and McGurk (1999) have suggested that in patients with schizophrenia risperidone may also improve the functioning of the visuospatial sketchpad as measured by a computerized delayed response task similar to that used by Goldman-Rakic with non-human primates. Finally, the performance of patients with schizophrenia on maze tasks, which require intact functioning of the SAS, has been found to be improved with risperidone. Thus, preliminary work indicates that various aspects of working memory may be improved by treatment with risperidone.

While no published studies have assessed the impact of olanzapine, quetiapine, or ziprasidone on working memory, large-scale studies by several different pharmaceutical companies currently are underway to test these effects, and results should be available soon. These studies will also serve to determine the differences among the novel antipsychotics in terms of their ability to improve working memory functions.

Summary and conclusion

This chapter has detailed the various methods that have been used to establish that patients with schizophrenia have working memory impairment. The following conclusions may be made about the data to date.

(i) Patients with schizophrenia demonstrate deficits in all aspects of working memory outlined by Baddeley, including the phonological loop, visuospatial sketchpad and the SAS.

(ii) Although there are conflicting results regarding the relative severity of impairment in the three aspects of working memory according to the Baddeley model, it appears as though the three types of working memory deficit are related to one another. At this point, there are more data to support the notion that an SAS impairment is primary to the deficits of the 'slave' systems, but the trend in this direction is weak.

(iii) Working memory impairment extends beyond patients with full-blown psychotic schizophrenia to less severe points along the schizophrenia spectrum, including patients with schizophrenia-related personalities, and possibly to the non-psychotic biological relatives of schizophrenic patients.

(iv) A host of areas of cognitive dysfunction in patients with schizophrenia appear to be correlated with working memory deficits. Tests sensitive to frontal dysfunction most frequently have been found to be correlated with working memory deficits, yet these are also those that have been investigated most often.

(v) Like other cognitive deficits, working memory impairment appears to be related to negative symptoms and formal thought disorder. I have argued that working memory impairment may indeed underlie some negative symptoms and formal thought disorder. Recent studies also suggest that unlike many other aspects of cognitive dysfunction in schizophrenia, working memory deficits may be associated with positive symptoms, particularly with regard to those positive symptoms that may derive from deficits in self-monitoring.

(vi) Recent functional imaging studies suggest that working memory tasks activate the prefrontal cortex in normal individuals, especially for tasks with high working memory loads. Patients with schizophrenia appear to demonstrate normal or greater than normal activation of the prefrontal cortex when the working memory load is low, yet demonstrate reduced activation compared with normals at high working memory loads.

(vii) While typical antipsychotic medication does little to improve working memory functions, atypical antipsychotic medication appears to improve various aspects of working memory functions in patients with schizophrenia. At the time of the completion of this chapter, risperidone appears to have particular benefit compared with clozapine. Data on the impact of olanzapine, quetiapine and ziprasidone on working memory are not yet available.

References

Addington, J., Addington, D. and Maticka-Tyndale, E. (1991) Cognitive functioning and positive and negative symptoms in schizophrenia. *Schizophrenia Research*, **4**, 123–134.

Allport, D.A. (1980) Patterns and actions: cognitive mechanisms are content-specific. In: Claxton, G. (ed.), *Cognitive Psychology: New Direction*. Routledge and Kegan Paul, London, pp. 26–64.

Andreasen, N.C. (1982) Negative symptoms in schizophrenia. *Archives of General Psychiatry*, **39**, 784–788.

Andreasen, N.C., Rezai, K., Alliger, R., Swayze, V.W., Flaum, M., Kirchner, P. *et al.* (1992) Hypofrontality in neuroleptic-naïve patients and in patients with chronic schizophrenia: assessment with Xenon 133 single-photon emission computed tomography and the Tower of London. *Archives of General Psychiatry*, **49**, 943–958.

Arnsten, A.F.T. and Goldman-Rakic, P.S. (1998) Noise stress impairs prefrontal cortical cognitive function in monkeys: evidence for a hyperdopaminergic mechanism. *Archives of General Psychiatry*, **55**, 362–368.

Atkinson, R.C. and Shiffrin, R.M. (1968) Human memory: a proposed system and its control processes. In: Spence, K.W. (ed.), *The Psychology of Learning and Motivation: Advances in Research and Theory Vol. 2*. Academic Press, New York, pp. 89–195.

Baddeley, A. (1986) *Working Memory*. Oxford Science Publications, Oxford.

Baddeley, A. (1992a) Working memory. *Science*, **255**, 556–559.

Baddeley, A. (1992b) Working memory: the interface between memory and cognition. *Journal of Cognitive Neuroscience*, **4**, 281–288.

Baddeley, A.D. and Hitch, G.J. (1974) Working memory. In: Bowers, G. (ed.), *Recent Advances in Learning and Motivation*. Academic Press, New York, Vol. VIII, pp. 47–90.

Baddeley, A.D. and Lewis, V.J. (1981) Inner active processes in reading: the inner voice, the inner ear and the inner eye. In: Lesgold, A.M. and Perfetti, C.A. (eds), *Interactive Processes in Reading*. Erlbaum, Hillsdale, NJ, pp. 107–129.

Baddeley, A.D. and Lieberman, K. (1980) Spatial working memory. In: Nickerson, R. (ed.), *Attention and Performance VIII*. Erlbaum, Hillsdale, NJ, pp. 521–539.

Baddeley, A.D., Thomson, N. and Buchanan, M. (1975) Word length and the structure of short-term memory. *Journal of Verbal Learning and Verbal Behavior*, **14**, 575–589.

Barnard, P. (1985) Interacting cognitive subsystems: a psycholinguistic approach to short-term memory. In: Ellis, A. (ed.), *Progress in the Psychology of Language Vol. 2*. Erlbaum, London, pp. 197–258.

Brebrion, G., Amador, X., Smith, M.J. and Gorman, J.M. (1998) Memory impairment and schizophrenia: the role of processing speed. *Schizophrenia Research*, **30**, 31–39.

Bressi, S., Miele, L., Bressi, C., Astori, S., Gimosti, E., Linciano, A.D. *et al.* (1996) Deficit of central executive component of working memory in schizophrenia. *New Trends in Experimental and Clinical Psychiatry*, **12**, 243–252.

Brown, J. (1958) Some tests of the decay theory of immediate memory. *Quarterly Journal of Experimental Psychology*, **10**, 12–21.

Byrne, B. (1974) Item concreteness vs. spatial organization as predictors of visual imagery. *Memory and Cognition*, **2**, 53–59.

Callicott, J., Ramsey, N.F., Tallent, K., Bertolino, A., Knable, M.B., Coppola, R. *et al.* (1998a) Functional magnetic resonance imaging brain mapping in psychiatry: methodological issues illustrated in a study of working memory in schizophrenia. *Neuropsychopharmacology*, **18**, 186–196.

Callicott, J.H, Bertolino, A., Mattay, V.S., Jones, K.M., Ellmore, T., Frank, J.A. *et al.* (1998b) Limited working memory capacity in schizophrenia. *Society of Neuroscience Abstracts*, 24, 1520.

Carpenter, P.A. and Just, M.A. (1977) Reading comprehension as the eye sees it. In: Just, M.A. and Carpenter, P. (eds), *Cognitive Processes in Comprehension*. Erlbaum, Hillsdale, NJ, pp. 109–139.

Carter, C., Robertson, L., Nordahl, T., Chaderjian, M., Kraft, L. and O'Shora-Celaya, L. (1996) Spatial working memory deficits and their relationship to negative symptoms in unmedicated schizophrenia patients. *Biological Psychiatry*, **40**, 930–932.

Carter, C.S., Perlstein, W., Ganguli, R., Brar, J., Mintun, M. and Cohen, J.D. (1998) Functional hypofrontality and working memory dysfunction in schizophrenia. *American Journal of Psychiatry*, **155**, 1285–1287.

Cassens, G., Inglis, A.K., Appelbaum, P.S. and Gutheil, T.G. (1990) Neuroleptics: effects on neuropsychological function in chronic schizophrenic patients. *Schizophrenia Bulletin*, **16**, 477–500.

Condray, R., Steinhauer, S.R., van Kammen, D.P. and Kasparek, A. (1996) Working memory capacity predicts language comprehension in schizophrenic patients. *Schizophrenia Research*, **20**, 1–13.

Conrad, R. (1964) Acoustic confusion in immediate memory. *British Journal of Psychology*, **55**, 75–84.

Craik, F.I.M. and Lockhart, R.S. (1972) Levels of processing: a framework for memory research. *Journal of Verbal Learning and Verbal Behavior*, **11**, 671–684.

Daneman, M. and Carpenter, P.A. (1980) Individual differences in working memory and reading. *Journal of Verbal Learning and Verbal Behavior*, **19**, 450–466.

Davis, K.L., Kahn, R.S., Ko, G. and Davidson, K.G. (1991) Dopamine in schizophrenia: a review and reconceptualization. *American Journal of Psychiatry*, **148**, 1474–1486.

Docherty, N.M., Hawkins, K.A., Hoffman, E.H., Rakfeldt, J. and Sledge, W.H. (1996) Working memory, attention, and communication disturbances in schizophrenia. *Journal of Abnormal Psychology*, **105**, 212–219.

Farah, M.J. (1988) Is visual imagery really visual? Overlooked evidence from neuropsychology. *Psychology Review*, **95**, 307–317.

Fleming, K., Goldberg, T.E., Gold, J.M. and Weinberger, D.R. (1995) Verbal working memory dysfunction in schizophrenia: use of a Brown–Peterson paradigm. *Psychiatry Research*, **56**, 155–161.

Fletcher, P.C., McKenna, P.J., Frith, C.D., Grasby, P.M., Friston, K.J. and Dolan, R.J. (1998) Brain activations in schizophrenia during a graded memory tack studied with functional neuroimaging. *Archives of General Psychiatry*, **55**, 1001–1008.

Frith C.D. (1992) *The Cognitive Neuropsychology of Schizophrenia*. Erlbaum, Hove, UK.

Frith, C. and Dolan, R. (1996) The role of the prefrontal cortex in higher cognitive functions. *Cognitive Brain Research*, **5**, 175–181.

Frith, C.D. and Done, D.J. (1988) Towards a neuropsychology of schizophrenia. *British Journal of Psychiatry*, **153**, 437–443.

Frith, C.D. and Done, D.J. (1989) Experiences of alien control in schizophrenia reflect a disorder in central monitoring of action. *Psychological Medicine*, **19**, 359–363.

Funahashi, S., Bruce, C.J. and Goldman-Rakic, P.S. (1993) Dorsolateral prefrontal lesion and oculomotor delayed response performance: evidence for mnemonic 'scotmas.' *Neuroscience*, **13**, 1479–1497.

Galletly, C.A., Clark, R.C., McFarlane, A.C. and Weber, D.L. (1997) The relationship between changes in symptom ratings, neuropsychological test performance, and quality of life in schizophrenic patients treated with clozapine. *Psychiatry Research*, **72**,161–166.

Gold, D.A. (1998) Attention, working memory and negative thought disorder in schizophrenia. Unpublished dissertation, New York University.

Gold, J.M. and Harvey, P.D. (1993) Cognitive deficits in schizophrenia. *Psychiatric Clinics of North America*, **16**, 295–312.

Gold, J.M., Carpenter, C., Randolph, C., Goldberg, T.E. and Weinberger, D.R. (1997) Auditory working memory and Wisconsin Card Sorting Test performance in schizophrenia. *Archives of General Psychiatry*, **54**, 159–165.

Goldberg, T.E. and Weinberger, D.R. (1996) Effects of neuroleptic medications on the cognition of patients with schizophrenia: a review of recent studies. *Journal of Clinical Psychiatry*, **57**, 62–65.

Goldberg, T.E., Weinberger, D.R., Berman, K.F., Pliskin, N.H. and Podd, M.H. (1987) Further evidence for dementia of the prefrontal type in schizophrenia? *Archives of General Psychiatry*, **44**, 1008–1014.

Goldberg, T.E., Gold, J.M., Greenberg, R., Griffin, S., Schulz, S.C., Pickar, D. *et al.* (1993) Contrasts between patients with affective disorders and patients with schizophrenia on a neuropsychological test battery. *American Journal of Psychiatry*, **150**, 1355–1362.

Goldberg, T.E., Patterson, K.J., Taqqu, Y. and Wilder, K. (1998) Capacity limitations in short-term memory in schizophrenia: tests of competing hypotheses. *Psychological Medicine*, **28**, 665–673.

Goldman, P.S. and Rosvold, H.E. (1970) Localization of function within the dorsolateral prefrontal cortex of the rhesus monkey. *Experimental Neurology*, **27**, 291–304.

Goldman-Rakic, P.S. (1987) Circuitry of primate prefrontal cortex and regulation of behavior by representative memory. In: Plum, E. and Mountcastle, V. (eds), *Handbook of Physiology. The Nervous System. Higher Functions of the Brain*. American Psychological Society, Bethesda, MD, Section I, Vol. V., Part 1, pp. 373–417.

Goldman-Rakic, P.S. (1994) Working memory dysfunction in schizophrenia. *Journal of Neuropsychiatry*, **6**, 348–357.

Grace, J., Bellus, S.P., Raulin, M.L., Herz, M.L., Priest, B.L., Brenner, V. *et al.* (1996) Long-term impact of clozapine and psychosocial treatment on psychiatric symptoms and cognitive functioning. *Psychiatric Service*, **4**, 41–45,

Granholm, E., Asarnow, R.F. and Marder, S.R. (1991) Controlled information processing resources and the development of automatic detection responses in schizophrenia. *Journal of Abnormal Psychology*, **100**, 22–30.

Granholm, E., Asarnow, R.F., Sarkin, A.J. and Dykes, K.L. (1996) Pupillary responses index cognitive resource limitations. *Psychophysiology*, **33**, 457–461.

Granholm, E., Morris, S.K., Sarkin, A.J., Asarnow, R.F. and Jeste, D.V. (1997) Pupillary responses index overload of working memory resources in schizophrenia. *Journal of Abnormal Psychology*, **106**, 458–467.

Gray, J.A., Feldon, J., Rawlins, J.N.P., Hemsley, D.R. and Smith, A.D. (1991) The neuropsychology of schizophrenia. *Behavioral and Brain Sciences*, **14**, 1–84.

Green, M.F. (1996) What are the functional consequences of neurocognitive deficits in schizophrenia? *American Journal of Psychiatry*, **153**, 321–330.

Green, M.F., Marshall, B.D., Wirshing, W.C., Ames, D., Marder, S.R., McGurk, S., Kern, R.S. and Mintz, J. (1997) Does risperidone improve verbal working memory in treatment-resistant schizophrenia? *American Journal of Psychiatry*, **154,** 799–804.

Hagger, C., Buckley, P., Kenny, J.T., Friedman, L., Ubogy, D. and Meltzer, H.Y. (1993) Improvement in cognitive functions and psychiatric symptoms in treatment-refractory schizophrenic patients receiving clozapine. *Biological Psychiatry*, **34,** 702–712.

Hashtroudi, S., Johnson, M.K. and Chrosniak, L.D. (1989) Aging and source monitoring. *Psychology and Aging*, **4**, 106–112.

Hirshman, E. and Bjork, R.A. (1988) The generation effect: support for a two-factor theory. *Journal of Experimental Psychology: Learning, Memory, and Cognition*, **14**, 484–494.

Hoffman, R.E. (1986) Verbal hallucinations and language production processes in schizophrenia. *Behavioral and Brain Sciences*, **9**, 503–548.

Hoffman, R.E., Stopek, S. and Andreasen, N.C. (1986) A comparative study of manic vs schizophrenic speech disorganization. *Archives of General Psychiatry*, **43**, 831–838.

Hutton, S.B., Puri, B.K., Duncan, L.-J., Robbins, T.W., Barnes, T.R.E. and Joyce, E.M. (1998) Executive function in first-episode schizophrenia. *Psychology Medicine*, **28**, 463–473.

Javitt, D.C., Doneshka, P., Grochowski, S. and Ritter, W. (1995) Impaired mismatch negativity generation reflects widespread dysfunction of working memory in schizophrenia. *Archives of General Psychiatry*, **52**, 550–558.

Johnson, M.K. and Raye, C.L. (1981) Reality monitoring. *Psychological Review*, **88**, 67–85.

Johnson, M.K., Hashtroudi, S. and Lindsay, D.S. (1993) Source monitoring. *Psychological Bulletin*, **114**, 3–28.

Keefe, R.S.E. (1995) The contribution of neuropsychology to psychiatry. *American Journal of Psychiatry*, **152**, 6–15.

Keefe, R.S.E. (1998) The neurobiology of disturbances of the self: autonoetic agnosia in schizophrenia. In: Amador, X.F. and David, A. (eds), *Insight and Psychosis*. Oxford University Press, New York, pp. 142–173.

Keefe, R.S.E. (2000) The assessment of neurocognitive treatment response and its relation to negative symptoms in schizophrenia. In: Keefe, R.S.E. and McEvoy, J.P. (eds), *Negative Symptom and Cognitive Deficit Treatment Response in Schizophrenia*. American Psychiatric Press, Washington, DC (in press).

Keefe, R.S.E., Lees Roitman, S.E., Harvey, P.D., DuPre, R.L., Prieto, D.M., Davidson, M. *et al.* (1995) A pen-and-paper human analogue of a monkey prefrontal cortex activation task: spatial working memory in patients with schizophrenia. *Schizophrenia Research*, **17**, 25–33.

Keefe, R.S.E., Lees Roitman, S.E., Dupre, R.L. and Harvey, P.D. (1996) Laboratory and clinical tests of spatial working memory. *Schizophrenia Research: Special Issue Abstracts*, **18**, 208–209.

Keefe, R.S.E., Silverman, J., Mohs, R.C., Siever, L.J, Harvey, P.D., Friedman, L. *et al.* (1997) Eye tracking, attention, and schizotypal personality symptoms in nonpsychotic relatives of patients with schizophrenia. *Archives of General Psychiatry*, **54**, 169–177 .

Keefe, R.S.E., Arnold, M.C., Bayen, U.J., McEvoy, J.P. and Wilso, W.H. (2000) Source monitoring deficits for self-generated stimuli schizophrenia: multinomial modeling of data from three sources. (in review).

Kendler, K.S., Gruenberg, A.M. and Strauss, J.S. (1981) An independent analysis of the Copenhagen sample of the Danish Adoption Study of Schizophrenia: III. The relationship between paranoid psychosis (Delusional Disorder) and the schizophrenia spectrum disorders. *Archives of General Psychiatry*, **38**, 985–987.

Kolb, B. and Whishaw, I.Q. (1983) Performance of schizophrenic patients on tests sensitive to left or right frontal, temporal, or parietal function in neurological patients. *Journal of Nervous and Mental Diseases*, **171**, 435–443.

Leahy, L. (1987) Sentence Span Test. Unpublished test.

Lee, M.A., Thompson, P.A. and Meltzer, H.Y. (1994) Effects of clozapine on cognitive function in schizophrenia. *Journal of Clinical Psychiatry*, **55**, 82–87.

Lees Roitman, S.E., Mitropoulou, V., Keefe, R.S.E., Silverman, J.M., Serby, M., Harvey, P.D. *et al* (2000) Visuospatial working memory in schizotypal personality disorder patients. *Schrizophrenia Research,* **41**, 447–455.

Leudar, I., Thomas, P. and Johnston, M. (1992) Self-repair in dialogues of schizophrenics: effects of hallucinations and negative symptoms. *Brain and Language*, **43**, 487–511.

Levy, B.A. (1971) The role of articulation in auditory and visual short-term memory. *Journal of Verbal Learning and Verbal Behavior*, **10**, 123–132.

Logie, R.H. (1986) Visuo-spatial processing in working memory. *Quarterly Journal of Experimental Psychology*, **38**, 229–247.

Logie, R.H. (1995) *Visuospatial Working Memory*. Erlbaum, Hove, UK.

Luciana, M., Depue, R. A., Arbisi, P. and Leon, A. (1992) Facilitation of working memory in humans by a D2 dopamine receptor agonist. *Journal of Cognitive Neuroscience*, **4**, 59–68.

Luria, R.A. (1965) *The Working Brain*. Basic Books, New York.

McCarthy, G. (1995) Functional neuroimaging of memory. *The Neuroscientist*, **1**, 155–163.

McCarthy, G., Blamire, A.M., Puce, A., Nobre, A.C., Bloch, G. and Hyder, F. *et al*. (1994) Functional MRI studies of frontal cortex activation during a spatial working memory task in humans. *Proceedings of the National Academy of Sciences of the United States of America*, **91**, 8690–8694.

Medalia, A., Gold, J.M. and Merriam, A. (1988) The effects of neuroleptics on neuropsychological test results of schizophrenics. *Archives of Clinical Neuropsychology*, **3**, 249–271.

Meltzer, H.Y. and McGurk, S.R. (1999) The effect of clozapine, risperidone, and olanzapine on cognitive function in schizophrenia. *Schizophrenia Bulletin*, **251**, 233–255.

Morris, R.H. (1986) Short-term forgetting in senile dementia of the Alzheimer's type. *Cognitive Neuropsychology*, **3**, 77–97.

Murphy, B.L., Roth, R.H. and Arnsten, A.F. (1997) Clozapine reverses the spatial working memory deficits induced by FG7142 in monkeys. *Neuropsychopharmacology*. **16**, 433–437.

Nestor, P.G., Shenton, M.E., Wible, C., Hokama, H., O'Donnell, B.F., Law, S. *et al*. (1998) A neuropsychological analysis of schizophrenic thought disorder. *Schizophrenia Research*, **29**, 217–225.

Norman, D.A. and Shallice, T. (1980) *Attention to Action. Willed and Automatic Control of Behavior*. University of California San Diego CHIP Report 99.

Pantelis, C., Barnes, T.R.E., Nelson, H.E., Tanner, S., Weatherley, L, Owen, A.M. *et al*. (1997) Frontal-striatal cognitive deficits in patients with chronic schizophrenia. *Brain*, **120**, 1823–1843.

Park, S. (1997) Association of an oculomotor delayed response test and the Wisconsin Card Sorting Test in schizophrenic patients. *International Journal of Psychophysiology*, **27**, 147–151.

Park, S. and Holzman, P.S. (1992) Schizophrenics show working memory deficits. *Archives of General Psychiatry*, **49**, 975–982.

Park, S. and Holzman, P.S. (1993) Association of working memory deficit and eye tracking dysfunction in schizophrenia. *Schizophrenia Research*, **11**, 55–61.

Park, S. and McTigue, K. (1997) Working memory and the syndromes of schizotypal personality. *Schizophrenia Research*, **26**, 213–220.

Park, S. and O'Driscoll, G. (1996) Components of working memory deficit in schizophrenia. In: Matthysse, S., Levy, D.L., Kagan, J. and Benes, F. (eds), *Psychopathology: The Evolving Science of Mental Disorder*. Cambridge University Press, New York, pp. 34–50.

Park, S., Holzman, P.S. and Lenzenweger, M.F. (1995a) Individual differences in spatial working memory in relation to schizotypy. *Journal of Abnormal Psychology*, **104**, 355–364.

Park, S., Holzman, P.S. and Goldman-Rakic, P.S. (1995b) Spatial working memory deficits in the relatives of schizophrenic patients. *Archives of General Psychiatry*, **52**, 821–828.

Perlick, D., Mattis, S., Stastny, P. and Silverstein, B. (1992) Negative symptoms are related to both frontal and nonfrontal neuropsychological measures in chronic schizophrenia. *Archives of General Psychiatry*, **49**, 245–246.

Raine, A. (1991) The SPQ: a scale for the assessment of schizotypal personality based on DSM-III-R criteria. *Schizophrenia Bulletin*, **17**, 555–564.

Reisberg, D. and Logie, R.H. (1993) The in's and out's of visual working memory. Overcoming the limits on learning from imagery. In: Intons-Peterson, M., Roskos-Ewoldsen, B. and Anderson, R. (eds), *Imagery, Creativity, and Discovery: A Cognitive Approach*. Elsevier, Amsterdam, pp. 39–76.

Renzi, E.D. and Vignolo, L.A. (1962) The token test: a sensitive test to detect receptive disturbances in aphasics. *Brain*, **85**, 665–678.

Rochester, S.R. (1978) Are language disorders in acute schizophrenia actually information processing problems? *Journal of Psychiatry Research*, **14**, 275–283.

Rossi, A., Mancini, F., Stratta, P., Mattei, P., Gismondi, R., Pozzi, F. and Casacchia, M. (1997) Risperidone, negative symptoms and cognitive deficit in schizophrenia: an open study. *Acta Psychiatrica Scandinavica*, 95, 40–43.

Sagar, H. J., Sullivan, E.V., Gabrieli, J.D.E., Corkin, S. and Growdon, J.H. (1988) Temporal ordering and short-term memory deficits in Parkinson's disease. *Brain*, **111**, 525–539.

Salame, P. and Baddeley, A.D. (1982) Disruption of short-term memory by unattended speech: implications for the structure of working memory. *Journal of Verbal Learning and Verbal Behavior*, **21**, 150–164.

Salame, P. and Baddeley, A.D. (1989) Effects of background music on phonological short-term memory. *Quarterly Journal of Experimental Psychology*, **41A**, 107–122.

Salame, P., Danion, J., Peretti, S. and Cuervo, C. (1998) The state of functioning of working memory in schizophrenia. *Schizophrenia Research*, **30**, 11–29.

Salthouse, T.A. and Babcock, T.L. (1991) Decomposing adult age differences in working memory. *Developmental Psychology*, **27**, 763–776.

Salway, A.F. and Logie, R.H. (1995) Visuospatial working memory, movement control and executive demands. *British Journal of Psychology*, **86**, 253–269.

Sawaguchi, T. and Goldman-Rakic, P.S. (1994) The role of D1-dopamine receptor in working memory: local injections of dopamine antagonists into the prefrontal cortex of rhesus monkeys performing an oculomotor delayed-response task. *Journal of Neurophysiology*, **71**, 515–528.

Schneider, K. (1959) Klinische Psychopathologie [Clinical psychopathology] (5th ed.), Grune & Stratton, New York.

Schooler, C., Neumann, E., Caplan, L.J. and Roberts, B.R. (1997) A time course analysis of Stroop interference and facilitation: comparing normal individuals and individuals with schizophrenia. *Journal of Experimental Psychology: General*, **126**, 19–36.

Serper, M.R., Bergman R.L. and Harvey, P.D. (1990) Medication may be required for the development of automatic information processing in schizophrenia. *Psychiatry Research*, **32**, 281–288.

Shallice, T. (1982) Specific impairments of planning. *Philosophical Transactions of the Royal Society of London*, **298**, 199–209.

Slamecka, N.J. and Graf, P. (1978) The generation effect: delineation of a phenomenon. *Journal of Experimental Psychology: Human Learning and Memory*, **4**, 592–604.

Spindler, K.A., Sullivan, E.V., Menon, V., Lim, K.O. and Pfefferbaum, A. (1997) Deficits in multiple systems of working memory in schizophrenia. *Schizophrenia Research*, **27**, 1–10.

Spitzer, M. (1993) The psychopathology, neuropsychology, and neurobiology of associative and working memory in schizophrenia. *European Archives of Psychiatry and Clinical Neuroscience*, **243**, 57–70.

Stevens, A.A., Goldman-Rakic, P.S., Gore, J.C., Fulbright, R.K. and Wexler, B.E. (1998) Cortical dysfunction in schizophrenia during auditory word and tone working memory demonstrated by functional magnetic resonance imaging. *Archives of General Psychiatry*, **55**, 1097–1103.

Stone, M., Gabrieli, J.D.E., Stebbins, G.T. and Sullivan, E.V. (1998) Working and strategic memory deficits in schizophrenia. *Neuropsychology*, **12**, 278–288.

Stratta, P., Daneluzzo, E., Prosperini, P., Bustini, M., Mattei, P. and Rossi, A. (1997) Is Wisconsin Card Sorting Test performance related to 'working memory' capacity? *Schizophrenia Research*, **27**, 11–19.

Strauss, M.E. (1993) Relations of symptoms to cognitive deficits in schizophrenia. *Schizophrenia Bulletin*, **19**, 215–231.

Stuss, D.T., Kaplan, E.F., Benson, D.F., Weir, W.S., Chiulli, S. and Sarazin, F.F. (1982) Evidence for the involvement of orbitofrontal cortex in memory functions: an interference effect. *Journal of Comparative and Physiological Psychology*, **96**, 913–925.

Sullivan, E.V., Shear, P.K., Zipursky, R.B., Sagar, H.J. and Pfefferbaum, A. (1997) Patterns of content, contextual, and working memory impairments in schizophrenia and nonamnesic alcoholism. *Neuropsychology*, **11**, 195–206.

Tracy, J.I., Monaco, C., McMichael, H., Tyson, K., Chambliss, C., Christensen, H.L. *et al.* (1998) Information-processing characteristics of explicit time estimation by patients with schizophrenia and normal controls. *Perceptual and Motor Skills*, **86**, 515–526.

Vallar, G. and Baddeley, A.D. (1982) Short-term forgetting and the articulatory loop. *Quarterly Journal of Experimental Psychology*, **34**, 53–60.

Van der Does, A.J.W. and Van den Bosh, R.J. (1992) What determines Wisconsin Card Sorting performance in schizophrenia? *Clinical Psychology Review*, **12**, 567–583.

Weinberger, D.R. (1987) Implications of normal brain development for the pathogenesis of schizophrenia. *Archives of General Psychiatry*, **44**, 660–669.

Weinberger, D.R. and Berman, K.F. (1996) Prefrontal function in schizophrenia: confounds and controversies. *Philosophical Transactions of the Royal Society of London*, **351**, 1495–1503.

Wexler, B.E., Stevens, A.A., Bowers, A.A., Sernyak, M.J. and Goldman-Rakic, P.S. (1998) Word and tone working memory deficits in schizophrenia. *Archives of General Psychiatry*, **55**, 1093–1096.

Wilson, F.A.O., O'Scalaidhe, S.P. and Goldman-Rakic, P.S. (1993) Dissociation of object and spatial processing domains in primate prefrontal cortex. *Science*, **260**, 1955–1958.

3 Executive dysfunction in schizophrenia

Barton W. Palmer and Robert K. Heaton

Introduction

Recognition of the potential importance of executive dysfunction in schizophrenia dates back to Kraepelin (1919). He noted that while many of the basic cognitive skills (such as memory/retention and general orientation) remain relatively intact in this disorder, apparent decrements in some skills, such as attention and judgement, appeared to reflect an underlying deficit in the process of volition. He further suggested that the deficits in 'higher intellectual abilities' (p. 219) might reflect a propensity for the disorder to involve the frontal brain regions. It appears that he was not using the term 'higher intellectual abilities' in the restricted sense as measured by contemporary IQ scales, but rather in a sense similar to contemporary notions of executive skills (Zec, 1995).

Kraepelin's (1919) comments anticipated (and partially catalyzed) the subsequent development of an immense literature regarding possible frontal lobe pathology in schizophrenia which continues to grow to this day. In just the past 8 years there have been over 500 publications related to this topic (as identified in the MEDLINE computer database with the subject search terms 'schizophrenia and frontal lobe').

Although some aspects of schizophrenia clearly relate to prefrontal dysfunction, this disorder does not appear to be explainable by a simple model of focal frontal lobe lesion(s) (Weinberger and Berman, 1996), and deficits in other, non-executive, domains of neuro-cognition (particularly learning) may be equally relevant to understanding schizophrenia (Saykin *et al.*, 1991). Nonetheless, executive deficits are quite common among schizophrenia patients, and careful consideration of the meaning of the construct of 'executive dysfunction', its operationalization and its relationship to other dimensions of this disorder may provide insight into factors underlying the wide heterogeneity among schizophrenia patients in terms of clinical presentation, functional disability and course/outcome.

The goal of the present chapter is to provide a general overview addressing the following questions. What are 'executive skills'? What neuropsychological tests are employed commonly to assess these skills? What is the relationship of executive dysfunction to the other clinical characteristics associated with schizophrenia? How do the findings of executive functioning relate to abnormalities in brain structure or function among schizophrenia patients? What is the impact of these executive deficits on patients' everyday functioning? Also, finally, what is the impact of treatment on executive deficits, and vice versa? As will be seen below, definitive answers to many of the above questions are still lacking. However, it is hoped that this overview may prove helpful to both clinicians and researchers in furthering attempts to understand schizophrenia and develop more effective interventions.

What are 'executive skills'?

Historical development

The term 'executive dysfunction' (or 'executive skills') is often used, but difficult to define specifically. Its historical roots include the attempts of neuropsychologists and behavioral neurologists to delineate the 'higher' functions of the prefrontal cortex (Milner, 1964; Luria, 1966; Stuss and Benson, 1986) and traditionally has been used synonymously with the term 'frontal skills'. However, the concept also has roots in cognitive psychology and computer science (Neisser, 1967; Logan, 1985) wherein it evolved initially without specific emphasis on any proposed neuroanotomical substrates.

Recent trends in neuropsychology and behavioral neurology have included a growing recognition of the importance of cortical–subcortical circuits in 'frontal' functions (Evarts *et al.*, 1984; Cummings, 1993), as well as observations of a lack of specificity for frontal lesions shown by common 'frontal tests' (Anderson *et al.*, 1991; Reitan and Wolfson, 1995; Axelrod *et al.*, 1996). Thus, contemporary conceptualizations of executive skills within the schizophrenia literature tend to place less emphasis on executive deficits as being synonymous with prefrontal cortex dysfunction, while maintaining a focus on the frontal–subcortical circuits believed to subserve many of these functions (e.g. Goldman-Rakic, 1991, 1994; Jones, 1997; Lewis, 1997; Pantelis *et al.*, 1997).

Okay, but what are they?

Since 'executive functioning' remains a somewhat elusive construct, it is helpful to consider some of the proposed definitions within the literature. For example, the *INS (International Neuropsychological Society) Dictionary of Neuropsychology* (Loring, 1999) provided the following definition of executive function:

> Cognitive abilities necessary for complex goal-directed behavior and adaptation to a range of environmental changes and demands. Executive function includes the ability to plan and anticipate outcomes (cognitive flexibility) and to direct attentional resources to meet the demands of nonroutine events. Many conceptualizations of executive function also include self-monitoring and self-awareness since these are necessary for behavioral flexibility and 'appropriateness.' Because of individual variability and changing task demands required to demonstrate executive functions, they are often difficult to assess with standardized measures. Cerebral localization also remains elusive and controversial. Regions of the prefrontal cortex may play a special role in recruiting other brain areas in a series of distributed networks that handle different components of executive functions, depending on the processing demands of the specific task. (p. 64)

Stuss and Benson (1986) defined executive functions as:

> [The] important activities that are almost universally attributed to the frontal lobes which become active in nonroutine, novel situations that require new solutions. . .[which include] at

least the following: anticipation, goal selection, preplanning..., monitoring, and use of feedback. (p. 244)

Similarly, Lezak (1995) defined such functions as:

those capacities that enable a person to engage successfully in independent, purposive, self-serving behavior. (p. 42)

Green (1998) offered the following definition:

Executive functioning refers to a host of neurocognitive activities that are associated with the prefrontal cortex such as planning, problem solving, shifting cognitive set, and alternating between two or more tasks. (p. 47)

Welsh *et al.* (1990) defined executive function as:

the ability to maintain an appropriate problem solving set for attainment of a future goal. .allow[ing] for strategic planning, impulse control, organized search, and flexibility of thought and action. (p. 1698–1699)

Logan (1985) included the following components among the executive functions:

(1) choice among different strategies for performing a task, (2) construction or instantiation of the chosen strategy to enable performance of the task, (3) execution and maintenance of the strategy to perform the task, and (4) inhibition or disablement of the strategy in response to changes in goals or changes in the task environment. (p. 194)

The historical link between the construct of executive skills and frontal lobe functioning is apparent in several of these definitions, although, as noted above, there recently has been increased awareness that executive skills may not be fully housed within the frontal lobes. Despite the subtle differences among some of the above definitions, each yields a sense of cognitive and behavioral control. Specifically, executive skills permit an adaptive balance of maintenance and shifting of cognitive or behavioral responses to environmental demands permitting longer term goal-directed behavior rather than reflexive or automated action. Such control requires consideration of current and probable future environmental circumstances, generation and evaluation of response alternatives, choice and implementation of a specific course, and monitoring/re-evaluation in response to environmental feedback. Abilities underlying such activities may include: search of knowledge, abstraction and planning, evaluation/decision-making skills, initiation, self-monitoring, mental flexibility and inhibition of immediate/reflex responses in pursuit of a longer term goal.

Although none of the above definitions explicitly mentioned the concept of 'working memory', this also appears to be a related construct (Shallice, 1982; Goldman-Rakic, 1991, 1994). Working memory may be thought of as a 'mental workbench', i.e. a mechanism for brief storage (usually of the order of moments or seconds) and manipulation of auditory and visual information. As Goldman-Rakic (1994) has stated "working memory confers the ability to guide behavior by representations of the outside world rather than by immediate stimulation, and thus to base behavior on ideas and thoughts" (p. 349).

One of the most influential models of 'working memory' has been Baddeley's (1992), which consists of a 'central executive' controlling and coordinating the attentional resources between two slave systems. These slave systems include a visual sketchpad (used to manipulate visual images) and a phonological loop (used to manipulate auditory/speech-based information). A detailed review of the construct of working memory and its relationship to schizophrenia is provided by Keefe (Chapter 2), but, given the overlap of this construct with executive skills, as well as the possible role of working memory in some executive tasks (Goldman-Rakic, 1994; Gold *et al.*, 1997), brief consideration within the context of the present discussion will be provided where appropriate.

Neuropsychological measures of executive skills

Another approach to understanding the meaning of the term 'executive functioning' is to consider the specific tasks that have been used to operationalize it within the schizophrenia literature. Although a large number of tests are available (Lezak, 1995), we have focused our review to some of the most commonly employed tests, including the Wisconsin Card Sorting Test (WCST), the Category Test, the Stoop task, the Tower of London/Hanoi/Toronto tasks, the Controlled Oral Word Association Test (COWAT) and the Trail Making Test. We will also briefly discuss a few working memory tasks.

None of these tests is a pure measure of executive functioning. As is true of virtually all neuropsychological tasks, each requires subjects to draw upon a range of neurocognitive abilities (as well as basic sensory motor skills), some more salient than others, subserved by a number of brain areas and systems. Yet, each traditionally has been categorized as an executive task because successful performance requires engagement of some form of executive control in addition to any of the more basic cognitive processes.

Wisconsin Card Sorting Test (WCST)

The WCST (Berg, 1948; Heaton *et al.*, 1993) is perhaps the single most widely used measure of executive functioning within the schizophrenia literature, as well as being widely used within general neuropsychological practice and research (Butler *et al.*, 1991). Since the original study of the WCST in schizophrenia patients by Fey (1951), a virtual cottage industry has developed around the WCST in schizophrenia [we located ~150 publications in the MEDLINE computer database (1966–1998) on the subject of schizophrenia in which the WCST was listed explicitly in the title or abstract, about half of which were published in the last 3 years]. As Green (1998) recently commented "the amount of emphasis on the WCST [in the schizophrenia literature] defies complete explanation" (p. 48). Since much of the research on executive dysfunction in schizophrenia specifically involved the WCST, the following descriptions of this task will be somewhat more detailed than that provided for other executive measures.

In the WCST, the patient is asked to match each in a series of response cards to one of four stimulus cards. The standard version of this task involves sorting of actual cards, although computerized versions are increasingly popular (Artiola i Fortuny and Heaton, 1996).

The WCST response and stimulus cards each vary along three dimensions: form/shape of the elements, number of elements and color of the elements on each card. The subject is not told explicitly which of these dimensions represents the correct sorting principle, but after each attempted match of a response card to a stimulus card, the examiner informs the subject whether or not his/her preceding response was correct. By generating hypotheses about the correct sorting principle, and testing these hypotheses through trial and error, the subject is able to determine whether he/she is to sort the cards according to color, form or number. Following 10 consecutive correct responses ('completion of a category'), the examiner covertly changes the correct sorting principle. This procedure is repeated several times (in the standard version, until six categories or 128 card sorts have been completed).

The WCST yields several scores which potentially can be examined (Heaton *et al.*, 1993), such as categories completed, number of errors, perseverative responses/errors, conceptual level responses and failures to maintain set. Those which tend to be analyzed most frequently in the schizophrenia literature include perseveration (responses or errors) and total categories completed. Results of factor analytic studies suggest that failures to maintain set and perseveration should be considered as separable factors within impaired subjects (Goldman *et al.*, 1996; Bell *et al.*, 1997), although perseverative responses may be the most sensitive and specific to the deficits shown by schizophrenia patients (Koren *et al.*, 1998).

The WCST generally is interpreted in terms of abstraction/problem-solving skills and ability to shift strategies efficiently in response to environmental feedback (Lezak, 1995). For example, most of the response cards do not exactly match any of the four stimulus cards (i.e. on all three sorting principles). On such trials, subjects cannot succeed through a direct match of the stimuli, but instead must abstract the underlying rule by considering the various dimensions which may underlie the sorting principle. Abandoning a successful strategy too soon (a 'failure to maintain set') or retaining a previously successful strategy after the rule has been changed covertly (perseveration) also hinder performance.

The tendency for schizophrenia patients to show deficient WCST performance has been known for half a century (Fey, 1951). There have been recent suggestions that these deficits may be related at least partially to working memory deficits in schizophrenia (Goldman-Rakic, 1994; Gold *et al.*, 1997), although some findings to the contrary have also been reported (Stratta *et al.*, 1997a).

Category Test

Although it has not received the attention that the WCST has in the schizophrenia literature, the Category Test (Reitan and Wolfson, 1993) seems to draw upon some similar executive skills. Although abbreviated forms have appeared, the standard form of the Category Test involves 208 visually presented items, grouped into seven sections. In each section, there is an underlying rule which the subject must discern to respond correctly with one of four choices. For example, the covert rule might be 'choose the one that is most different'. Subjects are informed that there is a rule underlying correct responses in each section, and that the rule may be different after each section. They are not told what the rule is, but after each response they are informed whether that response was correct or incorrect. Thus, similar to the WCST, subjects must generate hypotheses, test these hypotheses and adjust their performance in response to obtained feedback. They must also abandon old rules and adopt new ones as appropriate across sections.

The primary score obtained from the Category Test is the total number of errors. Numerous investigations have demonstrated that schizophrenics show an elevated number of errors relative to normal comparison subjects on this task (reviewed in Choca *et al.*, 1997).

Stroop Color Word Interference test

Another frequently used test of executive skills is the Stroop task. There are several versions of the Stroop task (reviewed in Lezak, 1995), however, most are guided by the same underlying principle. Specifically, in the Color Word Interference trial, subjects are shown a series of words which consist of names of colors. Each word is printed in colored ink; however, in the standard interference task, the content of each word conflicts with the color of the ink it is printed in. Subjects are required to ignore the content of each word, and tell the examiner the color of ink that it is printed in.

The Stroop task requires conscious effort and can be rather taxing, even for neurologically healthy normals. The precise reasons for this difficulty continue to be researched and debated (reviewed in MacLeod, 1991), but the most popular interpretations, dating back to the work of Cattell in the 1890s, emphasize the notion of response competition. On a perhaps over-simplified level, the task can be understood as requiring subjects actively to inhibit a more automatic (or more quickly processed) tendency to read the words in favor of the less automatic (or slower processed) color naming (Dyer, 1973). It is because of this need for active response inhibition (or 'selective attention') that the Stroop task is considered a measure of executive functioning.

There are numerous variations in format of the Stroop task (Lezak, 1995). In some versions (e.g. Golden, 1978), subjects are given a set period of time, and the number of successful trails (and in some versions, errors) in that time period is recorded. In other versions (e.g. Comalli *et al.*, 1962), the time that subjects require to complete a set number of trials is recorded. An increasingly popular alternative, particularly among researchers, is a 'single-trial' format (Perlstein *et al.*, 1998), wherein the individual stimuli are presented on a computer screen and response time (and accuracy) can be recorded for each trial, instead of over a series of trials.

Time on the interference task can be examined directly, or relative to performance on a non-interference naming task (e.g. wherein subjects are required to name colors of non-word ink patches). Some investigators also examine 'facilitation effects' by asking subjects to name colors from words with congruent ink content (such as the word 'red' printed in red ink). These comparisons are examined most frequently in terms of difference scores, although some authors suggest the use of ratios (Graf *et al.*, 1995).

Perlstein *et al.* (1998) recently reviewed the literature on the Stroop task in schizophrenia patients. In general, the studies they reviewed reported that relative to controls, schizophrenia patients have slower speed and a greater number of errors on the interference task. Schizophrenics also appear to show greater than normal facilitation (increased speed) when naming the ink color from color-congruent words. Perlstein *et al.* questioned the degree to which the results from traditional card versions (time summed over series of trials) could be interpreted definitively in terms of greater interference effects among schizophrenics, and suggested that error rates on single-trial versions of the task may be the among the most sensitive to the selective attention deficits of schizophrenia.

Tower tasks

Another dimension of executive functioning that is gaining increasing attention within the schizophrenia literature is planning ability. Tower tasks frequently are employed to measure the latter aspect of executive functioning (Shallice, 1982). As is true of the Stroop, there are several versions of the Tower task (reviewed in Lezak, 1995), but each relies on the same underlying principle—moving objects one at a time from a starting position to a goal position, with some type of restraint on movements requiring an indirect route to the goal. For example, in the Tower of London task (Shallice, 1982), subjects are presented with a board having three pegs and three beads, wherein each bead is a different color. The first (far left) peg can hold three beads, the middle can hold two beads, but the far right peg can hold only one bead at a time. The subjects' task is to move the beads one at a time from a starting position to a goal position in the fewest possible moves. Performance typically is judged in terms of the number of moves.

Physical trial and error movement of the beads, even if ultimately successful in leading to the goal, would tend to involve a relatively high number of moves for completion. Thus, efficient performance of Tower tasks appears to require subjects to envision different multistep routes to the goal, consider the number of moves required by each route and retain these evaluations within working memory for comparison.

The principles underlying the two most common alternative tower tasks (i.e. the Tower of Hanoi and the Tower of Toronto) are basically the same as in the Tower of London, with a few alterations in materials and the movement restrictions (Lezak, 1995). Specifically, rather than restricting movements by the length of pegs, the Tower of Hanoi involves disks of varying sizes; subjects are not permitted to place a larger disk on top of a smaller disk. In the Tower of Toronto, the disks are each equal in size, but vary with respect to color; subjects are restricted from placing darker disks on top of lighter ones. Although it would seem that these three tasks should be interchangeable, Humes et al. (1997) recently reported that the correlation between the London and Hanoi tasks was only $r = 0.37$, which they attributed to relatively poor reliability in the London task.

Until recently, there had been less research attention paid to Tower tasks relative to that given to the WCST and Stoop in the schizophrenia literature. However, several recent investigations indicated that schizophrenic patients have more difficulty on these tasks (requiring more moves) than do normal comparison subjects (Goldberg et al., 1990; Andreasen et al., 1992; Morris et al., 1995; Pantelis et al., 1997).

Controlled Oral Word Association Test (COWAT)

Word fluency tests have been used for over 60 years. In the 1930s, Thelma Thurstone devised a test called 'First and Last Letter' in which patients were given a 'first' and a 'last' letter and were asked to write as many words as they could think of with the given initial and terminal letters (L.L. Thurstone, 1938). In a more widely employed version of the Thurstone Word Fluency Task (described in Milner, 1964; Heaton et al., 1991), subjects are given 5 min to write words that start with the letter S, and then they are given 4 min to write four-letter words that start with the letter C.

Perhaps the most widely used fluency task is the Controlled Oral Word Association Test (COWAT; Benton, 1968; Lezak, 1995; Spreen and Strauss, 1998). In the COWAT (also known as the 'FAS test'), the subject is asked to say as many words as he or she can think of beginning with the letters F, A and S (some authors substitute the letters C, F and L), during three respective 1 min trials. The primary score obtained from the COWAT is the total number of words generated. Patients' performance on this task may be interpreted in comparison with that of healthy normals (Spreen and Strauss, 1998) or relative to their own performance on a 'Category Fluency' task, in which they are asked to generate words in a semantic category, such as animals (Goodglass and Kaplan, 1983).

Among non-aphasic individuals, performance on the COWAT is thought to reflect subjects' abilities to generate and utilize an efficient strategy for searching their lexicon. Thus, the COWAT is thought to exemplify the aspects of 'organized search' included in some authors' definition of executive skills (e.g. Welsh *et al.*, 1990). Recent findings reported by Joyce *et al.* (1996) are consistent with the notion that schizophrenics have relative difficulty with fluency tasks due to inefficient access to their semantic store.

Trail Making Test

Some authors interpret the Trail Making Test (Reitan and Wolfson, 1993), specifically Part B, as an executive task. This task consists of two parts. In Part A, subjects are required rapidly to connect a series of circles containing numbers in ascending order. Rapid performance in Part A appears to be dependent primarily on efficiency of visual scanning and psychomotor speed. In contrast, Part B consists of circles, some of which contain numbers and others letters. The subjects are required to connect the circles rapidly, alternating between two ascending sequences (going from 1 to A, A to 2, 2 to B, B to 3, and so on). This alternation between two sequences is thought to require executive control, specifically flexibility of thinking and a greater demand for working memory.

Standard scoring systems and published normative data for the Trail Making Test emphasize time to completion (Heaton *et al.*, 1991; Reitan and Wolfson, 1993). Numerous investigators have found that schizophrenia patients have slower performance on this task than do normals (e.g. Braff *et al.*, 1991; Franke *et al.*, 1993a). A difference score, subtracting the time on Part A from that on Part B, can be used to factor out the effects of simple psychomotor speed (Heaton *et al.*, 1981; see also Buchanan *et al.*, 1994). Although the latter approach has not been reported widely within studies of schizophrenia patients, it may be helpful in isolating the effects of mental flexibility deficits since psychomotor slowing can be a side effect of some antipsychotic medications.

Working memory tasks

As mentioned above, working memory is a construct closely tied to that of executive dysfunction in schizophrenia (Goldman-Rakic, 1991, 1994). Goldman-Rakic provided a cogent argument for the role of working memory in many of the above-listed 'executive tests', and some empirical support has been reported with regard to WCST performance (Gold *et al.*, 1997), although others report negative findings (Stratta *et al.*, 1997a). Since

Keefe (Chapter 2) provides a detailed review of working memory, and its relationship to schizophrenia, we will only briefly mention some of the currently popular working memory tasks.

A commonly given example of auditory working memory is mental rehearsal of a telephone number prior to dialing (Goldman-Rakic, 1994). This simple task is analogous to the digit span subtest of the Wechsler scales (Wechsler, 1997a), wherein subjects are required to repeat a string of numbers of increasing length. While the first part of this task 'digits forward' requires only simple storage, the latter half 'digits backward' requires subjects to report the series of numbers in the reverse order from that in which they were presented. Thus, the latter task captures more clearly the idea of a 'mental workbench' wherein information is not only held temporarily, but manipulated.

The latest revisions of the Wechsler Adult Intelligence Scale (WAIS-III; Wechsler, 1997a) and the Wechsler Memory Scale (WMS-III; Wechsler, 1997b) both include an even more challenging measure of auditory working memory, the 'letter–number sequencing' subtest. In this task, subjects are told a string of intermixed letters and numbers, and then must repeat back the numbers and letters separately in ascending order. Gold *et al.* (1997) found performance on this task to be highly correlated with the number of categories achieved on the WCST.

The digit span and letter–number sequencing tasks appear most relevant to Baddeley's (1992) notion of a phonological loop (although envisioning the information with the visual sketchpad could be involved in some manipulations such as the digits backward). The WMS-III (Wechsler, 1997b) includes a visual analog to the digit span task (spatial span). Also, Park and her colleagues (1995) have developed several versions of a spatial working memory task which has been gaining popularity among schizophrenia researchers (see Chapter 2 for a more extensive review).

Relationship to psychiatric characteristics

The degree of neurocognitive dysfunction, including executive dysfunction, varies greatly among patients with schizophrenia (Braff *et al.*, 1991; Goldstein, 1994; Palmer *et al.*, 1997). Differences in levels of executive deficits, and the clinical and neurobiological factors which may be associated with these differences among schizophrenics, could be more important in understanding this disorder and its impact on patients' lives than are group differences between patients and normals.

Many investigators report no association between severity of psychopathology and executive deficits (Franke *et al.*, 1992; Hepp *et al.*, 1996; Abbruzzese *et al.*, 1997; Stratta *et al.*, 1997a), but there are some suggestions of a differential relationship depending upon the type of symptom. The severity of 'positive' symptoms (such as hallucinations and delusions) generally appears to have a minimal relationship to the severity of executive deficits in schizophrenia (Franke *et al.*, 1992; Morris *et al.*, 1995; Voruganti *et al.*, 1997). In contrast, 'negative' symptoms (those symptoms involving an absence of normal functions, such as affective flattening, alogia, social withdrawal or avolition; Andreasen and Olsen, 1982) may be associated more consistently with poor executive functioning. [Alernatively, those patients with poor executive functioning may be more likely to show consistent negative symptoms (Lysaker *et al.* 1997).]

Several investigators (e.g. Butler *et al.*, 1992; Capleton, 1996; Berman *et al.*, 1997; Rossi *et al.*, 1997; Voruganti *et al.*, 1997), albeit not all (Franke *et al.*, 1992; Abbruzzese *et al.*, 1997; Collins *et al.*, 1997), have reported an association between severity of negative symptoms and executive dysfunction as measured by the WCST, as well as the Trail Making Test and COWAT (Berman *et al.*, 1997). Also, using a computerized version of the Tower of London task, Morris *et al.* (1995) found that, while the number of moves did not correlate with either positive or negative symptoms, response times tended to be longer in those with more negative symptoms.

A related issue is the association between executive deficits and poor illness insight. Several investigators (Young *et al.*, 1993; Lysaker and Bell, 1994; Voruganti *et al.*, 1997), albeit again not all (Cuesta *et al.*, 1996; Collins *et al.*, 1997), report an association between worse WCST performance and lack of insight or awareness of illness. Young *et al.* (1998) further reported that the relationship between lack of illness insight and WCST performance was stronger among schizophrenia patients than among a small sample of patients with bipolar affective disorder, suggesting some specificity to schizophrenia.

Results of comparisons among diagnostic subtypes of schizophrenia have yielded inconsistent findings. For example, some studies show those with paranoid subtype to have relatively better performance on the WCST (Seltzer *et al.*, 1997), and Steindl and Boyle (1995) reported that patients with delusions had better performance on the Category Test than did those without delusions. Yet, other investigators (Abbruzzese *et al.*, 1997) have found those with paranoid subtype to have worse WCST performance than other schizophrenia patients. Consistent with the tendency for negative symptoms and poor insight to be associated with worse executive skills, Buchanan *et al.* (1994) reported that patients with 'deficit syndrome' had poorer performance on the Stroop interference task and Trail Making Part B, as well as on a visuospatial task, relative to other schizophrenia patients. On the other hand, no significant differences between 'deficit' and 'non-deficit' schizophrenics were observed on the WCST or the COWAT in the latter study.

An enduring and unresolved question has been whether neurocognitive deficits in schizophrenia reflect factors associated with the presence of the disorder itself, or neurobiological vulnerability. Results of 'at risk' populations have been inconsistent, with some studies indicating deficits in executive skills (usually assessed with the WCST) among unaffected first-degree relatives (Franke *et al.*, 1993b), or undergraduates scoring high on a perceptual aberration scale (Suhr, 1997), or those with schizotypal personality disorder (Trestman *et al.*, 1995). In contrast, other researchers report no deficits on the WCST among unaffected first-degree relatives of schizophrenics (Stratta *et al.*, 1997b) or people with schizotypal personality disorder (Battaglia *et al.*, 1994).

Relationship to neuroimaging findings

Most of the studies that have focused on the relationship of executive deficits to brain pathology have used functional imaging techniques, although there is also some evidence of an association between structural abnormalities and worse executive performance. For example, Stratta *et al.* (1997c) found that poorer WCST performance was associated with decreased striatal volume on MRI.

There have been numerous functional neuroimaging studies (predominantly SPECT studies) of prefrontal function in schizophrenia patients. Findings from resting paradigms, wherein brain function is evaluated while patients are at rest, have been inconsistent. Some investigators report that schizophrenic patients have resting prefrontal hyperperfusion (e.g. Parellada *et al.*, 1994), whereas others find that schizophrenics have lower resting prefrontal blood flow relative to normal comparison subjects (e.g. Rubin *et al.*, 1994) (for detailed reviews, see Andreasen *et al.*, 1992; Weinberger and Berman, 1996).

Results from activation paradigms have been much more consistent. A large number of studies (e.g. Weinberger *et al.*, 1986; Parellada *et al.*, 1994; Steinberg *et al.*, 1996; Volz *et al.*, 1997) reveal a failure of schizophrenia patients to demonstrate normal increases in prefrontal activation while performing the WCST. Similar results have been observed in the anterior cingulate gyrus for the Stroop task (Carter *et al.*, 1997) and in the mesial frontal region for the Tower of London test (particularly among those patients with more negative symptoms) (Andreasen *et al.*, 1992). A primary controversy in the activation literature has been whether the findings of hypoactivation among schizophrenics reflect their poor task performance or their neuropathology. Studies in which schizophrenics were matched to normals or those with other disorders in terms of level of WCST performance do not seem to support the performance-based interpretation (for detailed reviews, see Taylor 1996; Weinberger and Berman, 1996).

Overall, the neuroimaging studies are consistent with the historical interest in the potential role of abnormalities in frontal or frontal–subcortical circuitry in the genesis of schizophrenia. In the absence of a simple neurological model of schizophrenia, however, clinicians are faced with two more practical concerns: do these deficits impact patients everyday functioning and, moveover, are there any present or potential future effective interventions for these deficits?

Impact of executive impairment on everyday functioning

As Siris (1991) has noted, the WCST involves subjects in a somewhat ambiguous challenge that approximates real life social interactions in many ways. Indeed, given the emphasis on self-regulatory, goal-directed behavior in the definitions of 'executive skills' provided above, it is difficult to imagine that executive deficits would not impact patients' everyday functioning.

The literature on factors impacting everyday functioning among schizophrenics presently is small, and often methodologically flawed (reviewed in Green 1996, 1998). However, there is tentative evidence that performances on standard tests of executive skills are associated with at least some aspects of everyday functioning. For example, Lysaker *et al.* (1995) found that better WCST performance was related to higher levels of work functioning, and this relationship appeared to be at least partially independent of differences in age, education and overall intelligence. On the other hand, negative findings have been reported with regard to patients' self-ratings of quality of life. Heslegrave *et al.* (1997) found no significant relationship between WCST deficits and self-ratings of quality of life. It is possible that objectively measured differences in the adequacy of patients' everyday functioning do not translate into meaningful differences in self-perceived well being.

The degree of association between executive skills and everyday functioning may be partially dependent on the specific domain of functioning, and/or the methods used to assess those domains. For example, Brekke *et al.* (1997) found a significant correlation between two executive measures (Stroop and COWAT) and levels of independence in living, but not with ratings of work or social functioning. The latter negative finding in terms of occupational functioning appears to conflict with those of Lysaker *et al.* (1995). However, Brekke *et al.* used a relatively broad rating of employment, whereas Lysaker *et al.* examined more specific subcomponents of occupational functioning.

In his recent reviews of the literature regarding neurocognitive correlates of functional status among schizophrenia patients, Green (1996, 1998) noted that WCST performance is associated consistently with global measures of community functioning and may be associated with skill acquisition in psychosocial training programs, but does not appear to be associated with social problem solving. In addition, verbal working memory has been related to acquisition of psychosocial skills in rehabilitation programs, and may also be related to social problem solving. It must be noted, however, that Green's reviews also suggested that verbal learning or memory, presumably non-executive skills, consistently were related to all three functional domains.

Further research is needed to explore the degree to which specific executive skills impact upon specific aspects of everyday functioning. For example, it may be important to assess not only patients' degree or level of employment, but also the quality of their job performance. Also, specific executive skills (as well as other specific neurocognitive skills) may be related differentially to specific aspects of everyday living.

Impact of treatment for schizophrenia on executive skills

Antipsychotic medications

Traditional neuroleptics, such as haloperidol, do not appear to have either an adverse or a beneficial impact on most neurocognitive abilities, except for partial normalization of some aspects of attention (reviewed in Spohn and Strauss, 1989; Cassens *et al.*, 1990). Similarly, chronic administration of neuroleptics appears to have no clear effect on abstraction or problem solving (Cassens *et al.*, 1990). There may be an adverse or beneficial impact on the more attentional aspects of executive functioning. Verdoux *et al.* (1995) found improvements on the Stroop task (but not the WCST) after initiation of neuroleptic treatment. In contrast, findings from a recent study from our research center (involving older psychotic patients) suggested that Stroop performance may improve when neuroleptics are tapered to the lowest effective dose (Harris *et al.*, 1997). Further investigations are needed to reconcile these different findings; however, it seems possible that there is a non-linear relationship between neuroleptic dose and Stroop performance.

Recent findings suggest that some of the newer 'atypical' (serotonin–dopamine-blocking) antipsychotics may have a beneficial impact on some neurocognitive skills, including some aspects of executive functioning (reviewed in Fujii *et al.*, 1997). Clozapine appears to have a positive impact on verbal fluency (COWAT) (Hagger *et al.*, 1993; Lee *et al.*, 1994), although any effect on other executive skills is less robust. In a longitudinal study of 13 patients treated with clozapine for ~15 months, Goldberg *et al.* (1993) found no significant improvements on WCST performance, Category Test scores or Trails B, in spite of marked improvements in psychiatric symptoms. However, Fujii *et al.* (1997) found a trend toward improved WCST performance among eight schizophrenics treated with clozapine for 12 months.

In one of the few double-blind studies, Green *et al.* (1997) found improvements in verbal working memory following several weeks of treatment with risperidone as compared with haloperidol. He has also reported finding similar improvements in spatial working memory, as well as psychomotor speed, in currently unpublished studies (reviewed in Green, 1998). The potential impact of such improvements on patients' everyday functioning awaits investigation. Further research is also needed to investigate the relationship between the specific pharmacodynamic properties of the various medications and changes in executive and other neurocognitive skills.

Non-pharmacological interventions for executive dysfunction

The large majority of research pertaining to non-pharmacological interventions for executive deficits in schizophrenia has been focused on effects of training, incentives and modified instructions for the WCST. For example, Summerfelt *et al.* (1991) found that schizophrenics' performance on the WCST improved when monetary reinforcements for correct responses were provided, suggesting that WCST perseverative errors may partially reflect motivational factors. On the other hand, other investigators have found that modified instructions and training can improve WCST performance in the absence of monetary reinforcement, although a combination of increased incentives and training appears to be most effective (e.g. Green *et al.*, 1992). The degree to which these improvements represent durable improvements in executive functioning, rather than enhancement of performance on a particular test paradigm alone, remains a point of controversy (reviewed in Goldberg and Weinberger, 1994; Green, 1998).

There has also been recent interest in the possibility of modifying executive deficits in schizophrenia through 'cognitive rehabilitation'. For example, Delahunty and Morice (1996) describe a cognitive rehabilitation program, designed to exercise specific neural network processes theoretically linked to frontal/prefrontal functioning. The idea underlying such programs appears to be that the functioning of specific neural circuits can be improved through exercise. Empirical demonstration of the validity of the latter assumption, and the effectiveness of their program, is still needed.

Summary and conclusions

A simple definition of executive skills remains elusive, but in general this construct appears to involve those cognitive processes which permit an adaptive balance of initiation, maintenance and shifting of responses to environmental demands permitting goal-directed behavior. The construct also appears closely linked to that of 'working memory' (Goldman-Rakic, 1991, 1994). Although these processes have been attributed historically to frontal cortical functioning, there has been growing recognition of the importance of cortical–subcortical connections in these functions (Cummings, 1993; Evarts *et al.*, 1984). Some of the most commonly used neuropsychological tests of executive skills include the WCST (for abstraction, maintenance and adaptive shifting of cognitive set), the Category Test (abstraction, problem solving and set shifting), the Stroop test (response inhibition or selective attention), Tower of London/Hanoi/Toronto (planning), COWAT (strategic search of the lexicon) and Part B of the Trail Making Test (mental flexibility and working memory).

Despite some lingering conceptual vagueness regarding the construct itself, performance on neuropsychological measures of executive skills seems to be associated with differences in certain types of psychiatric symptoms among schizophrenia patients, i.e. those patients with greater executive impairment tend to have more severe or stable negative symptoms, and may have less independence in at least some aspects of everyday functioning. Although the primary focus of the present review was not on neuropathology, functional neuroimaging studies also suggest that schizophrenics lack normal patterns of frontal activation while performing these executive tasks. Schizophrenics may lack the ability to organize brain activity efficiently in response to environmental demands for executive control (Taylor, 1996).

Traditional neuroleptic medications appear to have minimal impact on executive skills, although they may be helpful in partially improving attentional aspects of executive functioning (Spohn and Strauss, 1989; Cassens *et al.*, 1990). Recent studies involving treatment with atypical antipsychotic medications suggest that at least some of these may be helpful in partially normalizing certain aspects of executive functioning and working memory. Yet, these atypical antipsychotic medications are themselves a heterogeneous class of compounds with varying pharmacodynamic profiles, and further research is needed to evaluate the extent to which improved executive functioning may be associated with the specific pharmacodynamic properties of each of these medications. There has also been growing interest in non-pharmacological interventions, although research examining the degree to which such interventions lead to generalizable improvements in everyday functioning is still needed.

Although this large literature contains many contradictory findings and controversies, the overall picture that emerges is reminiscent of attempts to identify subtypes of schizophrenia patients based on the relative predominance of negative or deficit symptoms, such as 'Type II syndrome' (Crow, 1980), 'negative symptom syndrome' (Andreasen and Olsen, 1982) or 'deficit syndrome' (Carpenter *et al.*, 1988). Although the validity of strict dichotomies between positive and negative symptom groups, or between deficit and non-deficit syndromes may be questioned, studies of such subtypes suggest that a predominance of chronic negative or deficit symptoms may be associated with more obvious neuropathology, involving more prominent structural and functional brain abnormalities, greater cognitive impairment and poorer everyday functioning. In the context of executive dysfunction, as reviewed above, it appears that those patients with worse executive functioning tend to have more negative symptoms (including less illness insight), and poorer functioning in at least some aspects of everyday living skills. Whether these reflect differences in type versus degree of schizophrenic neuropathology remains unknown.

One question that has not been addressed adequately is the issue of specificity. To what degree are the relationships described specific to executive skills, as opposed to general neurocognitive impairment? It is clear that the neurocognitive deficits of schizophrenia are not limited to executive skills. For example, the WCST is not more sensitive to the neurocognitive deficits of schizophrenia than many non-executive neuropsychological measures, and those patients with impaired WCST scores may show similar deficits in general neurocognitive functioning (Braff *et al.*, 1991; Goldstein *et al.*, 1996; Dieci *et al.*, 1997).

Studies by Saykin *et al.* (1991) and Heaton *et al.* (1994), as well as our examination of 'neuropsychologically normal' schizophrenics (Palmer *et al.*, 1997), suggest that impairment on learning measures (i.e. wherein patients are required to learn and immediately recall word lists, short passages or visually presented figures) may be the most commonly or severely impaired neuropsychological ability among schizophrenia patients. However, learning impairment among schizophrenics may at least partially reflect a form of impairment in executive functioning or working memory, perhaps reflecting disruption in cortical–subcortical circuits (Paulsen *et al.*, 1995). Furthermore, even if executive deficits are less sensitive than other neurocognitive skills to schizophrenia in general, they may be particularly sensitive to the pathology underlying certain subsyndromes, such as the negative symptom/deficit syndrome subtypes discussed above (Buchanan *et al.*, 1994).

Whether or not other (non-executive) neurocognitive skills prove to be more universally impaired in schizophrenia patients, executive skills are an important dimension of functioning on which schizophrenia patients vary widely. As noted above, given the role of these skills in self-regulation of thoughts and behavior, it is almost inconceivable that executive deficits would not adversely impact patients' everyday functioning, and the current literature, albeit relatively small and methodologically troubled, tends to support their functional importance. Further research is needed to examine the relationships between specific executive deficits and specific aspects of impairment in everyday living, i.e. what types of difficulties in everyday living do schizophrenia patients typically encounter, and how do these relate to their neurocognitive strengths and weaknesses. Clarification of the links between specific executive and other neurocognitive deficits and specific impairments in everyday functioning will provide obvious potential targets for (pharmacological and rehabilitative) interventions.

References

Abbruzzese, M., Ferri, S. and Scarone S. (1997) The selective breakdown of frontal functions in patients with obsessive–compulsive disorder and in patients with schizophrenia: a double dissociation experimental finding. *Neuropsychologia*, **35**, 907–912.

Anderson, S.W., Damasio, H., Jones, R.D. and Tranel, D. (1991) Wisconsin Card Sorting Test performance as a measure of frontal lobe damage. *Journal of Clinical and Experimental Neuropsychology*, **13**, 909–922.

Andreasen, N.C. and Olsen, S. (1982) Negative versus positive schizophrenia: definition and validation. *Archives of General Psychiatry*, **39**, 789–794.

Andreasen, N.C., Rezai, K., Alliger, R., Swayze, V.W., II, Flaum, M., Kirchner, P., Cohen, G. and O'Leary, D.S. (1992) Hypofrontality in neuroleptic-naive patients and in patients with chronic schizophrenia: assessment with xenon 133 single-photon emission computed tomography and the Tower of London. *Archives of General Psychiatry*, **49**, 943–958.

Artiola i Fortuny, L. and Heaton, R.K. (1996) Standard versus computerized administration of the Wisconsin Card Sorting Test. *The Clinical Neuropsychologist*, **10**, 419–424.

Axelrod, B.N., Goldman, R.S., Heaton, R.K., Curtiss, G., Thompson, L.L., Chelune, G.J. and Kay, G.G. (1996) Discriminability of the Wisconsin Card Sorting Test using the standardization sample. *Journal of Clinical and Experimental Neuropsychology*, **18**, 338–342.

Baddeley, A. (1992) Working memory. *Science*, **255**, 556–559.

Battaglia, M., Abbruzzese, M., Ferri, S., Scarone, S., Bellodi, L. and Smeraldi, E. (1994) An assessment of the Wisconsin Card Sorting Test as an indicator of liability to schizophrenia. *Schizophrenia Research*, **14**, 39–45.

Bell, M.D., Greig, T.C., Kaplan, E. and Bryson, G. (1997) Wisconsin Card Sorting Test dimensions in schizophrenia: factorial, predictive, and divergent validity. *Journal of Clinical and Experimental Neuropsychology*, **19**, 933–941.

Benton, A.L. (1968) Differential behavioral effects of frontal lobe disease. *Neuropsychologia*, **6**, 53–60.

Berg, E.A. (1948) A simple objective test for measuring flexibility in thinking. *Journal of General Psychology*, **39**, 15–22.

Berman, I., Viegner, B., Merson, A., Allan, E., Pappas, D. and Green, A.I. (1997) Differential relationships between positive and negative symptoms and neuropsychological deficits in schizophrenia. *Schizophrenia Research*, **25**, 1–10.

Braff, D.L., Heaton, R.K., Kuck, J., Cullum, M. Moranville, J., Grant, I. and Zisook, S. (1991) The generalized pattern of neuropsychological deficits in outpatients with chronic schizophrenia with heterogeneous Wisconsin Card Sorting Test results. *Archives of General Psychiatry*, **48**, 891–898.

Brekke, J.S., Raine, A., Ansel, M., Lencz, T. and Bird, L. (1997) Neuropsychological and psychophysiological correlates of psychosocial functioning in schizophrenia. *Schizophrenia Bulletin*, **23**, 19–28.

Buchanan, R.W., Strauss, M.E., Kirkpatrick, B., Holstein, C., Breier, A. and Carpenter, W.T., Jr (1994) Neuropsychological impairments in deficit vs nondeficit forms of schizophrenia. *Archives of General Psychiatry*, **51**, 804–811.

Butler, M., Retzlaff, P.D.and Vanderploeg, R. (1991) Neuropsychological test usage. *Professional Psychology: Research and Practice*, **22**, 510–512.

Butler, R.W., Jenkins, M.A., Sprock, J. and Braff, D.L. (1992) Wisconsin Card Sorting Test deficits in chronic paranoid schizophrenia. Evidence for a relatively discrete subgroup? *Schizophrenia Research*, **7**, 169–176.

Carpenter, W.T., Jr, Heinrichs, D.W. and Wagman, A.M. (1988) Deficit and nondeficit forms of schizophrenia: the concept. *American Journal of Psychiatry*, **145**, 578–583.

Carter, C.S., Mintun, M., Nichols, T. and Cohen, J.D. (1997) Anterior cingulate gyrus dysfunction and selective attention deficits in schizophrenia: [^{15}O]H$_2$O PET study during single-trial Stroop task performance. *American Journal of Psychiatry*, **154**, 1670–1675.

Capleton, R.A. (1996) Cognitive function in schizophrenia: association with negative and positive symptoms. *Psychological Reports*, **78**, 123–128.

Cassens, G., Inglis, A.K., Appelbaum, P.S. and Gutheil, T.G. (1990) Neuroleptics: effects on neuropsychological function in chronic schizophrenic patients. *Schizophrenia Bulletin*, **16**, 477–499.

Choca, J.P., Laatsch, L., Wetzel, L. and Agresti, A. (1997) The Halstead Category Test: a fifty year perspective. *Neuropsychology Review*, **7**, 61–75.

Collins, A.A., Remington, G.J., Coulter, K. and Birkett, K. (1997) Insight, neurocognitive function and symptom clusters in chronic schizophrenia. *Schizophrenia Research*, **27**, 37–44.

Comalli, P.E, Jr., Wapner, S. and Werner, H. (1962) Interference effects of Stroop Colour-Word Test in childhood, adulthood and aging. *Journal of Genetic Psychology*, **100**, 47–53.

Crow, T.J. (1980) Molecular pathology of schizophrenia: more than one disease process? *British Medical Journal*, **12**, 66–68.

Cuesta, M.J., Peralta, V., Caro, F. and de Leon, J. (1996) Is poor insight in psychotic disorders associated with poor performance on the Wisconsin Card Sorting Test? *American Journal of Psychiatry*, **152**, 1380–1382.

Cummings, J.L. (1993) Frontal–subcortical circuits and human behavior. *Archives of Neurology*, **50**, 873–880.

Delahunty, A. and Morice, R. (1996) Rehabilitation of frontal/executive impairments in schizophrenia. *Australian and New Zealand Journal of Psychiatry*, **30**, 760–767.

Dieci, M., Vita, A., Silenzi, C., Caputo, A., Comazzi, M., Ferrari, L., Ghiringhelli, L., Mezzetti, M., Tenconi, F. and Invernizzi, G. (1997) Non-selective impairment of Wisconsin Card Sorting Test performance in patients with schizophrenia. *Schizophrenia Research*, **25**, 33–42.

Dyer, F.N. (1973) The Stroop phenomenon and its use in the study of perceptual, cognitive, and response processes. *Memory and Cognition*, **1**, 106–120.

Evarts, E.V., Kimura, M., Wurtz, R.H. and Hikosaka, O. (1984) Behavioral correlates of activity in basal ganglia neurons. *Trends in Neurosciences*, **7**, 447–453.

Fey, E.T. (1951) The performance of young schizophrenics and young normals on the Wisconsin Card Sorting Test. *Journal of Consulting Psychology*, **15**, 311–319.

Franke, P., Maier, W., Hain, C. and Klingler, T. (1992) Wisconsin Card Sorting Test: an indicator of vulnerability to schizophrenia? *Schizophrenia Research*, **6**, 243–249.

Franke, P., Maier, W., Hardt, J., Frieboes, R., Lichterman, D. and Hain, C. (1993a) Assessment of frontal lobe functioning in schizophrenia and unipolar depression. *Psychopathology*, **26**, 76–84.

Franke, P., Maier, W., Hardt, J. and Hain, C. (1993b) Cognitive functioning and anhedonia in subjects at risk for schizophrenia. *Schizophrenia Research*, **10**, 77–84.

Fujii, D.E.M., Ahmed, I., Jokumsen, M. and Compton, J.M. (1997) The effects of clozapine on cognitive functioning in treatment-resistant schizophrenic patients. *Journal of Neuropsychiatry and Clinical Neurosciences*, **9**, 240–245.

Gold, J.M., Carpenter, C., Randolph, C., Goldberg, T.E. and Weinberger, D.R. (1997) Auditory working memory and Wisconsin Card Sorting Test performance in schizophrenia. *Archives of General Psychiatry*, **54**, 159–165.

Goldberg, T.E. and Weinberger, D.R. (1994) Schizophrenia, training paradigms, and the Wisconsin Card Sorting Test redux. *Schizophrenia Research*, **11**, 291–296.

Goldberg, T.E., Saint-Cry, J.A. and Weinberger, D.R. (1990) Assessment of procedural learning and problem solving in schizophrenic patients by Tower of Hanoi type tasks. *Journal of Neuropsychiatry and Clinical Neurosciences*, **2**, 165–173.

Goldberg, T.E., Greenberg, R.D., Griffin, S.J., Gold, J.M., Kleinman, J.E., Pickar, D., Schulz, S.C. and Weinberger, D.R. (1993) The effects of clozapine on cognition and psychiatric symptoms in patients with schizophrenia. *British Journal of Psychiatry*, **162**, 43–48.

Golden, C.J. (1978), *Stroop Color and Word Test*. Stoelting, Chicago.

Goldman, R.S., Axelrod, B.N., Heaton, R.K., Chelune, G.J., Curtiss, G., Kay, G.G. and Thompson, L.L. (1996) Latent structure of the WCST with the standardization samples. *Assessment*, **3**, 73–78.

Goldman-Rakic, P.S. (1991) Prefrontal cortical dysfunction in schizophrenia: the relevance of working memory. In: Carroll, B.J. and Barrett, J.E. (eds), *Psychopathology and the Brain*. Raven Press, New York, pp. 1–23.

Goldman-Rakic, P.S. (1994) Working memory dysfunction in schizophrenia. *Journal of Neuropsychiatry and Clinical Neurosciences*, **6**, 348–357.

Goldstein, G. (1994) Cognitive heterogeneity in psychopathology: the case of schizophrenia. In: Veron, P.A. (ed.), *The Neuropsychology of Individual Differences*. Academic Press, San Diego, CA, pp. 209–233.

Goldstein, G., Beers, S.R. and Shemansky W.J. (1996) Neuropsychological differences between schizophrenic patients with heterogeneous Wisconsin Card Sorting Test performance. *Schizophrenia Research*, **21**, 13–18.

Goodglass, H. and Kaplan, E. (1983) *Boston Diagnostic Aphasia Examination*. Lea & Febiger, Philadelphia.

Graf, P., Uttl, B. and Tuokko, H. (1995) Color- and picture-word Stroop tests: performance changes in old age. *Journal of Clinical and Experimental Neuropsychology*, **17**, 390–415.

Green, M.F. (1996) What are the functional consequences of neurocognitive deficits in schizophrenia? *American Journal of Psychiatry*, **153**, 321–330.

Green, M.F. (1998) *Schizophrenia From a Neurocognitive Perspective: Probing the Impenetrable Darkness*. Allyn and Bacon, Boston.

Green, M.F., Satz, P., Ganzell, S. and Vaclav, J.F. (1992) Wisconsin Card Sorting Test performance in schizophrenia: remediation of a stubborn deficit. *American Journal of Psychiatry*, **149**, 62–67.

Green, M.F., Marshall, B.D., Wirshing, W.C., Ames, D., Marder, S.R., McGurk, S., Kern, R.S. and Mintz, J. (1997) Does risperidone improve verbal working memory in treatment-resistant schizophrenia? *American Journal of Psychiatry*, **154**, 799–804.

Hagger, C., Buckley, P., Kenny, J.T., Friedman, L., Ubogy, D. and Meltzer, H.Y. (1993) Improvement in cognitive functions and psychiatric symptoms in treatment-refractory schizophrenic patients receiving clozapine. *Biological Psychiatry*, **34**, 702–712.

Harris, M.J., Heaton, R.K., Schalz, A., Bailey, A. and Patterson, T.L. (1997) Neuroleptic dose reduction in older psychotic patients. *Schizophrenia Research*, **27**, 241–248.

Heaton, R.K., Nelson L.M., Thompson, D.S., Burks, J.S. and Franklin, G.M. (1981)

Neuropsychological findings in relapsing–remitting and chronic-progressive multiple sclerosis. *Journal Consulting and Clinical Psychology*, **53**, 103–110.

Heaton, R.K., Grant, I. and Matthews, C.G. (1991) *Comprehensive Norms for an Expanded Halstead–Reitan Battery: Demographic Corrections, Research Findings, and Clinical Applications.* Psychological Assessment Resources, Odessa, FL.

Heaton, R.K., Chelune, G.J., Talley, J.L., Kay, G.G. and Curtiss, G. (1993) *Wisconsin Card Sorting Test Manual: Revised and Expanded.* Psychological Assessment Resources, Inc., Odessa, FL.

Heaton, R.K., Paulsen, J.S., McAdams, L.A., Kuck, J., Zisook, S., Braff, D., Harris, M. J. and Jeste, D.V. (1994) Neuropsychological deficits in schizophrenia: relationship to age, chronicity, and dementia. *Archives of General Psychiatry*, **51**, 469–476.

Hepp, H.H., Maier, S., Hermle, L. and Spitzer, M. (1997) The Stroop effect in schizophrenic patients. *Schizophrenia Research*, **22**, 187–195.

Heslegrave, R.J., Awad, A.G. and Voruganti, L.N. (1997) The influence of neurocognitive deficits and symptoms on quality of life in schizophrenia. *Journal of Psychiatry and Neuroscience*, **22**, 235–243.

Humes, G.E., Welsh, M.C., Retzlaff, P. and Cookson, N. (1997) Towers of Hanoi and London: reliability of two executive function tasks. *Assessment*, **4**, 249–257.

Jones, E.G. (1997) Cortical development and thalamic pathology in schizophrenia. *Schizophrenia Bulletin*, **23**, 483–501.

Joyce, E.M., Collinson, S.L. and Crichton, P. (1996) Verbal fluency in schizophrenia: relationship with executive function, semantic memory and clinical alogia. *Psychological Medicine*, **26**, 39–49.

Koren, D., Seidman, L.J., Harrison, R.H., Lyons, M.J., Kremen, W.S., Caplan, B., Goldstein, J.M., Faraone, S.V. and Tsuang, M.T. (1998) Factor structure of the Wisconsin Card Sorting Test: dimensions of deficit in schizophrenia. *Neuropsychology*, **12**, 289–302.

Kraepelin, E. (1919) *Dementia Praecox and Paraphrenia.* (transl. R. M. Barclay, ed. G. M. Robertson). Robert E. Krieger Publishing Co. Inc., Huntington, NY.

Lee, M.A., Thompson, P.A. and Meltzer, H.Y. (1994) Effects of clozapine on cognitive function in schizophrenia. *Journal of Clinical Psychiatry*, **55** (Suppl B), 82–87.

Lewis, D.A. (1997) Development of the prefrontal cortex during adolescence: insights into vulnerable neural circuits in schizophrenia. *Neuropsychopharmacology*, **16**, 385–398.

Lezak, M.D. (1995) *Neuropsychological Assessment.* 3rd edn. Oxford University Press, New York.

Logan, G.D. (1985) Executive control of thought and action. *Acta Psychologica*, **60**, 193–210.

Loring, D.W. (ed.) (1999) *INS Dictionary of Neuropsychology.* Oxford University Press, New York.

Luria, A.R. (1966) *Higher Cortical Functions in Man.* (transl. B. Haigh) Basic Books, New York.

Lysaker, P. and Bell, M. (1994) Insight and cognitive impairment in schizophrenia. Performance on repeated administrations of the Wisconsin Card Sorting Test. *Journal of Nervous and Mental Disease*, **182**, 656–660.

Lysaker, P., Bell, M. and Beam-Goulet, J. (1995) Wisconsin Card Sorting Test and work performance in schizophrenia. *Psychiatry Research*, **56**, 45–51.

Lysaker, P.H., Bell, M.D., Bioty, S.M. and Zito, W.S. (1997) Cognitive impairment and substance abuse history as predictors of the temporal stability of negative symptoms in schizophrenia. *Journal of Nervous and Mental Disease*, **185**, 21–26.

MacLeod, C.M. (1991) Half a century of research on the Stroop effect: an integrative review. *Psychological Bulletin*, **109**, 163–203.

Milner, B. (1964) Some effects of frontal lobectomy in man. In: Warren, J.M. and Akert, K. (eds), *The Frontal Granular Cortex and Behavior.* McGraw-Hill, New York, pp. 313–334.

Morris, R.G., Rushe, T., Woodruffe, P.W. and Murray, R.M. (1995) Problem solving in schizophrenia: a specific deficit in planning ability. *Schizophrenia Research*, **14**, 235–246.

Neisser, U. (1967) *Cognitive Psychology.* Prentice-Hall, Englewood Cliffs, NJ.

Palmer, B.W., Heaton, R.K., Paulsen, J.S., Kuck, J., Braff, D., Harris, M.J., Zisook, S. and Jeste, D.V. (1997) Is it possible to be schizophrenic yet neuropsychologically normal? *Neuropsychology*, **11**, 437–446.

Pantelis, C., Barnes, T.R., Neslon, H.E., Tanner, S., Weahterley, L., Owen, A.M. and Robbins, T.W. (1997) Frontal–striatal cognitive deficits in patients with chronic schizophrenia. *Brain*, **120**, 1823–1840.

Parellada, E., Catafau, A.M., Bernardo, M., Lomena, F., Gonzalez-Monclus, E. and Setoain, J. (1994) Prefrontal dysfunction in young acute neuroleptic-naive schizophrenic patients: a resting and activation SPECT study. *Psychiatry Research*, **55**, 131–139.

Park, S., Holzman, P.S. and Goldman-Rakic, P.S. (1995) Spatial working memory deficits in relatives of schizophrenic patients. *Archives of General Psychiatry*, **52**, 821–828.

Paulsen, J.S., Heaton, R.K., Sadek, J.R., Perry, W., Delis, D.C., Braff, D., Kuck, J., Zisook, S. and Jeste, D.V. (1995) The nature of learning and memory impairments in schizophrenia. *Journal of the International Neuropsychological Society*, **1**, 88–99.

Perlstein, W.M., Carter, C.S., Barch, D.M. and Baird, J.W. (1998) The Stroop task and attention deficits in schizophrenia: a critical evaluation of card and single-trial stroop methodologies. *Neuropsychology*, **12**, 414–425.

Reitan, R.M. and Wolfson, D. (1993) *The Halstead–Reitan Neuropsychological Test Battery: Theory and Clinical Interpretation.* 2nd edn. Neuropsychology Press, South Tucson, AZ.

Reitan, R.M. and Wolfson, D. (1995) Category Test and Trail Making Test as measures of frontal lobe functions. *The Clinical Neuropsychologist*, **9**, 50–56.

Rossi, A., Mancini, F., Stratta, P., Mattei, P., Gismondi, R., Pozzi, F. and Casacchia, M. (1997) Risperidone, negative symptoms and cognitive deficit in schizophrenia: an open study. *Acta Psychiatrica Scandinavica*, **95**, 40–43.

Rubin, P., Holm, S., Madsen, P.L., Friberg, L., Videbech, P., Andersen, H.S., Bendsen, B.B., Stromso, N., Larsen, J.K. and Lassen, N.A. (1994) Regional cerebral blood flow distribution in newly diagnosed schizophrenia and schizophreniform disorder. *Psychiatry Research*, **53**, 57–75.

Saykin, A.J., Gur, R.C., Gur, R.E., Mozley, P.D., Mozley, L.H., Resnick, S.M., Kester, D.B. and Stafiniak, P. (1991) Neuropsychological function in schizophrenia: selective impairment in memory and learning. *Archives of General Psychiatry*, **48**, 618–624.

Seltzer, J., Conrad, C. and Cassens, G. (1997) Neuropsychological profiles in schizophrenia: paranoid versus undifferentiated distinctions. *Schizophrenia Research*, **23**, 131–138.

Shallice, T. (1982) Specific impairments of planning. *Philosophical Transactions of the Royal Society of London*, **298**, 199–209.

Siris, S.G. (1991) Is life a Wisconsin Card Sorting Test? *American Journal of Psychiatry*, **148**, 1413–1414.

Spohn, H.E. and Strauss, M.E. (1989) Relation of neuroleptic and anticholinergic medication to cognitive functions in schizophrenia. *Journal of Abnormal Psychology*, **98**, 367–380.

Spreen, O. and Strauss, E. (1998) *A Compendium of Neuropsychological Tests: Administration, Norms and Commentary*. 2nd edn. Oxford University Press, New York.

Steinberg, J.L., Devous, M.D., Sr and Paulman, R.G. (1996) Wisconsin card sorting activated regional cerebral blood flow in first break and chronic schizophrenic patients and normal controls. *Schizophrenia Research*, **19**, 177–187.

Steindl, S.R. and Boyle, G.J. (1995) Use of the Booklet Category Test to assess abstract concept formation in schizophrenic disorders. *Archives of Clinical Neuropsychology*, **10**, 205–210.

Stratta, P., Daneluzzo, E., Prosperini, P., Bustini, M., Mattei, P. and Rossi, A. (1997a) Is Wisconsin Card Sorting Test performance related to 'working memory' capacity? *Schizophrenia Research*, **27**, 11–19.

Stratta, P, Daneluzzo, E., Mattei, P., Bustini, M., Casacchia, M. and Rossi, A. (1997b) No deficit in Wisconsin Card Sorting Test performance of schizophrenic patients' first-degree relatives. *Schizophrenia Research*, **26**, 147–151.

Stratta, P., Mancini, F., Mattei, P., Daneluzzo, E., Casacchia, M. and Rossi, A. (1997c) Association between striatal reduction and poor Wisconsin Card Sorting Test performance in patients with schizophrenia. *Biological Psychiatry*, **42**, 816–820.

Stuss, D.T. and Benson, D.F. (1986) *The Frontal Lobes*. Raven Press, New York

Suhr, J.A. (1997) Executive functioning deficits in hypothetically psychosis-prone college students. *Schizophrenia Research*, **27**, 29–35.

Summerfelt, A.T., Alphs, L.D., Wagman, A.M., Funderburk, F.R., Hierholzer, R.M. and Strauss, M.E. (1991) Reduction of perseverative errors in patients with schizophrenia using monetary feedback. *Journal of Abnormal Psychology*, **100**, 613–616.

Taylor, S.F. (1996) Cerebral blood flow activation and functional lesions in schizophrenia. *Schizophrenia Research*, **19**, 129–140.

Thurstone, L.L. (1938) *Primary Mental Abilities*. University of Chicago Press, Chicago.

Trestman, R.L., Keefe, R.S., Mitropoulou, V., Harvey, P.D., deVegvar, M.L., Lees-Roitman, S., Davidson, M., Aronson, A., Silverman, J. and Siever, L.J. (1995) Cognitive function and biological correlates of cognitive performance in schizotypal personality disorder. *Psychiatry Research*, **59**, 127–136.

Verdoux, H., Magnin, E. and Bourgeois, M. (1995) Neuroleptic effects on neuropsychological test performance in schizophrenia. *Schizophrenia Research*, **14**, 133–139.

Volz, H.P., Gaser, C., Hager, F., Rzanny, R., Mentzel, H.J., Kreitschmann-Andermahr, I., Kaiser, W.A. and Sauer, H. (1997) Brain activation during cognitive stimulation with the Wisconsin Card Sorting Test—a functional MRI study on healthy volunteers and schizophrenics. *Psychiatry Research*, **75**, 145–157.

Voruganti, L.N., Heslegrave, R.J. and Awad, A.G. (1997) Neurocognitive correlates of positive and negative syndromes in schizophrenia. *Canadian Journal of Psychiatry*, **42**, 1066–1071.

Wechsler, D. (1997a) *Wechsler Adult Intelligence Scale—Third Edition (WAIS-III)*. The Psychological Corporation, San Antonio, TX.

Wechsler, D. (1997b) *Wechsler Memory Scale—Third Edition (WMS-III)*. The Psychological Corporation, San Antonio, TX.

Weinberger, D.R. and Berman, K.F. (1996) Prefrontal function in schizophrenia: confounds and controversies. *Philosophical Transactions of the Royal Society of London*, **351**, 1495–1503.

Weinberger, D.R., Berman, K.F. and Zec, R.F. (1986) Physiologic dysfunction of dorsolateral prefrontal cortex in schizophrenia. I. Regional cerebral blood flow evidence. *Archives of General Psychiatry*, **43**, 114–124.

Welsh, M.C., Pennington, B.F., Ozonoff, S., Rouse, B. and McCabe, E.R.B. (1990) Neuropsychology of early-treated phenylketonuria: specific executive function deficits. *Child Development*, **61**, 1697–1713.

Young, D.A., Davila, R. and Scher, H. (1993) Unawareness of illness and neuropsychological performance in chronic schizophrenia. *Schizophrenia Research*, **10**, 117–124.

Young, D.A., Zakzanis, K.K., Bailey, C., Davila, R., Griese, J., Sartory, G, and Thom, A. (1998) Further parameters of insight and neuropsychological deficit in schizophrenia and other chronic mental disease. *Journal of Nervous and Mental Disease*, **186**, 44–50.

Zec, R.F. (1995) Neuropsychology of schizophrenia according to Kraepelin: disorders of volition and executive functioning. *European Archives of Psychiatry and Clinical Neuroscience*, **245**, 216–223.

4 Learning and memory in schizophrenia

Ruben C. Gur, Stephen T. Moelter and J. Daniel Ragland

Introduction

Disordered cognitive functioning has long been considered a hallmark of schizophrenia. Early work concentrated on impairment in attention, abstraction and other prefrontal domains. Recent studies have focused on memory processes in schizophrenia, implicating temporo-limbic systems. An immediate and important question that arises in this context is the issue of 'differential deficit' as elucidated initially by Chapman and Chapman (1978). Is memory more impaired than other cognitive domains in schizophrenia? In order to establish differential impairment, it is necessary to show that patients are impaired in a specific domain more than other in domains on tasks in which normative samples perform equally (i.e. equivalent mean and true score variance). Demonstrating this can be a daunting task, yet is important prior to a more detailed examination of memory components in schizophrenia.

We therefore begin this chapter by examining evidence of differential memory impairment in schizophrenia. We then summarize several neuropsychological studies designed to elucidate the specific aspects of memory that appear compromised in schizophrenia. These studies have suggested that subgroups of people with schizophrenia may be more susceptible to such deficits. A brief overview of structural and functional neuroimaging data seems to confirm that both frontal and temporo-limbic regions that subserve the disrupted memory functions are abnormal in patients with schizophrenia. These anatomical and physiological abnormalities appear correlated with memory performance, strengthening our confidence that this line of research will help to identify core pathological processes in schizophrenia. We conclude by revisiting the issue of differential deficit, and propose that the differential deficit criterion, important as it may be, should not constrain the direction of neurocognitive research in schizophrenia. Several suggestions for future work are described.

Is there a differential deficit in memory?

Abundant evidence suggests that schizophrenia is characterized by generalized impairment across cognitive domains (for a meta-analysis, see Heinrichs and Zakzanis, 1998). Impairment in the ability to learn and recall information from previously experienced events, or episodic memory (Tulving, 1983), has been recognized as a central problem in schizophrenia (Koh, 1978; Calev *et al.*, 1983; Goldberg *et al.*, 1989; Levin *et al.*, 1989;

Yurgelun-Todd and Waternaux, 1991; Schwartz *et al.*, 1992). The magnitude of the memory impairment has led some investigators to characterize it as an area of differential deficit, distinct from generalized cognitive dysfunction (Rund, 1989; McKenna *et al.*, 1990; Saykin *et al.*, 1991, 1994; Gold *et al.*, 1992; Tamlyn *et al.*, 1992). However, others have argued that it represents a generalized deficit (Blanchard and Neale, 1994), and it has not been fully resolved as to whether the level of memory impairment in schizophrenia is such that it would qualify as an area of differential deficit by Chapman and Chapman's (1978) criteria.

In evaluating this issue, it may be helpful to parse the question into the following testable propositions. (i) Memory impairment is more severe than impairment in reliable estimates of general cognitive abilities (the 'weak' form of differential deficit). (ii) Memory impairment is more severe than that seen in any other behavioral domain measured with comparable assessment instruments (the 'strong' form). Chapman and Chapman's (1978) methodology would be useful for addressing both questions. Evaluation of generalized versus differential deficits depends greatly on how samples are matched (Resnick, 1992), and conclusions may vary with differences in age, chronicity, gender and medication effects.

Saykin *et al.* (1991) attempted to address the first question by administering a comprehensive battery of neuropsychological tests to a prospective sample of patients and sociodemographically matched healthy participants, who were screened for any comorbidity including substance abuse. All patients were evaluated off medication, and many were medication naive. The neuropsychological battery included several measures of verbal and non-verbal learning and memory [e.g. Logical Memory and Visual Reproduction from the Wechsler Memory Scale (WMS), and the California Verbal Learning Test (CVLT)]. Also measured were attention (digit span), abstraction (Wisconsin Card Sorting Test), language, spatial abilities, and sensory and motor functions. Patients' performance was at least one standard deviation below the control sample in all domains. However, a profile analysis demonstrated more severe impairments in memory function (Figure 4.1). These results support the weaker test of differential deficit, and also provide preliminary support to the proposition that memory impairment was significantly worse than any other domain.

This pattern of neuropsychological deficits was replicated in an investigation of first-episode neuroleptic-naive patients and previously treated patients (Saykin *et al.*, 1994). Thus, memory impairment did not appear to be a byproduct of neuroleptic treatment. The first-episode study also demonstrated that the pattern of deficit is stable with repeated measurements, even though the follow-up evaluations were obtained when patients were clinically improved. The stability of these neuropsychological deficits received further support in a study of the relationship between neuropsychological performance and symptom severity at intake and 1.5 year follow-up (Censits *et al.*, 1997). A subsequent follow-up magnetic resonance imaging (MRI) analysis found very small correlations between clinical improvement and change in neuropsychological measures (Gur *et al.*, 1998). It is unlikely that these small correlations reflected poor sensitivity of the neuropsychological instruments, since these measures have shown robust correlations with volumetric indices of brain parenchyma (Kareken *et al.*, 1995) and change in brain parenchymal volume (Gur *et al.*, 1998). Therefore, it seems that these neuropsychological measures may relate to stable neuroanatomical deficits, whereas symptoms may result from overcompensatory behavior and may fluctuate with clinical course. Thus, as Gur (1978) has pointed out, symptoms of schizophrenia may reflect

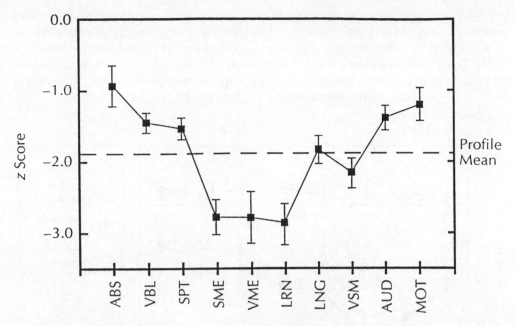

Figure 4.1. Neuropsychological profile (mean ± SEM) for patients with schizophrenia relative to controls whose performance is set to zero (±1 SD) Variables are abbreviated as follows: abstraction (ABS), verbal cognitive (VBL), spatial organization (SPT), semantic memory (SME), visual memory (VME), verbal learning (LRN), language (LNG), visual-motor processing and attention (VSM), auditory processing and attention (AUD), and motor speed and sequencing (MOT). From Saykin *et al.* (1991) with permission of the publishers..

not only the behavioral sequelae of structural lesions, but also 'overactivation' of the dysfunctional brain systems.

More robust correlations between neuropsychological performance and clinical measures, particularly for negative symptoms, have been reported from other centers (Harvey *et al.*, 1996, 1998; Zakzanis, 1998). Palmer *et al.* (1997) used expert ratings to classify patients as neuropsychologically normal or impaired, and found that the normal group demonstrated fewer negative symptoms, less extrapyramidal effects, more frequent socialization and were taking smaller doses of anticholinergic medications. Of particular note, however, is that the 'normal' group in this study maintained deficits in learning in comparison with a healthy control group; this was only one of nine cognitive factors found to be impaired in the normal patient group in comparison with the control group.

In addition to evaluations of learning and memory deficit in schizophrenia, attention has remained a primary candidate of differential impairment. For instance, a limitation of our previous battery (Saykin *et al.*, 1991) is that it did not include a continuous performance measure, which has been reported to be sensitive to attentional impairment in schizophrenia (Nuechterlein, 1991). When a measure of continuous performance was incorporated, attentional dysfunction emerged as an additional area of severe impairment (Censits *et al.*, 1997; Saykin *et al.*, 1994). As can be seen, memory retained its position as differentially impaired, still supporting the weak proposition, but attention was identified as a strong contender for differential deficit (see Figure 4.2). Differential impairment of attention has also been described on tasks that require switching of attention such as Trails A and B (Smith *et al.*, 1998). This finding is consistent with our results which found notable impairment of attention on those cognitive clusters that included tasks requiring attentional shifting and working memory (Saykin *et al.*, 1991, 1994; Censits *et al.*, 1997).

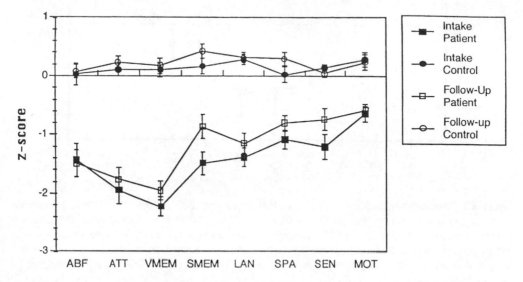

Figure 4.2. Neuropsychological profiles (mean ± SEM): *z*-scores of patients and controls tested at intake and at follow-up. Variables are abbreviated as follows: abstraction (ABF), attention (ATT), verbal memory (VMEM), spatial memory (SMEM), language ability (LAN), spatial ability (SPA), sensory functions (SEN) and motor function (MOT). From Censits *et al.* (1997) with permission of the publishers.

While Saykin *et al.* (1991) indicated that memory impairment remained pronounced following statistical removal of the contributions of attention, the issue of the relationship between attentional and memory deficit needs further empirical scrutiny. Because attentional processes mediate the selection of stimuli for further processing and storage, impairment in attention is likely to produce a deficit in information acquisition. Poor encoding strategies, conversely, may cause attentional disruption as a byproduct of failure to employ effective retrieval strategies and resultant failures of memory. In particular, investigations of working memory, as a construct at the intersection between attentional and mnemonic processes, may help to elucidate what is likely to be a very close relationship.

Other investigators using both meta-analytical and traditional methods have also found evidence of disproportionate memory impairment. In a meta-analysis of 204 studies, Heinrichs and Zakzanis (1998) reported a greater degree of impairment on measures of verbal memory than any other domain, but stopped short of identifying verbal memory as differentially impaired. Very similar effects have been reported in two other meta-analytical studies (Green, 1996; Aleman, 1999). However, as Heinrichs and Zakzanis correctly point out, the debate over the presence of a differential deficit will persist until cognitive tasks are developed that equate levels of difficulty and complexity between tasks; until this step is taken, findings of differential deficit must be interpreted cautiously. This challenge was taken up recently by Binks and Gold (1998) who utilized a battery of tasks conforming to the rigorous Chapman and Chapman (1978) requirements. This battery was administered to a sample of 30 patients with schizophrenia. The investigators concluded that the results generally confirmed the magnitude of memory problems reported by Saykin *et al.* (1994), although their data revealed less severe verbal learning deficits on the CVLT.

Heinrichs and Zakzanis' (1998) reservation notwithstanding, evidence is mounting that memory is impaired differentially, at least in the weak sense of the term, and that it is likely to be among the most impaired functions in the neurocognitive analysis of schizophrenia. It is evident, however, that memory is a complex construct affected by performance in other cognitive domains. Indeed, although the magnitude of memory impairment may exceed that of other functions, a small disturbance in a requisite domain may underlie extensive disruption in functions commanding higher levels of integration. While neuropsychological domains can be separated factorially, there are undoubtedly complex interactions among constructs that are yet to be well articulated. Thus, although memory impairment in schizophrenia is worthy of investigation because it is often severe, persistent and of functional importance, it may turn out that it is closely mediated by a more modest impairment in non-mnemonic abilities that are prerequisite for memory function. In the following section, we will examine which components of memory function appear most disrupted by schizophrenia.

Which aspects of memory are impaired?

Investigators have attempted to identify the specific memory components, stages of information processing and related anatomical networks that are compromised uniquely by schizophrenia. These studies have revealed several types of memory impairment, including a subgroup of patients who show relatively normal learning and memory (Heinrichs and Awad, 1993; Paulsen *et al.*, 1995). The method of subgrouping patients based on cognitive rather than clinical variables has contributed to a better understanding of the heterogeneity of schizophrenia. The CVLT (Delis *et al.*, 1987) has been a central tool in this approach (for a review of the CVLT, see Lezak, 1995).

CVLT studies of schizophrenia generally have found information storage processes to be relatively well preserved. For instance, Heinrichs and Awad (1993) combined the CVLT with measures of general intelligence, categorical reasoning and fine motor speed in order to subtype patients using a cluster analysis procedure. CVLT intrusion errors were examined as an index of short-term information storage related to hippocampal–diencephalic function. The investigators identified five distinct cognitive subtypes of schizophrenia. Low rates of CVLT intrusions in all subgroups, except for a generalized dementia subgroup, led the investigators to conclude that there was little evidence of a selective storage deficit. A similar conclusion was reached by Paulsen *et al.* (1995). They used multiple measures from the CVLT to stratify 175 patients with schizophrenia into subcortical versus cortical pathology groups using previously developed discriminant function analysis procedures (Massman *et al.*, 1992). The full sample had relatively mild recognition deficits and moderately to severely impaired recall, leading to the conclusion that information storage was relatively intact. These results did not replicate previous findings of recognition difficulties and increased forgetting rates (Calev *et al.*, 1983; Gold *et al.*, 1992; Beatty *et al.*, 1993; Clare *et al.*, 1993) that have been used to argue for an amnesia syndrome in schizophrenia.

There is growing evidence that rapid forgetting is not a core feature, and that retrieval and encoding problems are prominent. However, the relative contribution of post-encoding, long-term storage problems remains open to debate. Several investigators have proposed that such post-encoding recognition difficulties may be related to chronicity or severity of illness (Calev *et al.*, 1983; Paulsen *et al.*, 1995). Therefore, a plausible hypothesis is that encoding and retrieval deficits represent core features of memory impairment, and that post-encoding recognition deficits are due to generalized cognitive and intellectual impairment (Chapman and Chapman, 1978; McKenna *et al.*, 1994). Binks and Gold (1998), however, reported impairment of processing speed, visual processing and delayed memory greater than the degree of compromise elicited on other measures in their study. These authors also reported that initial learning was not impaired in their sample, contrary to other reports (Gold *et al.*, 1992).

In contrast, there is consistent evidence of prominent encoding and retrieval difficulties on the CVLT. The study by Paulsen *et al.* (1995) revealed marked retrieval deficits (severely impaired total recall and mildly impaired recognition discriminability). The discriminant analysis classified 50% of the sample into a subcortical profile memory impairment group characterized by prominent retrieval difficulties, suggesting frontostriatal dysfunction (Kramer *et al.*, 1988, 1989; Massman *et al.*, 1990; Buytenhuijs *et al.*, 1994). However, there was also evidence of less severe encoding difficulties including poor semantic clustering, and elevated rates of free recall intrusions and recognition false-positive errors, suggesting poor organization of the to-be-learned material. Failure to cluster or otherwise semantically organize information to facilitate learning and retrieval was also noted by Kareken *et al.* (1996) as perhaps contributing to the reduced level of proactive inhibition demonstrated by their sample. Furthermore, multiple encoding failures have been described previously (Gold *et al.*, 1992), and may be attributed to impaired executive aspects of working memory (Goldman-Rakic, 1994; Fleming *et al.*, 1995; Gold and Weinberger, 1995; Keefe, Chapter 2).

Stone *et al.* (1998) used forward digit span as a measure of immediate memory, and listening, comprehension and reverse digit span as measures of executive working memory. These variables were employed as covariates to determine whether they could account for patient–control differences on tests of strategic memory (free recall, temporal order and self-ordered pointing) and non-strategic memory (recognition). Forward digit span was not impaired and did not explain performance on other tasks. In contrast, measures of executive working memory were impaired and accounted for group differences in strategic memory, but did not explain group differences in recognition (non-strategic memory) performance. Thus, executive impairments in working memory appear related to poor self-generated organizational strategies, which can contribute to free recall deficits in schizophrenia. In this respect, the patients with schizophrenia appeared similar to patients with frontostriatal pathology. However, recognition performance was also impaired, leading the investigators to conclude that temporal–hippocampal networks might be disrupted as well.

Iddon *et al.* (1998) reached similar conclusions in their study of strategic memory processes during visuospatial sequence generation and verbal list learning tasks. The tasks were administered before, during and after training sessions that instructed patients in organizational strategies. Control subjects performed similarly on both tasks and benefited from training. Patients did not benefit from training and were impaired on both tasks, with more severe impairments on the verbal task. Patients also made a large number of perseverative errors, suggesting difficulties in central monitoring of their own action and mental activity (Frith and Done, 1989). As in the previous study (Stone *et al.*, 1998), patients were not impaired on an index of immediate memory. The patients in this study were judged similar to patients with Parkinson's disease (Buytenhuijs *et al.*, 1994) in that they used an externally mediated serial list-learning strategy rather than a more efficient, internally generated semantic clustering strategy. When semantic clustering was used as a covariate, there was no longer a group difference in list learning after the training session. However, semantic clustering did not fully explain verbal learning group differences prior to training. This evidence of residual post-encoding deficits led to the conclusion that impaired verbal learning was due to both encoding and storage or retrieval problems. Thus, both Stone *et al.* (1998) and Iddon *et al.* (1998) found that failure to generate or utilize an organizational strategy was the primary explanation of encoding and retrieval problems. Both studies, however, also provided evidence of post-encoding deficits, leading to the conclusion that learning and memory problems in schizophrenia may be related to both frontostriatal and temporal–hippocampal dysfunction.

Such failures to employ organizational strategies seem closely linked to disruption of semantic system functioning. Indeed, there is a growing body of evidence for semantic system impairment in schizophrenia (Kareken *et al.*, 1996; McKay *et al.*, 1996; Aloia *et al.*, 1998; Feinstein *et al.*, 1998; Goldberg *et al.*, 1998). For instance, McKay *et al.* administered tasks intended specifically to tap the semantic memory system (i.e. knowledge about words and their meanings, general factual information and the interrelationships between objects) and found evidence for semantic memory deficit approaching the level of impairment seen in patients with Alzheimer's dementia. The authors suggested that semantic memory might be an area of differential impairment because when they grouped patients according to preserved overall intellectual function, semantic memory remained consistently impaired—supporting the 'weak' form of differential deficit. Consistent with structural and functional imaging studies, the authors' point out that considerable evidence implicates the left temporal lobe in semantic memory.

It is also notable that a recent study identified the semantic system as differentially impaired on word list generation tasks, including both phonological and semantic fluency (Goldberg *et al.*, 1998). These tasks clearly require multiple cognitive processes, including strategic retrieval, for successful performance. Goldberg *et al.* (1998) found that clinically rated thought disorder was best discriminated by a discrepancy score between phonological and semantic fluency. In this study, the normal pattern of semantic greater than phonological output held for controls and patients without thought disorder. However, in those patients with thought disorder, this pattern was reversed so that phonological fluency output was greater than semantic word list generation. Moreover, Feinstein and colleagues (1998) concluded that this kind of semantic fluency deficit could not be explained as a retrieval failure because patients' performance did not improve significantly with superordinate cues intended to facilitate retrieval. Instead, these authors implicate degradation of semantic memory stores in temporal–parietal cortical regions. Other investigations, however, have not found such clear evidence for a storage deficit in schizophrenia, instead implicating both access and store disruption (Laws *et al.*, 1998).

Relationships between neuroanatomy and memory

The cognitive focus of this volume will not permit the comprehensive review of neuro-anatomical findings that the field deserves. We can only offer a general summary of evidence relating brain volume measures to neurocognitive performance, with specific attention to frontal and temporal regions implicated in memory.

Neuropsychological lesion and neuroimaging studies of human memory systems consistently have implicated the role of medial temporal, diencephalic and prefrontal regions (for reviews, see Squire and Zola, 1996; Gabrieli, 1998). Consistent with this approach, abnormalities in temporal (for a review, see Arnold, 1997) and frontal (for a review, see Goldman-Rakic and Selemon, 1997) structures in schizophrenia have been elucidated. More localized analyses of temporal structures, such as the hippocampus, have produced conflicting results. Arnold *et al.* (1995) described cellular abnormalities of hippocampal and para-hippocampal regions. In this investigation, reduced neuron size was found in subregions of the hippocampus, particularly in the subiculum, CA1 layer and layer II of the entorhinal cortex. Abnormality of the orientation of hippocampal cells has also been described (Conrad *et al.*, 1991). However, other studies have failed to uncover such cellular disarray (Christison *et al.*, 1989).

Volumetric studies with MRI have described global parenchymal volume reduction and increased cerebrospinal fluid (CSF), as well as more specific frontal and temporal lobe reduction in schizophrenia (Turetsky *et al.*, 1995). Several studies have reported correlations between performance on neuropsychological tasks and brain parenchymal volume both in healthy people and in participants with schizophrenia (e.g. Andreasen *et al.*, 1993; Kareken *et al.*, 1995; Turetsky *et al.*, 1995; R.E. Gur *et al.*, 1998; R.C. Gur *et al.*, 1999). Furthermore, Gur *et al.* (1998) reported correlations between volume change and neuropsychological performance, specific for frontal and temporal lobe volumes in relation to memory. Much like the cellular studies described above, however, localizing the association between temporal volume reduction and memory performance to the hippocampus has been problematic. In a meta-anaysis of hippocampal volumetric studies, Nelson *et al.* (1998) reported evidence of consistent bilateral hippocampal volume reduction across studies. Smaller hippocampal volumes in first-episode and chronic patients (Velakoulis *et al.*, 1999) and associations between volumetric reduction, particularly in the amygdala–hippocampal region, and familial risk for disease onset (Lawrie *et al.*, 1999) have been reported recently. Furthermore, our volumetric analysis found reduced volumes in hippocampus and temporal lobe cortex, which were correlated with memory deficits (Gur *et al.*, in press). Thus volumetric anatomical studies appear to demonstrate a convergence with the neuropsychological findings in implicating the frontotemporal memory network as impaired in schizophrenia.

Functional neuroimaging studies

Here again we restrict ourselves to very general statements about abnormalities in functional measures associated with schizophrenia, and focus on the issue of memory in relation to frontal and temporal measures. Those interested in a review of functional neuroimaging techniques are referred to Aine (1995) for a general overview and to Rauch and Renshaw (1995) and Callicott *et al.* (1998) for discussions of functional imaging techniques in psychiatry.

Several studies have suggested reduced resting metabolism and blood flow in frontal regions (Andreasen *et al.*, 1996, 1997; for a review, see Buchsbaum and Hazlett, 1998) in schizophrenia, although this effect has been challenged (Gur and Gur, 1995). In our sample of 42 patients and 42 healthy controls, we found identical metabolic rates for glucose in most brain regions (R.E. Gur *et al.*, 1995). The only significant difference was in the laterality gradient of the mid-temporal region, where patients had abnormally elevated left relative to right hemispheric metabolism. This lack of difference between patients and controls in resting metabolic rates does not reflect poor sensitivity of the metabolic measures as the groups demonstrated robust differences between men and women (R.C. Gur *et al.*, 1995).

To examine the implication of this lateralized temporal lobe abnormality for memory performance in schizophrenia, Mozley *et al.* (1996) divided a sample of 42 patients with schizophrenia into poor recall and preserved recall groups based on their WMS performance. Patients with more marked impairment demonstrated an increase in left-lateralized superior temporal, mid-temporal and inferior temporal metabolism, and also showed greater laterality for the inferior frontal region (Figure 4.3). This supports the notion that part of the neurobiology of schizophrenia involves not only hemispheric dysfunction but also pathological 'overactivation' (Gur, 1978).

Andreasen and colleagues have used functional imaging of memory challenge tasks to evaluate disruption in the cortical–cerebellar–thalamic circuitry (Andreasen *et al.*, 1996, 1997; Wiser *et al.*, 1998; Crespo-Facorro *et al.*, 1999). This series of studies has suggested that the neurocognitive profile in schizophrenia is characterized by relative decreases in cerebral blood flow (CBF) within regions of this circuit during word recall tasks. A model such as Andreasen's 'cognitive dysmetria' (for a review, see Andreasen *et al.*, 1998) is appealing for directing future investigations and providing a template on which neuroimaging studies can be based. However, given the results from several laboratories, including our own, the importance of intact temporal lobe functioning for cognitive task execution, particularly in memory, should not be discounted (Gur *et al.*, 1994; Mozley *et al.*, 1996; Fletcher *et al.*, 1998; Heckers *et al.*, 1998; Jennings *et al.*, 1998; Ragland *et al.*, 1998).

Disturbed activation of frontal and temporal regions in patients with schizophrenia has been reported in several studies using methods for measuring CBF. Consistent effects have been reported with ^{133}Xe clearance (Gur *et al.*, 1994) and ^{15}OH$_2$ positron emission tomography (PET) (Friston *et al.*, 1992; Heckers *et al.*, 1998; Ragland *et al.*, 1998), suggesting abnormal

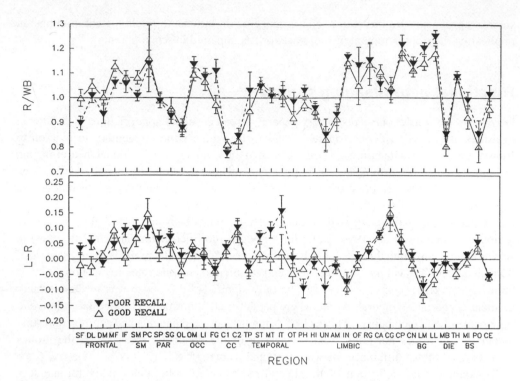

Figure 4.3. Mean (upper graph) and laterality (lower graph) data for patients divided on the basis of their WMS total recall performance. Patients with strong recall are represented by the open triangles; patients with poor performance by the filled triangles. Regions are marked using the following abbreviations: SF = superior frontal; DL = dorsal prefrontal—lateral; DM = dorsal prefrontal—medial; MF = medial frontal; IF = inferior frontal; SM = sensorimotor; PC = paracentral; SP = superior parietal; SG = supramarginal gyrus; OM = occipital cortex—medial; OL = occipital cortex—lateral; LI = lingual gyrus; FG = fusiform gyrus; OT = occipital temporal; ST = superior temporal; MT = mid-temporal; IT = inferior temporal; TP = temporal pole; PH = parahippocampal gyrus; HI = hippocampus; PP = pre-piriform (uncus); AM = amygdala; IN = insula; OF = orbital frontal; RG = rectal gyrus; CA = cingulate gyrus—anterior; CG = cingulate gyrus; CP = gingulate gyrus—posterior; C1 = corpus callosum—anterior; C2 = corpus callosum—posterior; CN = caudate nucleus; LM = lenticular—medial (globus pallidus); LL = lenticular—lateral (putamen); MB = mammillary body; TH = thalamus; MI = midbrain; PO = pons; CE = cerebellum. From Mozley *et al.* (1996) with permission of the publishers.

activation in these regions during memory challenge tasks. In the absence of task-specific effects on hypothesized regions of interest, Ragland *et al.* (1998) supported a model of generalized disruption of frontotemporal integration. However, evidence for reduced hippocampal activity during recollection and activation of dorsolateral prefrontal regions during effortful retrieval has also been obtained (Heckers *et al.*, 1998). The role of the prefrontal cortex in memory performance is a complex one that may be dependent on task difficulty and deployment of strategies to facilitate recall (Fletcher *et al.*, 1998). In their study, Fletcher and colleagues found that in a healthy control sample, prefrontal activation increased as the memory task became more difficult, whereas the patient group demonstrated initial increases that began to drop off with increasing task demands. Furthermore, patients failed to activate superior temporal and inferior parietal regions. Functional studies using PET have also been used to demonstrate disruption in frontal–temporal connections during a task requiring retrieval of semantic information (Jennings *et al.*, 1998). These results are in accord with neuropsychological investigations of semantic impairment in schizophrenia described previously (Kareken *et al.*, 1996; McKay *et al.*, 1996; Aloia *et al.*, 1998; Feinstein *et al.*, 1998; Goldberg *et al.*, 1998).

Another functional imaging method that can help to elucidate the metabolic abnormalities associated with schizophrenia is magnetic resonance spectroscopy (MRS). This method has been applied in neuropsychiatric research, and specifically in schizophrenia (for a review, see Kegeles *et al.*, 1998). Studies that employ MRS methodology have suggested a reduced ratio of *N*-acetyl-aspartate (NAA) to creatine (Cr), particularly in temporal regions, with some studies also showing frontal lobe reduction in this ratio. The NAA/Cr ratio is considered an index of neuronal integrity. In a sample of neuroleptic-naive first-episode patients, we examined NAA/Cr as well as choline (CHO) and amino acid (AA) ratios in both frontal and temporal regions (Cecil *et al.*, 1999). The pattern of metabolite ratios demonstrated some similarities but also some differences between the frontal and temporal lobes (Figure 4.4). Compared with healthy controls, reductions in the NAA/Cr ratio were evident in both frontal and temporal lobes. Both reduction in CHO and elevated AA ratios characterized the temporal lobe pattern. Such a pattern is consistent with metabolic overactivation, perhaps of the neurotransmitter glutamate. This study and others (Maier *et al.*, 1995; Bertolino *et al.*, 1996;

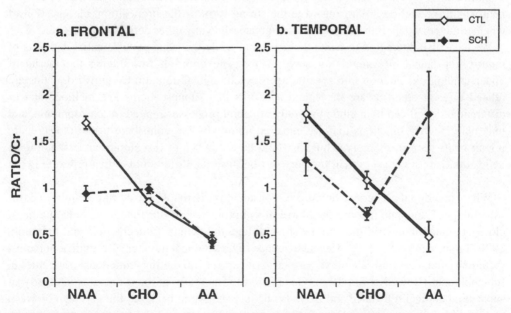

Figure 4.4. Metabolite ratios (mean ± SEM) for *N*-acetyl-aspartate (NAA), choline (CHO) and amino acids (AA) to creatine (Cr) in patients with schizophrenia (filled diamonds) and healthy controls (open diamonds) in the frontal (a) and the temporal lobes (b). From Cecil *et al.* (1999) with permission of the publishers.

Yurgelun-Todd *et al.*, 1996; Deicken *et al.*, 1998) suggest a disruption in temporal and frontal lobe neural circuity. Moreover, abnormality in these regions, as measured by MRS, may be associated with memory dysfunction (Buckley *et al.*, 1994).

Functional evaluation of memory in schizophrenia is now primed for rapid advancement with the emergence of functional MRI (fMRI) methods that offer spatial and temporal resolution superior to that of earlier techniques. Moreover, event-related fMRI analyses allow for the evaluation of individual behavioral trials without the constraints mandated by blocked designs in traditional PET and early fMRI studies (for a review of event-related fMRI, see D'Esposito *et al.*, 1999). Such investigations have offered a wealth of new insights in studies of healthy individuals, particularly in the study of memory using both blocked (Buckner *et al.*, 1998a) and event-related (Buckner *et al.*, 1998b) fMRI designs. Application of fMRI to the study of schizophrenia, however, has been slower to develop. Recent investigations by Weinberger and colleagues have added support for their hypothesis of reduced prefrontal activation during execution of a working memory task (Weinberger *et al.*, 1996; Callicott *et al.*, 1998).

Summary: differential deficit and beyond

The issue of whether memory impairment is an area of differential deficit in schizophrenia has occupied much of the research effort in the field, and accordingly consumed a large portion of this chapter. We conclude that considerable evidence supports a weak form of the differential impairment proposition, namely that memory is more impaired than global indices of general neurocognitive abilities. With regard to the strong form of the proposition, the question of whether memory deficit in schizophrenia is greater than any other deficit remains open.

We have also attempted to make the point that while the issue of differential deficit is of utmost importance, it should not serve as the sole criterion for judging the merits of understanding dysfunction in a specific neuropsychological domain. Cognitive domains are related to each other, as are the neural networks that support them. The methodology of differential deficit can help guide the study of neural processes related to schizophrenia, and may help identify functions that are impaired minimally but contribute to the more severe impairments seen in memory. Thus, it would be a mistake to discourage understanding of deficits that are less severe than memory just because the differential deficit criterion is not met.

What additional criteria should be considered? Perhaps most importantly, neuro-psychological domains that are predictive of symptom severity or functional outcome merit close examination even if they do not show differential deficits (Nuechterlein and Subotnik, 1996; Tamminga *et al.*, 1998). Recent evidence suggests that a number of cognitive domains, including memory and attention, appear critical for predicting functional outcome in schizophrenia (Bowen *et al.*, 1994; Green, 1996). The study of such domains is clearly of substantial clinical relevance and may also be informative in bridging the gap seen between one set of behaviors, measured by the neuropsychological tests, and behaviors measured by clinical and functional rating scales. Neuropsychological domains that show changes associated with medication also deserve attention even in the absence of evidence for differential deficits. Again, beyond clinical utility, such examination can help to illuminate the effects of changes in brain processes related to core symptomatology. Finally, it is necessary to continue to explicate carefully the relationship between cognitive neuropsychological theories of memory, the kinds of memory impairment demonstrated in schizophrenia, and neuroanatomical and neurofunctional studies of schizophrenia. Functional neuroimaging techniques, particularly event-related fMRI, appear to hold great promise for this purpose. In so doing, we may be able to trace the neural networks responsible for the range of abnormalities associated with schizophrenia.

References

Aine, C.J. (1995) A conceptual overview and critique of functional neuroimaging techniques in humans: I. MRI/fMRI and PET. *Critical Reviews in Neurobiology*, **9**, 229–309.

Aleman, A. (1999) Memory in schizophrenia: a meta-analysis. *Mt. Sinai Conference on Cognition in Schizophrenia: An Official Satellite of the International Congress on Schizophrenia Research*. April 16 and 17, 1999, Santa Fe, New Mexico.

Aloia, M.S., Gourovitch, M.L., Missar, D., Pickar, D., Weinberger, D.R. and Goldberg, T.E. (1998) Cognitive substrates of thought disorder, II: specifying a candidate cognitive mechanism. *American Journal of Psychiatry*, **155**, 1677–1684.

Andreasen, N.C., Flaum, M., Swayze, V.D., O'Leary, D.S., Alliger, R., Cohen, G., Ehrhardt, J. and Yuh, W.T. (1993) Intelligence and brain structure in normal individuals. *American Journal of Psychiatry*, **150**, 130–134.

Andreasen, N.C., O'Leary, D.S., Cizadlo, T., Arndt, S., Rezai, K., Boles Ponto, L.L., Watkins, G.L. and Hichwa, R.D. (1996) Schizophrenia and cognitive dysmetria: a positron-emission tomography study of dysfunctional prefrontal–thalamic–cerebellar circuitry. *Proceedings of the National Academy of Sciences of the United States of America*, **93**, 9985–9990.

Andreasen, N.C., O'Leary, D.S., Flaum, M., Nopoulos, P., Watkins, G.L., Boles Ponto, L.L. and Hichwa, R.D. (1997) Hypofrontality in schizophrenia: distributed dysfunctional circuits in neuroleptic-naïve patients. *Lancet*, **349**, 1730–1734.

Andreasen, N.C., Paradiso, S. and O'Leary, D.S. (1998) 'Cognitive dysmetria' as an integrative theory of schizophrenia: a dysfunction in cortical–subcortical–cerebellar circuitry. *Schizophrenia Bulletin*, **24**, 203–218.

Arnold, S.E. (1997) The medial temporal lobe in schizophrenia. *Journal of Neuropsychiatry and Clinical Neurosciences*, **9**, 460–470.

Arnold, S.E., Franz, B.R., Gur, R.C., Gur, R.E., Shapiro, R.M., Moberg, P.J. and Trojanowski, J.Q. (1995) Smaller neuron size in schizophrenia in hippocampal subfields that mediate cortical–hippocampal interactions. *American Journal of Psychiatry*, **152**, 738–748.

Beatty, W.W., Jocic, Z., Monson, N. and Staton, D. (1993) Memory and frontal lobe dysfunction in schizophrenia and schizoaffective disorder. *Journal of Nervous and Mental Disease*, **181**, 448–453.

Bertolino, A., Nawroz, S., Mattay, V.S., Barnett, A.S., Duyn, J.H., Moonen, C.T., Frank, J.A.,

Tedeschi, G. and Weinberger, D.R. (1996) Regionally specific pattern of neurochemical pathology in schizophrenia as assessed by multislice proton magnetic resonance spectroscopic imaging. *American Journal of Psychiatry*, **153**, 1554–1563.

Binks, S.W. and Gold, J.M. (1998) Differential cognitive deficits in the neuropsychology of schizophrenia. *The Clinical Neuropsychologist*, **12**, 8–20.

Blanchard, J.J. and Neale, J.M. (1994) The neuropsychological signature of schizophrenia. *American Journal of Psychiatry*, **151**, 40–48.

Bowen, L., Wallace, C.J., Glynn, S.M., Nuechterlein, K.H., Lutzker, J.R. and Kuehnel, T.G. (1994) Schizophrenic individuals' cognitive functioning and performance in interpersonal interactions and skills training procedures. *Journal of Psychiatric Research*, **28**, 289–301.

Buchsbaum, M.S. and Hazlett, E.A. (1998) Positron emission tomography studies of abnormal glucose metabolism in schizophrenia. *Schizophrenia Bulletin*, **24**, 343–364.

Buckley, P.F., Moore, C., Long, H., Larkin, C., Thompson, P., Mulvany, F., Redmond, O., Stack, J.P., Ennis, J.T. and Waddington, J.L. (1994) ¹H-magnetic resonance spectroscopy of the left temporal and frontal lobes in schizophrenia: clinical, neurodevelopmental, and cognitive correlates. *Biological Psychiatry*, **36**, 792–800.

Buckner, R.L., Koustall, W., Schacter, D.L., Wagner, A.D. and Rosen, B.R. (1998a) Functional–anatomic study of episodic retrieval using fMRI: I. Retrieval effort versus retrieval success. *Neuroimage*, **7**, 151–162.

Buckner, R.L., Koustall, W., Schacter, D.L., Dale, A.M., Rotte, M. and Rosen, B.R. (1998b) Functional–anatomic study of episodic retrieval: II. Selective averaging of event-related fMRI trials to test the retrieval success hypothesis. *Neuroimage*, **7**, 163–175.

Buytenhuijs, E.L., Berger, H.J.C, Van Spaendonck, K.P.M, Horstink, M.W.I.M., Borm, G.F. and Cools, A.R. (1994) Memory and learning strategies in patients with Parkinson's disease. *Neuropsychologia*, **32**, 335–342.

Calev, A., Venables, P.H. and Monk, A.F. (1983) Evidence for distinct verbal memory pathologies in severely and mildly disturbed schizophrenics. *Schizophrenia Bulletin*, **9**, 247.

Callicott, J.H., Ramsey, N.F., Tallent, K., Bertolino, A., Knable, M.B., Coppola, R., Goldberg, T., van Gelderen, P., Mattay, V.S., Frank, J.A., Moonen, C.T. and Weinberger, D.R. (1998) Functional magnetic resonance imaging brain mapping in psychiatry: methodological issues illustrated in a study of working memory in schizophrenia. *Neuropsychopharmacology*, **18**, 186–196.

Cecil, K.M., Lenkinski, R.E., Gur, R.E. and Gur, R.C. (1999) Proton magnetic resonance spectroscopy in the frontal and temporal lobes of neuroleptic naive patients with schizophrenia. *Neuropsychoparmacology*, **20**, 131–140.

Censits, D.M., Ragland, J.D., Gur, R.C. and Gur, R.E. (1997) Neuropsychological evidence supporting a neurodevelopmental model of schizophrenia: a longitudinal study. *Schizophrenia Research*, **24**, 289–298.

Chapman, L.J. and Chapman, J.P. (1978) The measurement of differential deficits. *Journal of Psychiatry Research*, **14**, 303–311.

Christison, G.W., Casanova, M.F., Weinberger, D.W., Rawlings, R. and Kleinman, J.E. (1989) A quantitative investigation of hippocampal pyramidal cell size, shape, and variability of orientation in schizophrenia. *Archives of General Psychiatry*, **46**, 1027–1032.

Clare, L., McKenna, P.J., Mortimer, A.M. and Baddeley, A.D. (1993) Memory in schizophrenia: what is impaired and what is preserved? *Neuropsychologia*, **31**, 1225–1241.

Conrad, A.J., Abebe, T., Austin, R., Forsythe, S. and Scheibel, A.B. (1991) Hippocampal pyramidal cell disarray in schizophrenia as a bilateral phenomenon. *Archives of General Psychiatry*, **48**, 413–417.

Crespo-Facorro, B., Paradiso, S., Andreasen, N.C., O'Leary, D.S., Watkins, L., Boles Pinto, L.L. and Hichwa, R.D. (1999) Recalling word lists reveals 'cognitive dysmetria' in schizophrenia: a positron emission tomography study. *American Journal of Psychiatry*, **156**, 386–392.

Deicken, R.F., Zhou, L., Schuff, N., Fein, G. and Weiner, M.W. (1998) Hippocampal neuronal dysfunction in schizophrenia as measured by proton magnetic resonance spectroscopy. *Biological Psychiatry*, **43**, 483–488.

Delis, D.C., Kramer, J.H., Kaplan, E. and Ober, B.A. (1987) *California Verbal Learning Test (CVLT) Manual: Research Edition*. The Psychological Corporation, New York.

D'Esposito, M., Zarahn, E. and Aguirre, G.K. (1999) Event-related functional MRI: implications for cognitive psychology. *Psychological Bulletin*, **125**, 155–164.

Feinstein, A., Goldberg, T.E., Nowlin, B. and Weinberger, D.R. (1998) Types and characteristics of remote memory impairment in schizophrenia. *Schizophrenia Research*, **30**, 155–163.

Fleming, K., Goldberg, T.E., Gold, J.M. and Weinberger, D.R. (1995) Verbal working memory dysfunction in schizophrenia: use of a Brown–Peterson paradigm. *Psychiatry Research*, **56**, 155–161.

Fletcher, P.C., McKenna, P.J., Frith, C.D., Grasby, P.M., Friston, K.J. and Dolan, R.J. (1998) Brain activations in schizophrenia during a graded memory task studied with functional neuroimaging. *Archives of General Psychiatry*, **55**, 1001–1008.

Friston, K.J., Liddle, P.F., Frith, C.D., Hirsch, S.R. and Frackowiak, R.S. (1992) The left medial temporal region and schizophrenia. A PET study. *Brain*, *115*, 367–382.

Frith, C.D. and Done, D.J. (1989) Experiences of alien control in schizophrenia reflect a disorder in the central monitoring of action. *Psychological Medicine*, **19**, 359–363.

Gabrieli, J.D.E. (1998) Cognitive neuroscience of human memory. *Annual Review of Psychology*, **49**, 87–115.

Gold, J.M. and Weinberger, D.R. (1995) Cognitive deficits and the neurobiology of schizophrenia. *Current Opinion in Neurobiology*, **5**, 225–230.

Gold, J.M., Randolf, C., Carpenter, C.J., Goldberg, T.E. and Weinberger, D.R. (1992) Forms of memory failure in schizophrenia. *Journal of Abnormal Psychology*, **101**, 487–94.

Goldberg, T.E., Weinberger, D.R., Pliskin, N.H., Berman, K.F. and Podd, M.H. (1989) Recall memory deficit in schizophrenia. A possible manifestation of prefrontal dysfunction. *Schizophrenia Research*, **2**, 251–257.

Goldberg, T.E., Aloia, M.S., Gourovitch, M.L., Missar, D., Pickar, D. and Weinberger, D.R. (1998) Cognitive substrates of thought disorder, I: the semantic system. *American Journal of Psychiatry*, **155**, 1671–1676.

Goldman-Rakic, P. (1994) Working memory dysfunction in schizophrenia. *Journal of Neuropsychiatry and Clinical Neurosciences*, **6**, 348–357.

Goldman-Rakic, P.S. and Selemon, L.D. (1997) Functional and anatomical aspects of prefrontal pathology in schizophrenia. *Schizophrenia Bulletin*, **23**, 437–458.

Green, M.F. (1996) What are the functional consequences of neurocognitive deficits in schizophrenia? *American Journal of Psychiatry*, **153**, 321–330.

Gur, R.C. and Gur, R.E. (1995) Hypofrontality in schizophrenia: RIP. *Lancet*, **345**, 1383–1384.

Gur, R.C., Mozley, L.H., Mozley, P.D., Resnick, S.M., Karp, J.S., Alavi, A., Arnold, S.E. and Gur, R.E. (1995) Sex differences in regional cerebral glucose metabolism during a resting state. *Science*, **267**, 528–531.

Gur, R.C., Turetsky, B.I., Matsui, M., Yan, M., Bilker, W., Hughett, P. and Gur, R.E. (1999) Sex differences in brain gray and white matter in healthy young adults: correlations with cognitive performance. *Journal of Neuroscience* (in press).

Gur, R.E. (1978) Left hemisphere dysfunction and left hemisphere overactivation in schizophrenia. *Journal of Abnormal Psychology*, **87**, 226–238.

Gur, R.E., Jaggi, J.L., Shtasel, D.L., Ragland, J.D. and Gur, R.C. (1994) Cerebral blood flow in schizophrenia: effects of memory processing on regional activation. *Biological Psychiatry*, **35**, 3–15.

Gur, R.E., Mozley, P.D., Resnick, S.M., Mozley, L.H., Shtasel, D.L., Gallacher, F., Arnold, S.E., Karp, J.S., Alavi, A., Reivich, M. and Gur, R.C. (1995) Resting cerebral glucose metabolism and clinical features of schizophrenia. *Archives of General Psychiatry*, **52**, 657–667.

Gur, R.E., Cowell, P., Turetsky, B.I., Galllacher, F., Cannon, T., Bilker, W. and Gur, R.C. (1998) A follow-up magnetic resonance imaging study of schizophrenia: relationship of neuroanatomical changes to clinical and neurobehavioral measures. *Archives of General Psychiatry*, **55**, 145–152.

Gur, R.E., Turetsky, B.I., Cowell, P.E., Finkelman, C., Maany, V., Grossman, R.I., Arnold, S.E., Bilker, W.B. and Gur, R.C. (in press) Temporolimbic volume reductions in schrizophrenia. *Archives of General Psychiatry*.

Harvey, P.D., Lombardi, J., Leibman, M., White, L., Parrella, M., Powchik, P. and Davidson, M. (1996) Cognitive impairment and negative symptoms in geriatric chronic schizophrenic subjects: a follow-up study. *Schizophrenia Research*, **22**, 223–231.

Harvey, P.D., Howanitz, E., Parrella, M., White, L., Davidson, M., Mohs, R.C., Hoblyn, J. and Davis K.L. (1998) Symptoms, cognitive functioning, and adaptive skills in geriatric patients with lifelong schizophrenia: a comparison across treatment sites. *American Journal of Psychiatry*, **155**, 1080–1086.

Heckers, S., Rauch, S. L., Goff, D., Savage, C. R., Schacter, D. L., Fischman, A.J. and Alpert, N.M. (1998) Impaired recruitment of the hippocampus during conscious recollection in schizophrenia. *Nature Neuroscience*, **1**, 318–323.

Heinrichs, R.W. and Awad, A.G. (1993) Neurocognitive subtypes of chronic schizophrenia. *Schizophrenia Research*, **9**, 49–58.

Heinrichs, R.W. and Zakzanis, K.K. (1998) Neurocognitive deficit in schizophrenia: a quantitative review of the evidence. *Neuropsychology*, **12**, 426–445.

Iddon, J.L., McKenna, P.J., Sahakian, B.J. and Robbins, T.W. (1998) Impaired generation and use of strategy in schizophrenia: evidence from visuospatial and verbal tasks. *Psychological Medicine*, **28**, 1049–1062.

Jennings, J.M., McIntosh, A.R., Kapur, S., Zipursky, R.B. and Houle, S. (1998) Functional network differences in schizophrenia: a rCBF study of semantic processing. *Neuroreport*, **9**, 1697–1700.

Kareken, D.A., Gur, R.C., Mozley, P.D., Mozley, L.H., Saykin, A.J., Shtasel, D.L. and Gur, R.E. (1995) Cognitive functioning and neuroanatomic volume measures in schizophrenia. *Neuropsychology*, **9**, 211–219.

Kareken, D.A., Moberg, P.J. and Gur, R.C. (1996) Proactive inhibition and semantic organization: relationship with verbal memory in patients with schizophrenia. *Journal of the International Neuropsychological Society*, **2**, 486–493.

Kegeles, L.S., Humaran, T.J. and Mann, J.J. (1998) *In vivo* neurochemistry of the brain in schizophrenia as revealed by magnetic resonance spectroscopy. *Biological Psychiatry*, **44**, 382–398.

Koh, S.D. (1978) Remembering of verbal materials by schizophrenic young adults. In: Schwartz, S. (ed.), *Language and Cognition in Schizophrenia*. Lawrence Earlbaum, Hillsdale, NJ.

Kramer, J.H, Delis, D.C., Blusewicz, M J., Brandt, J., Ober, B.A. and Strauss, M. (1988) Verbal memory errors in Alzheimer's and Huntington's dementias. *Developmental Neuropsychology*, **4**, 1–15.

Kramer, J.H, Levin, B., Brandt, J. and Delis, D.C. (1989) Differentiation of Alzheimer's, Huntington's, and Parkinson's diseases on the basis of verbal learning characteristics. *Neuropsychology*, **3**, 111–120.

Laws, K.R., McKenna, P.J. and Kondel, T. (1998) On the distinction between access and store disorders in schizophrenia: a question of deficit severity? *Neuropsychologia*, *36*, 313–321.

Lawrie, S. M., Whalley, H., Kestelman, J.N., Abukmeil, S.S., Byrne, M., Hodges, A., Rimmington, J.E., Best, J.J., Owens, D.G. and Johnstone, E.C. (1999) Magnetic resonance imaging of brain in people at high risk of developing schizophrenia. *Lancet*, **353**, 30–33.

Levin, S., Yurgelun-Todd, D. and Craft, S. (1989) Contributions of clinical neuropsychology to the study of schizophrenia. *Journal of Abnormal Psychology*, **98**, 341–346.

Lezak, M.D. (1995) *Neuropsychological Assessment*. 3rd edn. Oxford University Press, New York.

Maier, M., Ron, M.A., Barker, G.J. and Tofts, P.S. (1996) Proton magnetic resonance spectroscopy: an *in vivo* method of estimating hippocampal neuronal depletion in shizophrenia. *Psychological Medicine*, **26**, 1201–1209.

Massman, P.J., Delis, D.C., Butters, N., Levin, B.E. and Salmo, D.P. (1990) Are all subcortical dementias alike? Verbal learning and memory in Parkinson's and Huntington's disease patients. *Journal of Clinical and Experimental Neuropsychology*, **12**, 729–744.

Massman, P.J., Delis, D.C., Butters, N., Dupont, R.M. and Gillin, J.C. (1992) The subcortical dysfunction hypothesis of memory deficits in depression: neuropsychological validation in a subgroup of patients. *Journal of Clinical and Experimental Neuropsychology*, **14**, 687–706.

McKay, A.P., McKenna, P.J., Bentham, P., Mortimer, A.M., Holberry, A. and Hodges, J.R. (1996) Semantic memory is impaired in schizophrenia. *Biological Psychiatry*, **39**, 929–937.

McKenna, P.J., Tamlyn, D., Lund, C.E., Mortimer, A.M., Hammond, S. and Baddeley, A.D. (1990) Amnesic syndrome in schizophrenia. *Psychological Medicine*, **20**, 967–972.

McKenna, P.J., Mortimer, A.M. and Hodges, J.R. (1994) Semantic memory and schizophrenia. In: David, A.S. and Cutting, J.C. (eds), *The Neuropsychology of Schizophrenia*. Lawrence Erlbaum Associates, Mahwah, NJ, pp. 163–177.

Mozley, L.H., Gur, R.C., Gur, R.E., Mozley, P.D. and Alavi, A. (1996) The relationship between verbal memory performance and the cerebral distribution of FDG in patients with schizophrenia. *Biological Psychiatry*, **40**, 443–451.

Nelson, M.D., Saykin, A.J., Flashman, L.A. and Riordan, H.J. (1998) Hippocampal volume reduction in schizophrenia as assessed by magnetic resonance imaging: a meta-analytic study. *Archives of General Psychiatry*, **55**, 433–440.

Nuechterlein, K.H. (1991) Vigilance in schizophrenia and related disorders. In: Steinhauer, S.R., Gruzelier, J.H. and Zubin, J. (eds), *Handbook of Schizophrenia*. Elsevier, Amsterdam, pp. 397–433.

Nuechterlein, K.H. and Subotnik, K.L. (1996) The role of neurocognitive deficits in understanding adaptive functioning in severe psychiatric illness: commentary on Hawkins and Cooper. *Psychiatry*, **59**, 382–388.

Palmer, B.W., Heaton, R.K., Paulsen, J.S., Kuck, J.K., Braff, D. and Harris, M.J. (1997) Is it possible to be schizophrenic yet neuropsychologically normal? *Neuropsychology*, **11**, 437–446.

Paulsen, J.S., Heaton, R.K., Sadek, J.R., Perry, W., Delis, D.C., Braff, D., Kuck, J., Zisook, S. and Jeste, D.V. (1995) The nature of learning and memory impairments in schizophrenia. *Journal of the International Neuropsychological Society*, **1**, 88–99.

Ragland, J.D., Gur, R.C., Glahn, D.C., Censits, D.M., Smith, R.J., Lazarev, M.G., Alavi, A. and Gur, R.E. (1998) Frontotemporal cerebral blood flow change during executive and declarative memory tasks in schizophrenia: a positron emission tomography study. *Neuropsychology*, **12**, 399–413.

Rauch, S.L. and Renshaw, P.F. (1995) Clinical neuroimaging in psychiatry. *Harvard Review of Psychiatry*, **2**, 297–312.

Resnick, S.M. (1992) Matching for education in studies of schizophrenia. *Archives of General Psychiatry*, **49**, 246.

Rund, B.R. (1989) Distractibility and recall capability in schizophrenics: a four year longitudinal study of stability in cognitive performance. *Schizophrenia Research*, **2**, 265–275.

Saykin, A.J, Gur, R.C., Gur, R.E., Mozley, D., Mozley, L.H., Resnick, S.M., Kester, D.B. and Stafiniak, P. (1991) Neuropsychological function in schizophrenia: selective impairment in memory and learning. *Archives of General Psychiatry*, **48**, 618–624.

Saykin, A.J., Shtasel, D.L., Gur, R.E., Kester, D.B., Mozley, L.H., Stafiniak, P. and Gur, R.C. (1994) Neuropsychological deficits in neuroleptic naive patients with first-episode schizophrenia. *Archives of General Psychiatry*, **51**, 124–131.

Schwartz, B.L., Rosse, R.B. and Deutsch, S.I. (1992) Toward a neuropsychology of memory in schizophrenia. *Psychopharmacology Bulletin*, **28**, 341–351.

Smith, G.R., Large, M.M., Kavanagh, D.J., Karayanidis, F., Barrett, N.A., Michie, P.T. and O'Sullivan, B.T. (1998) Further evidence for a deficit in switching attention in schizophrenia. *Journal of Abnormal Psychology*, **107**, 390–398.

Squire, L.R. and Zola, S.M. (1996) Structure and function of declarative and nondeclarative memory systems. *Proceedings of the National Academy of Sciences of the United States of America*, **93**, 13515–13522.

Stone, M., Gabrieli, J.D.E., Stebbins, G.T. and Sullivan, E.V. (1998) Working and strategic memory deficits in schizophrenia. *Neuropsychology*, **12**, 278–288.

Tamlyn, D., McKenna, P.J., Mortimer, A.M., Lund, C.E., Hammond, S. and Baddeley, A.D. (1992) Memory impairment in schizophrenia: its extent, affiliations, and neuropsychological character. *Psychological Medicine*, **22**, 101–115.

Tamminga, C.A., Buchanan, R.W. and Gold, J.M. (1998) The role of negative symptoms and cognitive dysfuntion in schizophrenia outcome. *International Clinical Psychopharmacology*, **13**, S21–S26.

Tulving, E. (1983) *Elements of Episodic Memory*. Academic Press, New York.

Turetsky, B.I., Cowell, P.E., Gur, R.C., Grossman, R.I., Shtasel, D.L. and Gur, R.E. (1995) Frontal and temporal lobe brain volumes in schizophrenia: relationship to symptoms and clinical subtype. *Archives of General Psychiatry*, **52**, 1061–1070.

Velakoulis, D., Pantelis, C., McGorry, P. D., Dudgeon, P., Brewer, W., Cook, M., Desmond, P., Bridle, N., Tierney, P., Murrie, V., Singh, B. and Copolov, D. (1999) Hippocampal volume in first-episode psychoses and chronic schizophrenia. *Archives of General Psychiatry*, **56**, 133–140.

Weinberger, D.R., Mattay, V., Callicott, J., Kotrla, K., Santha, A., van Gelderen, P., Duyn, J., Moonen, C. and Frank, J. (1996) fMRI applications in schizophrenia research. *Neuroimage*, **4**, S118–S126.

Wiser, A.K., Andreasen, N.C., O'Leary, D.S., Watkins, G.L., Boles Ponto, L.L. and Hichwa, R.D. (1998) Dysfunctional cortico-cerebellar circuits cause 'cognitive dysmetria' in schizophrenia. *Neuroreport*, **9**, 1895–1899.

Yurgelun-Todd, D.A. and Waternaux, C.S. (1991) Cognitive deficits underlying verbal memory function in schizophrenic patients and controls. *Schizophrenia Research*, **4**, 396–397.

Yurgelun-Todd, D.A., Renshaw, P.F., Gruber, S.A., Ed, M., Waternaux, C. and Cohen, B.M. (1996) Proton magnetic resonance spectroscopy of the temporal lobes in schizophrenics and normal controls. *Schizophrenia Research*, **19**, 55–59.

Zakzanis, K.K. (1998) Neuropsychological correlates of positive vs. negative schizophrenic symptomatology. *Schizophrenia Research*, **29**, 227–233.

5 Information processing and attention in schizophrenia: clinical and functional correlates and treatment of cognitive impairment

Kristin S. Cadenhead and David L. Braff

Introduction

The study of information processing and attention abnormalities as core cognitive deficits in schizophrenia research has identified abnormalities in these domains and has clarified their relationship to neural substrate abnormalities and functional outcome in patients with schizophrenia (e.g. Braff, 1999). It has been hypothesized that the information processing and attentional deficits of schizophrenic patients are 'central' to the disorder and are strongly associated with the clinical and functional impairments of the illness (McGhie and Chapman, 1961; Steronko and Woods, 1978; Green, 1996; Braff, 1999). In addition, the study of information processing deficits in human research and animal models has increased our understanding of the neural circuit dysfunction of schizophrenia and provided means of assessing new treatments that 'normalize' these information processing deficits (e.g. Swerdlow *et al.*, 1994; Braff, 1999) . If information processing abnormalities are core and enduring deficits of patients with schizophrenia spectrum disorders and their relatives, they may also be useful intermediate phenotypic markers in genetic studies (Freedman *et al.*, 1997).

Since the time of Bleuler and Kraepelin, attention and information processing deficits have been identified as important features of schizophrenia (Braff, 1985). Many studies have been performed in order to understand the specific nature of cognitive deficits in patients with schizophrenia and to characterize whether specific information processing deficits are indeed central to the disorder. One strategy that has been used to evaluate the role of information processing deficits in schizophrenia is the use of studies that link cognitive deficits to clinical symptoms or the functional outcome of the disorder (Breier *et al.*, 1991; Strauss *et al.*, 1993; Corrigan and Toomey, 1995; Penn *et al.*, 1995). Additionally, studies that assess the state and trait contributions of information processing abnormalities add further insight into which measures best characterize the cognitive deficits of schizophrenic patients that are correlated with symptoms versus enduring schizophrenic-linked deficits

(Nuechterlein and Dawson, 1984; Braff, 1993). Once the measures of information processing deficits most closely linked to clinical symptoms and functional outcome are clarified, we may be able to utilize these measures in order to assess or even predict optimal treatment outcome.

In this chapter, we will first review the information processing literature that addresses the question of whether information processing abnormalities are central or core deficits that characterize schizophrenia. This section will also include studies of clinical and functional correlates of information processing disorders and outcome studies as well as studies that investigate information processing deficits as potential trait markers for schizophrenic spectrum illness. We will then address cognitive rehabilitation approaches that apply knowledge gained from information processing studies to the treatment of schizophrenia.

Information processing and clinical symptoms of schizophrenia

The 'pathway' by which information processing abnormalities might be associated with the psychotic and deficit symptoms of schizophrenic patients has, at times, been described in terms of an inhibitory failure or an impairment in stimulus gating or filtering (McGhie and Chapman, 1961; Frith, 1979, 1993; Braff and Geyer, 1990; Butler and Braff, 1991; Braff, 1999). If a schizophrenic patient lacks normal inhibitory functions, there may be an inundation or overload of normally inhibited external and internally generated stimuli that leads to the misinterpretation of words or events (Frith, 1979, 1993). Psychotic symptoms such as the auditory hallucinations might be explained by the intrusion of preconscious logogens (word roots) (Morton, 1979) secondary to misinterpreted sounds (Frith, 1979). In this context, delusions could be the result of efforts to explain misperceived information (Frith, 1979; Butler and Braff, 1991). Thus, if a schizophrenic patient is unable to inhibit the normally preconscious alternative meaning of words, they might be inundated with sensory stimuli with resulting thought disorder manifested by abnormal speech patterns (Frith, 1979).

Many information processing studies have shown consistent associations between information processing deficits and the so-called 'deficit' symptoms of schizophrenia (Green and Walker, 1984, 1986; Nuechterlein et al., 1986; Braff, 1989; Weiner et al., 1990; Katsanis and Iacono, 1991; Igata et al., 1994; Sweeney et al., 1994; Javitt et al., 1995; Buchanan et al., 1997; Cadenhead et al., 1997; Freedman et al., 1998) but the degree of these associations, while important and meaningful, typically are modest. These modest effects may be accounted for by the proposed complex heterogeneity of a mixture of both primary and secondary deficit symptoms in most schizophrenic patients (Castellon et al., 1994). The primary deficit symptoms reflect such factors as frontal hypoactivity and decreased frontal dopamine tone (Weinberger and Gallhofer, 1997), while the secondary symptoms are related to the effects of medication, psychotic symptoms and social isolation (Carpenter et al., 1988, 1993). If information processing deficits are related causally to an underlying neural structural and/or corresponding functional process, they are likely to be related to the enduring (primary) rather than transitory (secondary) deficit symptoms. In this context, some information processing studies have attempted to differentiate schizophrenic patients with persistent (and presumably primary) deficit symptoms from those with transitory (and presumably secondary) symptoms and found evidence that the persistent deficit symptoms are associated more robustly with information processing deficits (Thaker *et al.*, 1988; Castellon *et al.*, 1994; Buchanan *et al.*, 1997; Ross *et al.*, 1997). Thus, some studies that differentiate primary from secondary deficit symptoms offer indirect but interesting support for the hypothesis that information processing deficits are 'core' features of schizophrenia since they are strongly linked to persistent, deficit symptoms. Given the association between the deficit syndrome and information processing abnormalities, it is possible and worth exploring if the same or similar pathophysiological processes may underlie both sets of abnormalities. In support of this convergent strategy, neuroimaging studies demonstrate decreased metabolism in both the frontal and parietal association cortices in deficit patients (Tamminga *et al.*, 1992; Buchanan *et al.*, 1994) and those with abnormal smooth pursuit eye movements (Ross *et al.*, 1995) or impaired performance on the Continuous Performance Task (CPT) (Buchsbaum *et al.*, 1990; Pardo *et al.*, 1991; Corbetta *et al.*, 1993). These interlocking information processing and imaging studies, framed in terms of specific symptoms, strengthen the value of using information processing abnormalities as 'markers' to understand brain pathology in schizophrenia.

The association between information processing abnormalities, thought disorder and positive symptoms (hallucinations and delusions) has also been demonstrated in schizophrenic patients (Holzman *et al.*, 1974; Cornblatt *et al.*, 1985; Solomon *et al.*, 1987; Strauss *et al.*, 1993; Perry and Braff, 1994; Higashima *et al.*, 1998). Again, investigators have linked the positive symptoms in schizophrenia with neural substrate dysfunction of this disorder. It is striking that thought disorder is a hallmark of schizophrenia and that increased levels of thought disorder have been shown to be associated with a range of information processing dysfunctions including abnormal CPT performance (Cornblatt *et al.*, 1985; Strauss *et al.*, 1993), eye movement dysfunction (Holzman *et al.*, 1974; Solomon *et al.*, 1987), impaired visual backward masking performance (Perry and Braff, 1994), reduced prepulse inhibition of the startle response (VBM) (Perry and Braff, 1994) and reduced P300 amplitude (Higashima *et al.*, 1998). The neural substrates of at least some information processing deficits in patients with schizophrenia have been identified via neuroimaging studies that reveal a significant association between thought disorder and hallucinations and reduced total thalamic volumes (Portas *et al.*, 1998). These data also add support to the idea that the thalamus plays a central role in normal sensory gating (Jones, 1985, 1997) and the integration of cortical processing and behavior (Sherman and Koch, 1986; Crosson and Hughes, 1987; Livingstone and Hubel, 1987; Alexander *et al.*, 1990; Swerdlow *et al.*, 1992; Van Essen *et al.*, 1992; Cadenhead *et al.*, 1998) and that these functions may be impaired specifically due to thalamic abnormalities in schizophrenia.

Information processing: state versus trait issues

If, as hypothesized (Braff, 1999), information processing measures comprise a core and persistent, trait-linked deficit of schizophrenic patients, we might expect to see information processing deficits in remitted versus acute patients, 'non-affected' relatives of schizophrenic patients (who may carry a genetic predisposition to schizophrenia) and schizotypal personality disordered (SPD) patients who are phenomenologically, and perhaps phenotypically, linked to schizophrenia. In fact, the information processing literature supports the hypothesis that the schizophrenia diathesis carries with it a vulnerability to attentional and information processing dysfunction, supporting this 'trait interpretation' (Miller *et al.*, 1979; Braff, 1981, 1993, 1999; Nuechterlein and Dawson, 1984; Saccuzzo and Braff, 1986; Waldo *et al.*, 1991; Cadenhead *et al.*, 1993, 1996b, 2000, in press; Cannon *et al.*, 1994; Dawson *et al.*, 1994; Strandburg *et al.*, 1994; Clementz *et al.*, 1995; Lieb *et al.*, 1996; Green *et al.*, 1997; Freedman *et al.*, 1998). Evidence supporting the existence of trait-linked deficits comes form several sources.

(i) Remitted schizophrenic patients have been shown to have information processing deficits when assessed using VBM (Miller *et al.*, 1979; Saccuzzo and Braff, 1986), CPT (Nuechterlein *et al,.* 1986) and other measures including visual-evoked potential and P300 event-related potential (ERP) paradigms (Rao *et al.*, 1995; Matsuoka *et al.*, 1996).

(ii) The findings of information processing deficits in clinically unaffected relatives of schizophrenic patients (Cadenhead *et al.*, in press; Cornblatt and Erlenmeyer-Kimling, 1985; Waldo *et al.*, 1991; Green *et al.*, 1997; Young *et al.*, 1998) suggests that these measures are trait related and ultimately can provide intermediate phenotypes for genetic linkage analyses (Freedman *et al.*, 1997), increasing the probability of finding candidate genes for specific deficits (e.g. prepulse inhibition or P50 gating) that are phenotypic markers found to be defective in schizophrenia.

(iii) SPD patients, who are found at high rates in families of schizophrenic patients and may share a common genetic abnormality with schizophrenic patients, have also been shown to have deficits in information processing in a number of paradigms (Cornblatt and Erlenmeyer-Kimling, 1985; Lyons *et al.*, 1991; Cadenhead *et al.*, 1993, 1996a, 2000, in press; Clementz *et al.*, 1995; Trestman *et al.*, 1995; Salisbury *et al.*, 1996; Lees Roitman *et al.*, 1997). The findings of information processing abnormalities in a population of SPD patients who do not have the potential confounding variables seen in schizophrenia (e.g. chronic neuroleptic treatment, chronic hospitalization and the other effects of a debilitating illness) are important because they provide insight into what may be a non-artifactual abnormality of schizophrenic spectrum disease. SPD, like schizophrenia, is a heterogeneous disorder and meeting the criteria for SPD does not necessarily identify a schizophrenic phenotype. Schizotypal patients as well as schizophrenic patients with a family history of schizophrenia are more likely to demonstrate information processing abnormalities assessed by eye movement dysfunction (Schwartz *et al.*, 1995; Thaker *et al.*, 1996). Additionally, schizotypal symptoms in relatives of schizophrenia patients do not predict eye movement abnormalities, suggesting that the clinical manifestations and the eye movement dysfunction of the schizophrenia spectrum illness are independent factors (Keefe *et al.*, 1997). The data from familial studies of SPD and schizophrenia add support to the concept of identifying vulnerability markers to specific aspects of schizophrenia spectrum disorder and then understanding the genetic and neural basis of those markers to add insight into the multidimensional syndrome.

The relationship of information processing to functional and symptomatic outcome

Neurocognitive measures of information processing

Increasing interest has been focused on the functional consequences (e.g. community functioning, social skills, work functioning and independent living) of the information processing deficits assessed using neurocognitive measures (Wykes, 1994; Penn *et al.*, 1995; Green, 1996; Brekke *et al.*, 1997; Velligan *et al.*, 1997). In this view, the functional status of schizophrenic patients largely determines their quality of life. Green (1996) reviewed studies that assessed the functional consequences of neurocognitive deficits in schizophrenic patients. In his review, Green (1996) identified secondary verbal memory and vigilance as strong predictors of functional outcome (community outcome, social problem solving and social skill acquisition) in at least two separate studies. Card Sorting was found to be associated with community functioning but not social skill acquisition. More recently, Brekke *et al.* (1997) have reported associations between better community outcome (independent living), as assessed by the Role Functioning Scale (Goodman *et al.*, 1993), and better visuomotor (digit–symbol) and verbal processing (verbal fluency and Stroop), while better social skill acquisition (work functioning), assessed by the Strauss and Carpenter Outcome Scale (Strauss and Carpenter, 1974), was associated with better complex visuospatial processing (block design). Green also noted that deficit symptoms showed consistent associations with social problem solving but inconsistent associations with community functioning, while psychotic symptoms were not associated with these functional outcome measures. This lack of a robust relationship between clinical symptoms and functional outcome suggests that the prominent impairments in social functioning observed in schizophrenia cannot be explained by the clinical symptoms alone (Penn *et al.*, 1995). It is possible that information processing deficits do make independent contributions to functional outcome that explain some of this unaccounted for variance, but only future studies that directly assess the relationship of information processing to various outcome measures will clarify this issue.

Psychophysiological measures of information processing

Overall, a small but increasing number of studies have assessed the relationship between psychophysiological measures of information processing and functional outcome (Ohman *et al.*, 1989; Wieselgren *et al.*, 1994; Wykes, 1994; Ikebuchi *et al.*, 1996; Brekke *et al.*, 1997). Using indices of skin conductance, Brekke *et al.* (1997) found that those schizophrenic patients with better social functioning (assessed using the Strauss and Carpenter Outcome Scale) had higher resting arousal, lower stress reactivity and a greater number of responses to orienting stimuli. The findings of Brekke *et al.* (1997) are consistent with previous reports of low responsivity being associated with worse social and occupational outcome (Ohman *et al.*, 1989) but differ from a study by Wieselgren *et al.* (1994) that reported poorer functioning to be associated with high resting arousal in female patients, which suggests that gender may also be a factor in functional outcome. Gender differences in information processing have also been noted by Cadenhead *et al.* (1997), who reported that female patients with schizophrenia perform less well than male patients in a reaction time paradigm. These reports of gender differences in information processing as well as the predictability of outcome of these measures (Penn *et al.*, 1996) in patients with schizophrenia emphasize the need to continue to assess gender differences in these paradigms.

The consistent findings of a connection between high responsivity and better social functioning suggest that increased attentional allocation to the environment may lead to an ability to respond accurately to social cues (Brekke *et al.*, 1997). In this context, using an ERP paradigm, Ikebuchi *et al.* (1996) found that non-verbal social skills were related to N1 amplitude, which is thought to be based on either automatic discriminating processes or selective attention. Wykes (1994) reports that patients with schizophrenia who have information processing deficits, as assessed by a reaction time test, do less well in the community (as assessed by social behavior and the ability to live in a more independent setting) at 3 year follow-up, while those without reaction time deficits showed differential improvement in community functioning.

In terms of the relationship between information processing measures and symptomatic outcome, the physiological literature has produced mixed results (Zahn *et al.* 1981; Dawson *et al.*, 1992a; Wykes, 1994; Hegerl *et al.*, 1995; Brekke *et al.*, 1997). The most consistent finding in the skin conductance literature has been an association between high resting arousal in schizophrenic patients and poor symptomatic outcome (Zahn *et al.* 1981; Dawson *et al.*, 1992b; Brekke *et al.*, 1997). Wykes (1994) found that cognitive impairment (as measured by a reaction time paradigm) accounted for 23% of the variance in total symptom score at 3 year follow-up.

The relationship of functional outcome to information processing and symptomatology

In a model that directly addresses the functional importance of information processing deficits, Velligan *et al.* (1997) proposed that cognitive deficits contribute to both symptomatology and functional deficits and that the relationship between symptomatology and functional deficits can be attributed to their shared relationship with information processing deficits. This model is consistent with theories proposed by Frith (1993) who posits strong associations between information processing deficits and clinical symptoms as well as functional outcome. Supporting these hypotheses, Velligan *et al.* (1997) showed that cognitive functioning (assessed using the Cognitive Factor Score from the Negative Symptom Assessment, NSA; Alphs and Summerfelt, 1989) accounted for >40% of the variance in functional outcome (as measured by the Functional Needs Assessment; Dombrowski *et al.* 1990), while symptomatology [assessed with the NSA and Brief Psychiatric Rating Scale (BPRS)] was not associated with outcome. Similarly, Lysaker and Bell (1995) report that the degree of cognitive impairment, not positive or negative symptoms, was associated with improvement in insight during a vocational rehabilitation program. In different reports, Lysaker *et al.* (1995a,b) found that poor cognitive performance was associated with less symptomatic improvement and persistence of social skills deficits at follow-up.

A distinctive model proposed by Meehl (1989) states that neurological indicators (such as attention and information processing deficits) combined with potentiating factors (such as social dysfunction and hypoanhedonia) predict clinical decompensation. Freedman *et al.* (1998) tested Meehl's model as part of the New York High Risk Project. They found that while attentional deficits predicted deficits in social outcome variables such as 'Suspicious Solitude', they also predicted high scores for hypothesized potentiating factors such as physical anhedonia. The significant correlations between physical anhedonia and other social outcome measures were thought to represent an indirect relationship between attention and outcome measures mediated through anhedonia.

Implications for treatment and rehabilitation

Because attention and information processing deficits play an important, and perhaps central, role in the disabling clinical and functional aspects of schizophrenia, the notion of targeting treatment of these specific deficits to alter the course of the illness has gained increasing support (Brenner *et al.*, 1992; Penn *et al.*, 1995; Green, 1996). Although cognitive rehabilitation strategies have evolved to become of increasing interest in the treatment of schizophrenic patients (Flesher, 1990; Stuve *et al.*, 1991; Delahunty and Morice, 1996), it is necessary to identify those 'target' cognitive deficits that have an impact on social functioning in order to develop maximally effective rehabilitation programs (Hogarty and Flesher, 1992; Liberman and Green, 1992; Penn *et al.*, 1995). It is also true that cognitive rehabilitation strategies are generally expensive and time consuming, so a clear benefit must be shown in order to justify the additional cost of these potentially useful therapeutic approaches versus the use of antipsychotic medication alone (Braff, 1992). The information processing literature is concerned increasingly with the functional and symptomatic outcome associated with information processing abnormalities as well as the nature and theoretical direction (if one exists) of the causal relationships of these variables. For example, in 'generalization studies', a specific attentional or information processing deficit is targeted while the effects of the intervention are assessed in a clinical or functional outcome domain (Green, 1996) . An essential component of a generalization study is that there is a clear association between the information processing deficit and the outcome measure. For example, Medalia *et al.* (1998) assessed the effect of attention training on schizophrenic symptomatology. Schizophrenic patients were assessed on the CPT at baseline, then half participated in individual sessions utilizing computerized attention remediation while the other half had individual sessions during which they watched documentary films. These investigators found that those patients who received the attention training had both improved CPT performance and concurrent improvements on the BPRS (primarily somatization, emotional withdrawal and hallucinatory behavior) relative to those who did not receive this training. They concluded that it is possible to use practice and behavioral learning to remediate a core attention deficit in schizophrenic patients. The improvement in psychiatric status was thought to be a generalization of the attention training, but the exact duration of improvement and underlying mechanisms remain largely undefined and are subjects for future research efforts.

Conclusions

Information processing deficits are a prominent feature of schizophrenia. Deficits in information processing are found in acute and remitted patients with schizophrenia and their relatives, suggesting that information processing may be a phenotypic marker linked to specific information processing dysfunction (i.e. not the whole syndrome) of schizophrenia (Freedman *et al.*, 1997). Because information processing deficits appear to be at least partial predictors of both functional and symptomatic outcome, it appears that these deficits are important and even crucial features in understanding schizophrenia. Further work is needed to determine exactly which information processing deficits are linked to which domains of symptomatic and functional outcome (Green, 1996). We also need to utilize outcome measures with better ecological validity (Penn *et al.*, 1995) that will tell us something about an individual's functioning on an everyday basis and how individuals navigate through our complex, stimulus-laden environment. Once we determine which deficits are linked to various specific measures of functional, social and vocational outcome, we can determine whether those deficits are selectively remediable via medications and psychosocial treatments and whether the rehabilitation of specific deficits generalizes to clinical or functional outcome. It is possible that the subtypes of schizophrenia could be redefined using an information processing model that can better predict underlying neural circuit dysfunction as well as response to rehabilitation. Genetic studies of information processing deficits in schizophrenia, rather than cumbersome and low yield studies of the entire syndrome as defined by DSM-IV, appear to be most likely to yield a linkage to a gene or genes responsible for these information processing deficits which appear to be central to the neuropathology, symptoms and functional outcome of schizophrenia.

Acknowledgements

This work was supported by grants from the National Institute of Mental Health (MH01124 and MH42228), and a grant from the Department of Veterans Affairs (VISN 22, Mental Illness Research Education and Clinical Center, MIRECC)

References

Alexander, G.E., Crutcher, M.D. and DeLong, M.R. (1990) Basal ganglia–thalamocortical circuits: parallel substrates for motor, oculomotor, 'prefrontal' and 'limbic' functions. *Progress in Brain Research*, **85**, 119–146.

Alphs, L.D. and Summerfelt, A. (1989) The Negative Symptom Assessment. *Psychopharmacology Bulletin*, **25**, 159–163.

Braff, D.L. (1981) Impaired speed of information processing in non-medicated schizotypal patients. *Schizophrenia Bulletin*, **7**, 499–508.

Braff, D.L. (1985) Attention, habituation, and information processing in psychiatric disorders. In: Michels, R., Brodie, H.K., Cooper, A.M., Guze, S.B., Judd, L.L., Klerman, G. and Solnit, A.J. *Psychiatry*. J.B. Lippincott, Philadelphia, PA, Vol. 3, pp. 1–13.

Braff, D.L. (1989) Sensory input deficits and negative symptoms in schizophrenic patients. *American Journal of Psychiatry*, **146**, 1006–1011.

Braff, D.L. (1992) Reply to cognitive therapy and schizophrenia. *Schizophrenia Bulletin*, **18**, 37–38.

Braff, D. L. (1993) Information processing and attention dysfunctions in schizophrenia. *Schizophrenia Bulletin*, **19**, 233–259.

Braff, D.L. (1999) Psychophysiological and information processing approaches to schizophrenia. In: Charney, D.S., Nestler, E. and Bunney, B.S. (eds), *Neurobiological Foundation of Mental Illness*. Oxford University Press, New York, pp. 258–271.

Braff, D. L. and Geyer, M. A. (1990) Sensorimotor gating and schizophrenia. Human and animal model studies [see comments]. *Archives of General Psychiatry*, **47**, 181–188.

Breier, A., Schreiber, J.L., Dyer, J. and Pickar, D. (1991) National Institute of Mental Health longitudinal study of chronic schizophrenia: prognosis and predictors of outcome. *Archives of General Psychiatry*, **48**, 239–245.

Brekke, J.S., Raine, A., Ansel, M., Lencz, T. and Bird, L. (1997) Neuropsychological and psychophysiological correlates of psychosocial functioning in schizophrenia. *Schizophrenia Bulletin*, **23**, 19–28.

Brenner, H.D., Hodel, B., Roder, V. and Corrigan, P. (1992) Treatment of cognitive dysfunctions and behavioral deficits in schizophrenia. *Schizophrenia Bulletin*, **18**, 21–26.

Buchanan, R.W., Strauss, M.E., Kirkpatrick, B., Holstein, C., Breier, A. and Carpenter, W.T. (1994) Neuropsychological impairments in deficit vs nondeficit forms of schizophrenia. *Archives of General Psychiatry*, **52**, 804–811.

Buchanan, R.W., Strauss, M.E., Breier, A., Kirkpatrick, B. and Carpenter, W.T. (1997) Attentional impairments in deficit and nondeficit forms of schizophrenia. *American Journal of Psychiatry*, **154**, 363–370.

Buchsbaum, M.S., Neuchterlein, K.H., Haier, R.J., Wu, J., Sicotte, N., Hazlett, E. *et al*. (1990) Glucose metabolic rate in normals and schizophrenics during the continuous performance test assessed by positron emission tomography. *British Journal of Psychiatry*, **156**, 216–227.

Butler, R.W. and Braff, D.L. (1991) Delusions: a review and integration. *Schizophrenia Bulletin*, **17**, 633–647.

Cadenhead, K., Geyer, M. and Braff, D. (1993) Impaired startle prepulse inhibition and habituation in schizotypal personality disordered patients. *American Journal of Psychiatry*, **150**, 1862–1867.

Cadenhead, K.S., Perry, W. and Braff, D.L. (1996a) The relationship of information-processing deficits and clinical symptoms in schizotypal personality disorder. *Biological Psychiatry*, **40**, 853–858.

Cadenhead, K.S., Kumar, C. and Braff, D. (1996b) Clinical and experimental characteristics of 'hypothetically psychosis prone' college students. *Journal of Psychiatry Research*, **30**, 331–340.

Cadenhead, K.S., Geyer, M.A., Butler, R.W., Perry, W., Sprock, J. and Braff, D.L. (1997)

Information processing deficits of schizophrenia patients: relationship to clinical ratings, gender and medication status. *Schizophrenia Research*, **28**, 51–62.

Cadenhead, K.S., Geyer M.A., Swerdlow, N.R., Shafer, K., Diaz, M., Clementz, B.A. and Braff, D.L. (1998) Sensorimotor gating deficits in schizophrenic patients and their relatives. *Biological Psychiatry*, **43**, 10S.

Cadenhead, K., Light, G., Geyer, M., Braff, D. (2000) P50 event-related-potential sensory gating deficits in schizotypal personality disordered subjects. *American Journal of Psychiatry*, **157**, 55–59.

Cadenhead, K.S., Swerdlow, N.R., Schafer, K., Diaz, M., Braff, D.L. (in press) Modulation of the startle response and startle laterality in relatives of schizophrenia patients and schizotypal personality disordered subjects: Evidence of inhibitory deficits. *American Journal of Psychiatry*.

Cannon, T.D., Zorrilla, L.E., Shtasel, D., Gur, R.E., Gur, R.C., Marco, E.J. *et al.* (1994) Neuropsychological functioning in siblings discordant for schizophrenia and healthy volunteers. *Archives of General Psychiatry*, **51**, 651–666.

Carpenter, W.T., Heinrichs, D.W. and Wagman, A.M. (1988) Deficit and nondeficit forms of schizophrenia: the concept. *American Journal of Psychiatry*, **145**, 578–583.

Carpenter, W.T.J., Buchanan, R.W., Kirkpatrick, B., Tamminga, C. and Wood, F. (1993) Strong inference, theory testing, and the neuroanatomy of schizophrenia. *Archives of General Psychiatry*, **50**, 825–831.

Castellon, S.A., Asarnow, R.F., Goldstein, M.J. and Marder, S.R. (1994) Persisting negative symptoms and information-processing deficits in schizophrenia: implications for subtyping. *Psychiatry Research*, **54**, 59–69.

Clementz, B.A., Reid, S.A., McDowell, J.E. and Cadenhead, K.S. (1995) Abnormality of smooth pursuit eye movement initiation: specificity to the schizophrenia spectrum? *Psychophysiology*, **32**, 130–134.

Corbetta, M., Miezin, F.M., Shulman, G.L. and Petersen, S.E. (1993) A PET study of visuospatial attention. *Journal of Neuroscience*, **13**, 1202–1226.

Cornblatt, B.A. and Erlenmeyer-Kimling, L. (1985) Global attentional deviance as a marker of risk for schizophrenia: specificity and predictive validity. *Journal of Abnormal Psychology*, **94**, 470–486.

Cornblatt, B.A., Lenzenseger, M.F., Dworkin, R.H. and Erlenmeyer-Kimling, L. (1985) Positive and negative schizophrenic symptoms, attention, and information processing. *Schizophrenia Bulletin*, **11**, 397–408.

Corrigan, P.W. and Toomey, R. (1995) Interpersonal problem solving and information processing in schizophrenia. *Schizophrenia Bulletin*, **21**, 395–403.

Crosson, B. and Hughes, C.W. (1987) Role of the thalamus in language: is it related to schizophrenic thought disorder? *Schizophrenia Bulletin*, **13**, 605–621.

Dawson, M.E., Nuechterlein, K.H. and Schell, A.M. (1992a) Electrodermal anomalies in recent-onset schizophrenia: relationships to symptoms and prognosis. *Schizophrenia Bulletin*, **18**, 295–311.

Dawson, M.E., Neuchterlein, K.H., Schell, A.M. and Mintz, J. (1992b) Concurrent and predictive electrodermal correlates of symptomatology in recent-onset schizophrenic patients. *Journal of Abnormal Psychology*, **101**, 153–164.

Dawson, M.E., Neuchterlein, K.H., Schell, A.M., Gitlin, M. and Ventura, J. (1994) Autonomic abnormalities in schizophrenia: state or trait indicators? *Archives of General Psychiatry*, **51**, 813–824.

Delahunty, A. and Morice, R. (1996) Rehabilitation of frontal/executive impairments in schizophrenia. *Australian and New Zealand Journal of Psychiatry*, **30**, 760–767.

Dombrowski, S.B., Kane, M., Tuttle, N.B. and Kincaid, W. (1990) *Functional Needs Assessment Program for Chronic Psychiatric Patients*. Communications Skill Builders, Tucson, AZ.

Flesher, S. (1990) Cognitive habilitation in schizophrenia: a theoretical review and model of treatment. *Neuropsychology Review*, **1**, 223–246.

Freedman, R., Coon, H., Myles-Worsley, M., Orr-Urtreger, A., Olincy, A., Davis, A. *et al.* (1997) Linkage of a neurophysiological deficit in schizophrenia to a chromosome 15 locus. *Proceedings of the National Academy of Sciences of the United States of America*, **94**, 587–592.

Freedman, L.R., Rock, D., Roberts, S.A., Cornblatt, B.A. and Erlenmeyer-Kimling, L. (1998) The New York high-risk project: attention, anhedonia and social outcome. *Schizophrenia Research*, **30**, 1–9.

Frith, C. (1979) Consiousness, information processing and schizophrenia. *British Journal of Psychiatry*, **134**, 225–235.

Frith, C.D. (1993) *The Cognitive Neuropsychology of Schizophrenia*. Lawrence Erlbaum Associates, Hillsdale, NJ.

Goodman, S.H., Sewell, D.R., Cooley, E.L. and Leavitt, N. (1993) Assessing levels of adaptive functioning: the role functioning scale. *Community Mental Health Journal*, **29**, 119–131.

Green, M.F. (1996) What are the functional consequences of neurocognitive deficits in schizophrenia? *American Journal of Psychiatry*, **153**, 321–330.

Green, M.F. and Walker, E. (1984) Susceptibility to backward masking in schizophrenic patients with positive versus negative symptoms. *American Journal of Psychiatry*, **141**, 1273–1275.

Green, M.F. and Walker, E. (1986) Symptom correlates of vulnerablility to backward masking in schizophrenia. *American Journal of Psychiatry*, **143**, 181–186.

Green, M.F., Nuechterlein, K.H. and Breitmeyer, B. (1997) Backward masking performance in unaffected siblings of schizophrenia patients: evidence for a vulnerability indicator. *Archives of General Psychiatry*, **54**, 465–472.

Hegerl, U., Juckel, G., Muller-Schubert, A., Pietzcker, A. and Gaebel, W. (1995) Schizophrenics with small P300: a subgroup with a neurodevelopmental disturbance and a high risk for tardive dyskinesia. *Acta Psychiatrica Scandinavica*, **91**, 120–125.

Higashima, M., Urata, K., Kawasaki, Y., Maeda, Y., Sakai, N., Mizukoshi, C. *et al.* (1998) P300 and the thought disorder factor extracted by factor-analytic procedures in schizophrenia. *Biological Psychiatry*, **44**, 115–120.

Hogarty, G.E. and Flesher, S. (1992) Cognitive remediation in schizophrenia: proceed. . .with caution. *Schizophrenia Bulletin*, **18**, 51–57.

Holzman, P.S., Proctor, L.R., Levy, D.L., Yasillo, N.J., Meltzer, H.Y. and Hurt, S.W. (1974) Eye-tracking dysfunctions in schizophrenic patients and their relatives. *Archives of General Psychiatry*, **31**, 143–151.

Igata, M., Ohta, M., Hayashida, Y. and Abe, K. (1994) Missing peaks in auditory brainstem responses and negative symptoms in schizophrenia. *Japanese Journal of Psychiatry and Neurology*, **48**, 571–578.

Ikebuchi, E., Nakagome, K., Tugawa, R., Asada, Y., Mori, K., Takahashi, N. *et al.* (1996) What influences social skills in patients with schizophrenia? Preliminary study using the role play test, WAIS-R and event-related potential. *Schizophrenia Research*, **22**, 143–150.

Javitt, D.C., Doneshka, P., Grochowski, S. and Ritter, W. (1995) Impaired mismatch negativity generation reflects widespread dysfuntion of working memory in schizophrenia. *Archives of General Psychiatry*, **52**, 550–558.

Jones, E.D. (1985) *The Thalamus*. Plenum Press, New York.

Jones, E.G. (1997) Cortical development and thalamic pathology in schizophrenia. *Schizophrenia Bulletin*, **23**, 483–501.

Katsanis, J. and Iacono, W. (1991) Clinical, neuropsychological, and brain structural correlates of smooth-pursuit eye tracking performance in chronic schizophrenia. *Journal of Abnormal Psychology*, **100**, 526–534.

Keefe, R.S., Silverman, J.M., Mohs, R.C., Siever, L.J., Harvey, P.D., Friedman, L. *et al.* (1997) Eye tracking, attention, and schizotypal symptoms in nonpsychotic relatives of patients with schizophrenia. *Archives of General Psychiatry*, **54**, 169–176.

Lees Roitman, S.E., Cornblatt, B.A., Bergman, A., Obuchowski, M., Mitropoulou, V., Keefe, R.S.E. *et al.* (1997) Attentional functioning in schizotypal personality disorder. *American Journal of Psychiatry*, **154**, 655–660.

Liberman, R.P. and Green, M.F. (1992) Whither cognitive-behavioral therapy for schizophrenia? *Schizophrenia Bulletin*, **18**, 27–35.

Lieb, K., Denz, E., Hess, R., Schuttler, R., Kornhuber, H.H. and Schreiber, H. (1996) Preattentive information processing as measured by backward masking and texton detection tasks in adolescents at high genetic risk for schizophrenia. *Schizophrenia Research*, **21**, 171–182.

Livingstone, M.S. and Hubel, D.H. (1987) Psychophysical evidence for separate channels for the perception of form color movement and depth. *Journal of Neuroscience*, **7**, 3416–3468.

Lyons, M., Merla, M., Young, L. and Kremen, W.S. (1991) Impaired neuropsychological functioning in symptomatic volunteers with schizotypy: preliminary findings. *Biological Psychiatry*, **30**, 424–426.

Lysaker, P. and Bell, M. (1995) Work rehabilitation and improvements in insight in schizophrenia. *Journal of Nervous and Mental Disease*, **183**, 103–106.

Lysaker, P.H., Bell, M.D. and Goulet, J.L. (1995a) The Wisconsin Card Sorting Test and work performance in schizophrenia. *Schizophrenia Research*, **11**, 45–51.

Lysaker, P.H., Bell, M.D., Zito, W.S. and Bioty, S.M. (1995b) Social skills at work: Deficits and predictors of improvement in schizophrenia. *Journal of Nervous and Mental Disease*, **183**, 688–692.

Matsuoka, H., Saito, H., Ueno, T. and Sato, M. (1996) Altered endogenous negativities of the visual event-related potential in remitted schizophrenia. *Electroencephalography and Clinical Neurophysiology*, **100**, 18–24.

McGhie, A. and Chapman, J. (1961) Disorders of attention and perception in early schizophrenia. *British Journal of Medical Psychology*, **34**, 103–116.

Medalia, A., Aluma, M., Tryon, W. and Merriam, A.E. (1998) Effectiveness of attention training in schizophrenia. *Schizophrenia Bulletin*, **24**, 147–152.

Meehl, P.E. (1989) Schizotaxia revisited. *Archives of General Psychiatry*, **46**, 935–944.

Miller, S., Saccuzzo, D.P. and Braff, D.L. (1979) Information processing deficits in remitted schizophrenics. *Journal of Abnormal Psychology*, **88**, 446–449.

Morton, J. (1979) Word recognition. Morton, J. and Marshall, J.C. (eds), *Psycholinguistics, 2: Structures and processes*. MIT Press, Cambridge, Massachusetts. pp. 107–156.

Nuechterlein, K.H. and Dawson, M.E. (1984) Information processing and attentional functioning in the developmental course of schizophrenic disorders. *Schizophrenia Bulletin*, **10**, 160–203.

Nuechterlein, K.H., Edell, W.S., Norris, M. and Dawson, M.E. (1986) Attentional vulnerability indicators, thought disorder, and negative symptoms. *Schizophrenia Bulletin*, **12**, 408–426.

Ohman, A., Nordby, H. and D'Elia, G. (1989) Orienting in schizophrenia: habituation to auditory stimuli of constant and varying intensity in patients high and low in skin conductance responsivity. *Psychophysiology*, **26**, 48–61.

Pardo, J.V., Fox, P.T. and Raichle, M.E. (1991) Localization of a human system for sustained attention by positron emission tomography. *Nature*, **349**, 61–64.

Penn, D.L., Mueser, K.T., Spaulding, W., Hope, D.A. and Reed, D. (1995) Information processing and social competence in chronic schizophrenia. *Schizophrenia Bulletin*, **21**, 269–281.

Penn, D.L., Mueser, K.T. and Spaulding, W. (1996) Information processing, social skill, and gender in schizophrenia. *Psychiatry Research*, **59**, 213–220.

Perry, W. and Braff, D.L. (1994) Information-processing deficits and thought disorder in schizophrenia. *American Journal of Psychiatry*, **151**, 363–367.

Portas, C.M., Goldstein, J.M., Shenton, M.E., Hokama, H.H., Wible, C.G., Fischer, I. *et al.* (1998) Volumetric evaluation of the thalamus in schizophrenic male patients using magnetic resonance imaging. *Biological Psychiatry*, **43**, 649–659.

Rao, K.M., Ananthnarayanan, C.V., Gangadhar, B.N. and Janakiramaiah, N. (1995) Smaller auditory P300 amplitude in schizophrenics in remission [see comments]. *Neuropsychobiology*, **32**, 171–174.

Ross, D.E., Thaker, G.K., Holcomb, H.H., Cascella, N.G., Medoff, D.R. and Tamminga, C.A. (1995) Abnormal smooth pursuit eye movements in schizophrenic patients are associated with cerebral glucose metabolism in oculomotor regions. *Psychiatry Research*, **58**, 53–67.

Ross, D.E., Thaker, G.K., Buchanan, R.W., Kirkpatrick, B., Lahti, A.C., Medoff, D. *et al.* (1997) Eye tracking disorder in schizophrenia is characterized by specific ocular motor defects and is associated with the deficit syndrome. *Biological Psychiatry*, **42**, 781–796

Saccuzzo, D.P. and Braff, D.L. (1986) Information-processing abnormalities: trait- and state-dependent components. *Schizophrenia Bulletin*, **12**, 447–459.

Salisbury, D.F., Voglmaier, M.M., Seidman, L.J. and McCarley, R.W. (1996) Topographic abnormalities of P3 in schizotypal personality disorder. *Biological Psychiatry*, **40**, 165–172.

Schwartz, B.D., O'Brien, B.A., Evans, W.J., Sautter, F.J., Jr and Winstead, D.K. (1995) Smooth pursuit eye movement differences between familial and non-familial schizophrenia. *Schizophrenia Research*, **17**, 211–219.

Sherman, S.M. and Koch, C. (1986) The control of retinogeniculate transmission in the mammalian lateral geniculate nucleus. *Experimental Brain Research*, **63**, 1–20.

Solomon, C.M., Holzman, P.S., Levin, S. and Gale, H.J. (1987) The association between eye-tracking dysfunctions and thought disorder in psychosis. *Archives of General Psychiatry*, **44**, 31–35.

Steronko, R. and Woods, D. (1978) Impairment in early stages of visual information processing in non-psychotic schizotypal individuals. *Journal of Abnormal Psychology*, **87**, 481–490.

Strandburg, R.J., Marsh, J.T., Brown, W.S., Asarnow, R.F. and Guthrie, D. (1994) Information-processing deficits across childhood- and adult-onset schizophrenia. *Schizophrenia Bulletin*, **20**, 685–695.

Strauss, J.S. and Carpenter, W.T., Jr (1974) The prediction of outcome in schizophrenia: I. Characteristics of outcome. *Archives of General Psychiatry*, **27**, 739–746.

Strauss, M.E., Buchanan, R.W. and Hale, J. (1993) Relations between attentional deficits and clinical symptoms in schizophrenic outpatients. *Psychiatry Research*, **47**, 205–213.

Stuve, P., Erickson, R.C. and Spaulding, W. (1991) Cognitive rehabilitation: the next step in psychiatric rehabilitation. *Psychosocial Rehabilitation Journal*, **15**, 9–26.

Sweeney, J., Haas, G., Clementz, B., Escobar, M., Drake, K. and Francis, A. (1994) Eye tracking dysfunction in schizophrenia: characterization of component eye movement abnormalities, diagnostic specificity and the role of attention. *Journal of Abnormal Psychology*, **103**, 222–230.

Swerdlow, N., Caine, S., Braff, D. and Geyer, M. (1992) The neural substrates of sensorimotor gating of the startle reflex: a review of recent findings and their implications. *Journal of Neuropsychopharmacology*, **6**, 176–190.

Swerdlow, N.R., Braff, D.L., Taaid, N. and Geyer, M.A. (1994) Assessing the validity of an animal model of deficient sensorimotor gating in schizophrenic patients. *Archives of General Psychiatry*, **51**, 139–154.

Tamminga, C.A., Thaker, G.K., Buchanan, R., Kirkpatrick, B., Alphs, L.D., Chase, T.N. *et al.* (1992) Limbic system abnormalities identified in schizophrenia using positron emission tomography with fluorodeoxyglucose and neocortical alterations with deficit syndrome. *Archives of General Psychiatry*, **49**, 522–530.

Thaker, G.K., Buchanan, R.W., Kirkpatrick, B. and Tamminga, C. (1988) Eye movements in schizophrenia: clinical and neurobiological correlates. *Society for Neuroscience*, **14**, 339.

Thaker, G.K., Cassady, S., Adami, H., Moran, M. and Ross, DE. (1996) Eye movements in spectrum personality disorders: comparison of community subjects and relatives of schizophrenic patients. *American Journal of Psychiatry*, **153**, 362–368.

Trestman, R.L., Keefe, R.S.E., Mitropoulou, V., Harvey, P.D., deVegvar, M.L., Lees-Roitman, S. *et al.* (1995) Cognitive function and biological correlates of cognitive performance in schizotypal personality disorder. *Psychiatry Research*, **59**, 127–136.

Van Essen, D.C., Anderson, C.H. and Felleman, D.J. (1992) Information processing in the primate visual system: an integrated systems perspective. *Science*, **255**, 419–423.

Velligan, D.I., Mahurin, R.K., Diamond, P.L., Hazleton, B.C., Eckert, S.L. and Miller, A.L. (1997) The functional significance of symptomatology and cognitive function in schizophrenia. *Schizophrenia Research*, **25**, 21–31.

Waldo, M.C., Carey, G., Myles-Worsley, M., Cawthra, E., Adler, L.E., Nagamoto, H.T. *et al.* (1991) Codistribution of a sensory gating deficit and schizophrenia in multi-affected families. *Psychiatry Research*, **39**, 257–268.

Weinberger, D.R. and Gallhofer, B. (1997) Cognitive function in schizophrenia. *International Clinical Psychopharmacology*, **12** Suppl. 4, S29–S36.

Weiner, R.U., Opler, L.A., Stanley, R.K., Merriam, A.E. and Papouchis, N. (1990) Visual information processing in positive, mixed and negative schizophrenic syndromes. *Journal of Nervous and Mental Disease*, **178**, 616–626.

Wieselgren, I., Ohlund, L.S., Lindstrom, L.H. and Ohman, A. (1994) Electrodermal activity as a predictor of social functioning in female schizophrenics. *Journal of Abnormal Psychology*, **103**, 570–575.

Wykes, T. (1994) Predicting symptomatic and behavioural outcomes of community care. *British Journal of Psychiatry*, **165**, 486–492.

Young, D.A., Waldo, M., Rutledge, J.H. 3rd and Freedman, R. (1998) Heritability of inhibitory gating of the P50 auditory-evoked potential in monozygotic and dizygotic twins. *Neuropsychobiology*, **33**, 113–117.

Zahn, T.P., Carpenter, W.T., Jr and McGlashan, T.H. (1981) Autonomic nervous system activity in acute schizophrenia. *Archives of General Psychiatry*, **38**, 260–266.

6   Formal thought disorder in schizophrenia: characteristics and cognitive underpinnings

Philip D. Harvey

Introduction

Abnormalities in communication have been noted on the part of patients with schizophrenia since the first definitions of the illness. Both Kraepelin (1919) and Bleuler (1911) noted these impairments and described them in detail. While Bleuler believed that these disorders and their cognitive causes were a fundamental feature of schizophrenia, Kraepelin's perspective was that they were one of the important features of the illness but not necessarily pathognomonic. Regardless of whether disorders in communication are seen to be the central feature of the illness or only one its many symptoms, the importance of this symptom is not in question.

One of the issues involved in the study of communication disorders has involved terminology. The very term 'formal thought disorder' contains several assumptions, not all of which may be valid. Referring to disorders in spoken language as a thinking disorder is inferential and not necessarily accurate. Many of the older terms formerly used to describe aspects of disorders of communication are affected by this concern. For example, referring to verbal underproductivity as 'poverty of thought' makes the possibly unwarranted assumption that someone who speaks very little does not think much. In fact, conventional wisdom suggests that less speech sometimes is associated with more thought, as evidenced by the proverb 'Still waters run deep'. Thus, inferences regarding the amount of thought based on the amount of speech should be made with caution.

There are many reasons to believe that spoken language and thinking processes diverge with regularity. For example, in aphasia, an individual may be able to comprehend spoken language and write without errors, but be unable to speak. Another example is deception, where what is said is clearly not what the person thinks. This issue has been the focus of much debate in years past (Lanin-Kettering and Harrow, 1985; Chaika, 1990), but most would now agree that listening to an individual speak under spontaneous conditions is not the same as measuring the cognitive processes that determine competent and incompetent language use. In this chapter, abnormalities of spoken language will be described in detail and the research on the cognitive processes that potentially cause these problems in language will be evaluated. Recent developments in the study of cognition in schizophrenia may provide some new insights into the causes of this common and striking symptom in schizophrenia.

Research perspectives on formal thought disorder.

There are three main research methods for evaluating disorders of cognition and communication in schizophrenia. These methods include the clinical method, linguistic method and cognitive–neuropsychological method. Each of these methods has slightly different perspectives and goals. The best research typically has integrated several of these methods in order to provide a multidimensional approach to understanding communication impairments. As described below, these are complementary approaches to the study of the characteristics and causes of language abnormalities in schizophrenia. The study of the cognitive underpinnings is particularly important, because new pharmacological interventions aimed at cognitive impairments in schizophrenia may have the potential to alter communication disorders in schizophrenia at this level.

The clinical method

This approach applies formal diagnostic criteria to aspects of spoken language, identifying aspects of language that meet criteria for different types of abnormality. As a result, this approach is similar to that adopted with a structured diagnostic assessment of aspects of communication disorder. The researchers using contemporary approaches to the study of formal thought disorder have developed well-detailed and reliable criteria for rating the presence and severity of communication impairments.

The clinical method is the oldest tradition in the study of communication disorders and dates back to the descriptions of Kraepelin and Bleuler. There are many different aspects of impaired communication in schizophrenia, with some systems identifying as many as 18 distinct signs of communication disturbance. The disorders of communication noted in patients with schizophrenia tend to fall into three general types: impairments in the amount of speech, impairments in the level of integration or amount of interconnection of speech, and the production of extremely idiosyncratic language that is never produced by normal individuals (Berenbaum *et al.*, 1985; Harvey *et al.*, 1992; Peralta *et al.*, 1992). These dimensions of communication disorder are not always independent, in that speech can be both overproductive and poorly connected. Similarly to the different dimensions of communication disorder, the individual elements of communication disorder are also overlapping: one segment of language can meet criteria for several different communication disorders.

Much of the recent research on clinical communication disorders in schizophrenia has utilized the Scale for Assessment of Thought, Language and Communication (TLC; Andreasen, 1979a). This scale represents a comprehensive definition of 18 different aspects of impaired communication, which are rated for their severity on either a 5-point or 4-point severity scale. Table 6.1 presents a brief description of the major aspects of communication disorder as rated by this scale. Studies using this scale generally have been able to achieve adequate reliability for features of communication disorder that are common and severe enough to produce adequate variability (Andreasen, 1979a; Oltmanns *et al.*, 1985; Harvey *et al.*, 1997). The initial studies of the TLC both documented its reliability and presented preliminary data regarding the prevalence of each of these subtypes of disorders of communication (Andreasen, 1979b).

Table 6.1 Selected types of formal thought disorder and their definitions

Abnormalities in the amount of speech	
Poverty of speech	Reduced amount of spontaneous or elicited speech
Pressure of speech	Increase in the amount of spontaneous speech
Abnormalities in the connectedness of speech	
Poverty of content of speech	Speech that is adequate in amount but low in information
Derailment	Poorly interconnected speech
Tangentiality	Inadequate responses to questions
Circumstantiality	Wandering and over-detailed speech
Loss of goal	Speech where the point of the utterance is lost
Particularly unusual speech	
Neologisms	Individually created words with a special meaning
Word approximations	Old words assigned new meaning by the speaker
Clanging	Speech connected by rhymes or other phonological mechanisms
Echolalia	Speech where the words of the other speaker are repeated verbatim

Several important findings have emerged from studies using the TLC. The general prevalence of some form of communication disorder in patients with schizophrenia ranges from 50 to 90% (Andreasen, 1979a; Harvey, 1983). The prevalence of different aspects of communication disturbance varies considerably, with some features being present in as many as 60% of patients and other being much more rare, occurring at a rate of ~10% of patients or fewer (Andreasen, 1979b; Andreasen and Grove, 1986; Cuesta and Peralta, 1993; Harvey *et al.*, 1997). Factor analytic studies consistently have identified two reliable dimensions of communication disorder, i.e. verbal productivity and disconnection in speech (Harvey *et al.*, 1992). Some studies have also found evidence of a third factor, comprised of rare aspects of communication disorder such as neologisms and word approximations (Peralta *et al.*, 1992).

The results of these studies of formal thought disorder with clinical methods have answered several basic questions about schizophrenia. First, no recent report has ever indicated that every schizophrenic subject that they examined manifested formal thought disorder. This finding argues against the Bluelerian concept that thought disorder is a pathognomonic sign of the illness. Second, some signs of communication disorder are very rare, such as neologisms, limiting their potential usefulness as a potential diagnostic indicator. Third, different aspects of thought disorder vary considerably in their stability over time, with some signs being stable even after clinical remission and others being variable in their severity on a day to day basis (Harvey *et al.*, 1984, 1988; Earle-Boyer *et al.*, 1986). For example, the severity of aspects of disconnected speech, such as derailment or tangentiality, is reduced markedly when patients with schizophrenia no longer meet the active phase of illness criteria for schizophrenia (Docherty *et al.*, 1989; Harvey *et al.*, 1990). The severity of underproductivity of speech is much more stable, even in patients who no longer meet criteria for an active phase of illness (Harvey *et al.*, 1990).

Some additional insight into the nature of schizophrenia and its potential distinctness from other psychotic illnesses has emerged from clinical studies of formal thought disorder. Several different studies have suggested that patients with schizophrenia could be discriminated from patients with affective disorders, including both mania and depression, on the basis of the profile of their communication disorders (Andreasen, 1979b; Andreasen and Grove, 1986). Manic patients have been found to be discriminable from patients with schizophrenia on the basis of increased verbal productivity, with manic patients more likely to have pressured speech and less likely to have poverty of speech than patients meeting diagnostic criteria for schizophrenia (Cuesta and Peralta, 1993). Patients with depression have been found to be less likely to have disconnected language than patients with schizophrenia and to be less likely to have verbal overproductivity when compared with patients with mania (Andreasen, 1979b; Andreasen and Grove, 1986).

Poverty of speech has proven to be a particularly important aspect of communication disorder in patients with schizophrenia. Patients with poverty of speech early in the course of their illness are more likely to have a more adverse course of illness over time (Andreasen and Grove, 1986). For example, patients with poverty of speech early in the course of their illness are more likely to be found to be psychotic at follow-up, regardless of the follow-up interval, than patients without poverty of speech. Geriatric poor outcome patients with poverty of speech were reported to have Mini-Mental State Examination (MMSE) scores 10 points lower on average than patients without poverty of speech (Harvey *et al.*, 1997). These data indicate that poverty of speech may be related to the types of global cognitive impairment seen in the subset of patients with a deteriorating course of illness and a particularly poor functional outcome (Davidson *et al.*, 1995). No longitudinal data have been produced to indicate that poverty of speech is a definitive indicator of poor functional outcome and deterioration over the lifespan, but cross-sectional and short-term longitudinal data consistently have suggested that poverty of speech was related to functional outcome.

Factor analytic studies have found poverty of speech to be related to affective flattening and reduced vocal inflection in speech, suggesting that it may be a part of some underlying dimension that reflects a reduction in emotional and language production (Liddle, 1987; Arndt *et al.*, 1991; Andreasen *et al.*, 1995). Since these aspects of schizophrenia are also related to poor prognosis (Keefe *et al.*, 1987), poverty of speech may be seen as part of a constellation of indicators of risk for poor functional outcome. In contrast, these same studies have found that aspects of disconnection in speech are statistically related to aspects of disorganized symptoms such as inappropriate affect and bizarre behavior. These data suggest that disconnection in speech has more in common with disorganization in schizophrenia than with positive symptoms of the illness. Since both disconnected and underproductive speech tend to be more persistent over time, less episodic and less responsive to treatment with conventional antipsychotics than positive symptoms, these purely clinical data may suggest that communication disorders in schizophrenia may have causes different from those of positive symptoms of the illnesses.

Clinically rated communication disorders have been found to be associated in a global manner with functional deficits, in that one of the cross-sectional clinical discriminators of very poor outcome patients from those patients with a better functional outcome has been found to be the overall severity of TLC scores (Keefe *et al.*, 1987, 1996). In poor outcome patients, there are considerable age-related changes in formal thought disorder, in terms of both underproductivity and disconnection features. In a study of 393 patients with schizophrenia who ranged in age from 19 to 96 years, the severity of poverty of speech was found to increase linearly with age while the severity of disconnection thought disorders decreased with age (Harvey *et al.*, 1997). Interestingly, the severity of these two aspects of communication disorder was uncorrelated across the whole age range. Greater global cognitive impairment was associated with more severe poverty of speech, but not more severe disconnection thought disorders.

In summary, clinical studies of communication disorder in schizophrenia have provided several different pieces of information regarding the characteristics of communication disorders in schizophrenia and their importance in the illness. They have clarified the prevalence of overall communication impairment, as well as specific aspects of communication disorders. These studies have shown that the most common types of formal thought disorder, other than verbal underproductivity, are best conceptualized as symptoms of disorganization in schizophrenia and not as some aspect of positive symptoms. They have also identified aspects of the diagnostic specificity, age-related changes and the relationship of formal thought disorder to the outcome of the illness.

There are limitations to the clinical method that require the use of other complementary methods in order to understand the phenomenon and its causes more fully. Since clinical studies examine only language as an overt behavior, they do not measure directly the cognitive functions that underlie language. As a result, studies of the specific cognitive impairments that correlate with disturbed speech are required in order to identify potential causes of communication impairments in the cognitive domain. A second issue is more methodological in nature. Clinical ratings of communication disorders allow for the same speech to meet criteria for more than one category of impairment. Thus, severity ratings of the individual aspects of communication disorders are not independent and cannot be used to calculate differential correlations with some criterion measure, such as cognitive functioning. For example, the same language can meet criteria for derailment and loss of goal, meaning that the differential correlation between the severity of these two indices and a measure of, for example, attention, cannot be calculated validly. In order to perform those types of analyses, ratings of language on a unit-by-unit basis, such as in linguistically oriented research, is required. Finally, clinically rated communication disorders are often very global in their definitions and subsume many different aspects of impaired communication under the same heading. For example, in the TLC's definition of 'poverty of content of speech', aspects of speech that are overabstract or overconcrete both meet criteria for the same communication disorder. While this broad definition will probably increase the reliability of ratings, it is also unlikely that any single cognitive impairment simultaneously could produce speech that is both overabstract and overconcrete.

Linguistic studies of communication disorders in schizophrenia

Linguistic studies of communication disorders in schizophrenia examine the frequency of occurrence of aspects of language production that can occur in both normal and abnormal speech. In contrast to clinical studies, where the language unit of analysis is the severity of language events that are by definition rare in normal individuals, linguistic research traditionally has focused on defining abnormal language in terms of the frequencies of events that can be produced by any speakers. Linguistic research examines speech on a unit-by-unit basis, breaking language down into sentences or even smaller stand-alone units such as clauses. The genesis of contemporary linguistic research in schizophrenia can be traced to the research done by Rochester and Martin (1979) that culminated in the publication of the influential book 'Crazy Talk'. This book presented the results of a comprehensive study of language performance in schizophrenic and normal speakers based on the linguistic cohesion system initially published by Halladay and Hasan (1976).

The main focus of 'Crazy Talk' was on the patterns of impairment in linguistic cohesion and reference processes that lead listeners to become confused when they hear a schizophrenic speaker. Cohesion and reference are the set of processes involved in providing connections to previously presented language so that the entire chain of discourse has a coherent flow. One of the major innovations of the Rochester studies was the initial characterization of patients into groups of those patients who met clinical criteria for formal thought disorder and those who did not. Thus, this study had the benefit of being able to identify the linguistic aspects of impaired speech, on a unit-by-unit basis, that led a clinician to consider the patient 'thought-disordered'. As a result, the basic spoken language processes that led a listener to become confused and to label the patient's speech as deviant were identified on a preliminary basis.

The central finding of this study was the discovery that two types of failures in reference processes, unclear and ambiguous references to previously presented verbal material, were elevated in their frequency in schizophrenic speakers, particularly in those who met clinical criteria for 'thought disorder'. These two patterns of references, labeled 'reference failures' or 'incompetent references' by subsequent researchers (e.g. Harvey, 1983), have proven to be quite informative in understanding the linguistic representation of unclear speech in patients with schizophrenia. For example, elevated frequencies of these two types of unclear references characterize the speech of patients with both schizophrenia and mania who meet clinical criteria for 'thought disorder' (Wykes and Leff, 1982; Harvey, 1983; Harvey and Brault, 1986). The frequency of these reference failures also correlates with the severity ratings of two different types of disconnection thought disorders: derailment and tangentiality (Harvey and Brault, 1986). Differential correlations with reference failures can discriminate between the speech of both schizophrenic and manic patients who manifest derailment. In this study, the clinical impression (Kraepelin, 1921; Hoffman *et al.*, 1986) that manic patients were more fluent in their communication impairments than patients with schizophrenia was examined (McPherson and Harvey, 1996). The speech of manic and schizophrenic patients was divided into segments that met criteria for derailment, segments that met criteria for other types of communication disorder and segments that were unimpaired. 'Derailed' segments on the part of patients with schizophrenia had a higher frequency of unclear references than 'derailed' segments of patients with mania, suggesting that even the impaired speech of patients with mania was more coherent than that of patients with schizophrenia. In fact, derailed segments on the part of patients with mania were elevated in their level of discourse connectedness, relative to segments that did not meet criteria for derailment. These findings confirm the impression that communication with manic patients is difficult because of the tendencies of these patients to conduct several simultaneous conversations with the listener.

Some language abnormalities may reflect processes that are markers of vulnerability to the illness. For years, subtle communication disorder has been believed to be a reflection of vulnerablity processes. The best example is Meehl's (1989) conceptualization of 'cognitive slippage', reflected in subtle communication abnormalities, as the central identifying feature of the 'schizotype'. Subtle communication disorders, as evidenced by reference failures, are present in the children of schizophrenic parents (Harvey *et al.*, 1982), as well as in the parents of schizophrenic patients (Docherty, 1993, 1995), and are also present in patients with schizophrenia who are in clinical remission (Docherty *et al.*, 1989). Thus, these impairments are present both in individuals who may carry a genetic vulnerability to the illness and in individuals with the illness who currently have no other major symptoms of the illness.

These language abnormalities may be linked to the other aspects of the illness and vulnerability to the illness, such as affective abnormalities. In a series of studies, Docherty and colleagues demonstrated that patients with schizophrenia are more likely to manifest disorganization in their speech when discussing emotionally charged topics than normal individuals or their own relatives (Docherty *et al.*, 1998). These investigators concluded that the inability to manage and regulate affective experience had the potential to influence directly the competence with which schizophrenic individuals communicated. This finding may also suggest a direct linkage between some of the different symptoms of schizophrenia that are associated with poor prognosis: communication disorders and affective disturbances.

A problem with this particular linguistic method, however, is that reference failures are themselves a heterogeneous concept. Several different linguistic processes are subsumed under the concept of reference failures. Another recent series of studies by Docherty and colleagues has refined the linguistic ratings of failures in reference processes (Docherty *et al.*, 1996a). Docherty noted that references in speech that are unclear could be so characterized for a variety of reasons. For example, information referred to in previously presented speech may be ambiguous, in that more than one possible referent exists. The language can also be unclear because it contains references to information that apparently has never been presented previously in any recent speech. These references are referred to as 'missing information references'. Docherty and colleagues have demonstrated that missing information references are the most powerful discriminators of schizophrenic and non-schizophrenic speakers. These data suggest that patients with schizophrenia are more likely than other speakers to refer to completely non-existent information that was never presented before, confusing the listener because of the misleading linkages to prior speech. This pattern of communication deviance suggests a number of different cognitive processes that could be responsible, with these models reviewed below.

In summary, linguistic research has been successful in terms of more clearly delineating the language processes that lead listeners to become confused when listening to patients with schizophrenia. Linguistic research also has the benefit of clearly delineating specific aspects of language that can be examined in terms of their frequency of occurrence in normal and schizophrenic individuals. The more specifically the language impairments can be defined, the more likely it is that component cognitive impairments that contribute to these impairments can be identified. As a result, linguistic research, as shown below, can be a tool to identify small components of language failure that can then be related, on a correlational basis, to discrete cognitive deficits. This approach has the potential to be more specific than clinical ratings, because reference process analysis examines smaller units of language that are defined in terms of highly specific aspects of language production.

Like clinical research, linguistic research does not measure cognition directly, so it represents only a part of the process of identification of the causes of communication disorders. Linguistic research is also complemented by clinical methods. Clinical methods have proven highly successful in developing operational definitions for the aspects of impaired communication in schizophrenia that are obvious to clinicians and the public. Linguistic research is very useful in then determining exactly which unit-by-unit aspects of impairment in speech cause the impression that patients with schizophrenia are communicating poorly. The combination of clinical and linguistic methods in studies of the cognitive processes that may underlie language failures has the potential to be the most effective way to increase understanding of communication failures in schizophrenia.

Cognitive impairments and communication disorders.

The first 50 years of psychological research on cognitive deficits in schizophrenia was summarized 25 years ago by Chapman and Chapman (1973). Their comprehensive book on thought disorder in schizophrenia was a landmark in terms of the comprehensiveness of the review of the previous literature and their thorough description of the multitude of methodological problems that plagued the research up to that time. One of the features of the majority of the early research studies was the general failure of the researchers to link the cognitive deficits that they studied to the presence and severity of the 'formal thought disorder' or any of the other symptoms of the illness. Many of the early studies simply examined the severity of cognitive impairment in patients with a diagnosis of schizophrenia, operating with the Bleulerian assumption that studying schizophrenia was tantamount to studying thought disorder. As reviewed above, only ~50% of patients with schizophrenia have communication disorders, identified clinically, that are moderate or greater in their severity. Any study of cognitive functions that examines patients with schizophrenia without dividing them on the basis of the severity of their communication disorder cannot, therefore, identify the correlates of 'formal thought disorder' in schizophrenia.

Studies conducted since the publication of the Chapmans' book generally have had more methodological sophistication and have related the severity of theoretically selected cognitive impairments to the presence and severity of either linguistically or clinically evaluated communication disorder in schizophrenia. In the following section, the recent research that has examined cognitive functions that might be related to communication disorders in schizophrenia will be evaluated. The amount of this research has been increasing in the recent past and now involves studies in several different general domains.

Information processing and cognitive capacity

The study of information processing in schizophrenia has a 30 year history. Patients with schizophrenia have been demonstrated to have impairments in their ability to perform a variety of effort-demanding cognitive tasks (Neale and Oltmanns, 1980; Callaway and Naghdi, 1982). Some studies have also demonstrated that the ability of patients with schizophrenia to perform tasks with multiple cognitive demands is reduced relative to normal individuals and that the ability to divide or effectively allocate cognitive resources is also reduced in these patients (Serper *et al.*, 1990; Granholm *et al.*, 1991, 1996). One of the manifestations of this reduced cognitive capacity is that patients with schizophrenia are often vulnerable to influences of irrelevant distracting information and they perform very poorly in the presence of distractors that they are instructed to ignore (e.g. Oltmanns *et al.*, 1979; Harvey *et al.*, 1990).

The first study that directly examined the relationship between information processing and formal thought disorder dates back 20 years. In that study, performance on a test measuring memory span in the presence and absence of irrelevant distracting information was evasluated in patients with schizophrenia (Oltmanns *et al.*, 1979). Performance was found to be correlated with a global clinical severity rating of formal thought disorder, in that the extent to which patients deteriorated in their performance when distractors were present was related significantly to the severity of their thought disorder. The authors interpreted these results as suggesting that impairments in resource-dependent information processing capacity were related to the inability effectively to maintain coherence in speech. This finding has been replicated several times (e.g. Harvey and Pedley, 1989; Harvey *et al.*, 1990). Performance deficits in the processing of target information during distraction have been found to relate to the global severity of thought disorder as measured by the TLC and to the frequency of reference failures. Formal thought disorder has been found to be correlated more specifically with distractibility than with other schizophrenic symptoms such as hallucinations, delusions or negative symptoms (Walker and Harvey, 1986). The relationship between distractibility and communication disorder has also been found to persist in patients who are experiencing partial remission of their psychotic symptoms (Harvey *et al.*, 1990).

The initial theoretical interpretation of these findings was that impairments in overall information processing capacity lead to reductions in the ability to divide attention and ignore distractors, and that this same reduction in processing capacity also leads to deficits in the ability to plan and monitor discourse. It is, of course, possible that there is no direct relationship between reduced processing capacity or distractibility and communication disorders, because there is some third variable that causes both of these symptoms of the illness. In order to rule out that possibility and to demonstrate a direct relationship between the information processing in the presence of irrelevant information and the generation of impaired speech, two studies examined the ability of patients to produce coherent speech while ignoring concurrent distracting information. In the first study, concurrent distraction was examined for its ability to interfere with competent speech production (Hotchkiss and Harvey, 1990). Patients talked with an interviewer while they were exposed to alternating simultaneous blocks of spoken text, random words, white noise and silence. The interviewer was unaware of the distraction condition to which the speaker was exposed. It was found that the presence of all of the different types of irrelevant information, even if it was only white noise, led to a significant increase in the production of reference failures on the part of patients with schizophrenia. Normal individuals were not affected by any of the distraction conditions. The authors suggested that even simple perceptual overload could stress the information processing capacity of patients with schizophrenia to the extent that their language production processes suffered. The second study, using identical methodology, found that this effect was even more pronounced in patients who had been washed out from antipsychotic medication for a 2 week period before their assessment (Moskowitz *et al.*, 1991). The authors suggested that even conventional antipsychotic medication had a beneficial effect on information processing capacity in some patients with schizophrenia. Similarly to previous studies examining distractibility and conventional antipsychotic medications, a reduction of the adverse effects of irrelevant distracting information was found with antipsychotic treatment.

In a study examining normal college undergraduates, Barch and Berenbaum (1994) found that performance of a concurrent information processing task led to specific reductions in language competence. Specifically, length of pausing, syntactic complexity and overall language production were all reduced while the subjects were performing the concurrent processing task. A demonstration of the specific relationship between information processing capacity and language production was provided by the finding that there was a specific correlation between performance on the information processing task and reductions in language performance variables. Those individuals whose performance was worse during the information processing task manifested the greatest reduction in their concurrent language performance.

In a study that used non-verbal tests of information processing (i.e. the ability to respond when lines moving at variable speeds approached a border on a computer screen), Serper (1993) found that patients with more severe global clinical ratings of formal thought disorder had poorer performance than normal individuals. The performance of patients with more severe formal thought disorder also deteriorated more with higher processing loads than that of schizophrenic patients without formal thought disorder. Serper concluded that deficient information processing resources were a contributory factor in the production of formal thought disorder.

One of the limitations of all of these studies is one of specificity of the mechanism between reduced information processing capacity and formal thought disorder. It is not clear why formal thought disorder would be the result of reduced information processing capacity. After all, those normal individuals who perform 1 to 2 standard deviations below the population mean on indices of information processing capacity do not routinely demonstrate formal thought disorder. Thus, several studies have examined more specific aspects of cognitive functioning for their ability to predict the severity of communication disorders in schizophrenia. These aspects of cognitive functioning are resource dependent, meaning that reduced processing capacity would adversely affect these aspects of cognitive functioning and might cause impairments in language functions dependent on the intactness of these aspects of cognitive functioning.

Working memory and source monitoring

Working memory is the ability to hold information in mind while it is being used for other operations, while source monitoring is the ability to identify the origin of information that presently is held in short-term memory. Deficits in both of these domains have been identified consistently in patients with schizophrenia (see Keefe, Chapter 2). Both of these cognitive functions have a clear face-valid relationship with the production of competent speech. For example, if a discourse plan cannot be held in mind until the language that it calls for can be generated, then the spoken language is likely to implement the plan poorly. In a similar vein, if a speaker cannot discriminate whether information in their short-term memory is a part of the discourse plan or a recollection of previously produced speech, then the language about to be produced could be affected as a result. It would be easy for a speaker who confused planned and spoken discourse to confuse a listener as well, by referring to the planned speech as if it had already been produced and already presented to the listener.

A number of studies have examined abnormalities in working memory and source monitoring and related these cognitive impairments to difficulties in language production. In the first of these studies, Harvey (1985) reported that schizophrenic patients who met criteria for 'definite formal thought disorder' had more severe deficits in monitoring the difference between information that they had said versus that they had only thought than schizophrenic patients without thought disorder. An additional issue is that of response bias. If a speaker is confused about whether or not they have presented some information, then if they acted as if it was not yet presented and presented it again, their speech might be redundant but would not be disconnected. In a follow-up study, patients who had deficits in both the ability to monitor their working memory and specific response biases were shown to have more severe formal thought disorder than patients who did not have these deficits (Harvey et al., 1988). These patients also had clear response biases that were different from those of normal individuals. While normal individuals (and schizophrenic patients without communication disorders) typically responded that they had thought, but not said, information when they were uncertain of the source, the schizophrenic patients who manifested formal thought disorder routinely responded that they had said information that in reality they had thought. These impairments were found to persist at an 8 month follow-up assessment (Harvey et al., 1990), where those patients who were psychotic and manifested formal thought disorder also had deficits in source monitoring and atypical response biases when they made errors. The importance of both monitoring competence and response bias was also demonstrated by Brebion et al. (1997), who found that response biases in patients with schizophrenia tended to be in the direction of reporting that information presented by an external source was in actuality self-generated. In another study (Brebion et al., 1996), this same research group reported that reality monitoring failures were also related to performance on the Stroop color word test. They suggested that this finding indicated that selective attention is an important feature of reality monitoring and that general deficits in selection attention may also influence the ability to attend selectively to information in short-term memory.

In an additional study on the components of discourse production, Barch and Berenbaum (1997) found that impairments in discourse planning were related to the production of reference failures. While these findings do not bear directly on monitoring-based models of communication disorders, they do support the idea that planning processes and impairments in these planning processes may be linked intrinsically to the production of unclear language. Thus, the inability to create and monitor the progress of a discourse plan may be a crucial element in the effective generation of competent communication.

Studies of the relationship of other aspects of working memory and communication disorders have also indicated that impairments in these domains are also related to communication disorders. In a study by Docherty et al. (1996b), aspects of both attentional performance and working memory were correlated with the severity of communication disorders in patients with schizophrenia. Docherty *et al.* used an approach of extracting the working memory components of other tasks that have working memory as a task demand. Similar approaches have led to comparable findings.

For example, studies performed by McGrath (1991) had demonstrated that performance on measures of executive functioning (the Wisconsin Card Sorting Test, WCST; Heaton *et al.*, 1993) was correlated with the severity of formal thought disorder. The WCST is a multifactorial task and it has both executive operations and basic working memory demands (Gold *et al.*, 1997). In a later study by Vinogradov *et al.* (1997), however, source monitoring performance was only correlated with measures of executive functioning through their joint correlation with intelligence. These findings suggest a very complex relationship between different aspects of functioning that require working memory.

In summary, both normal and schizophrenic speakers generate unclear speech in situations where their information processing capacity is exceeded; this cognitive function potentially is very important in understanding the cognitive impairments that may underlie communication disorders. Since recent studies have indicated that capacity-limited working memory processes in schizophrenia have a distinct signature of cortical activation in patients with schizophrenia, functional magnetic resonance imaging (fMRI) studies of working memory performance may identify aspects of brain functions that are linked to communication disorders.

Context processing.

In a series of articles that began with theoretical formulations, progressed to computer simulations and then moved on to compelling empirical tests of the theories, Cohen and colleagues (Cohen and Servan-Schreiber, 1992; Cohen *et al.*, 1996; Servan-Schreiber *et al.*, 1996) presented their perspective that schizophrenia is a disorder where the primary cognitive deficit is an abnormality in the maintenance of awareness of environmental context. This process is hypothesized further to be localized to the anterior regions of the frontal lobe and to be dependent on the intact functioning of the dopamine system. Since the maintenance of contact with environmental context is a central feature of many previous models of communication disorder, this may be an important topic for later study. The current main importance of these models for the study of communication disorders lies in the highly elaborate nature of the models and the fact that they can be tested quite clearly with straightforward cognitive measures.

In a linguistic study that tested the importance of maintenance of environmental context, Barch and Berenbaum (1997) reported that patients with schizophrenia could be reliably influenced to produce different types of impaired speech as a function of the type of context processing manipulation to which they were exposed. In situations where the level of context for the question was low, patients generated impoverished discourse plans. When provided with queries that provided little structure to guide their answers, the patients generated responses that were poorly connected to the question, with evidence of the types of disconnection communication disorders discussed above. Thus, there may be some direct linguistic support for cognitive models suggesting that impaired, dopamine-dependent cortico-cortical connections lead to deficits in the ability to maintain and utilize context, which then in turn cause impairments in communication in schizophrenia.

Abnormalities of the structure of semantic memory

Related to the point of impaired context processing, an extensive line of research has developed that examines the ability of patients with schizophrenia to access information contained in their semantic memory. The basic cognitive neuroscience perspective on semantic memory is that semantic information is stored in an interactive network of modifiable representations. These representations are connected hypothetically in a dynamic and fluid manner, with new connections developed as new information is acquired and connections that are used more frequently being accessed more efficiently. Connections are based on conventions of semantic relatedness of information, combined with experiential influences to which the individual is exposed.

There were several pieces of information that initially led to the suggestion that patients with schizophrenia have abnormalities in the structure of their semantic storage and in their ability to access this storage. For instance, schizophrenic patients produce some utterances that are grossly out of line with normative semantic standards. These utterances often involve words that are created uniquely by the patient (neologisms) or old words with a new meaning assigned to them by the patient (word approximations). Another abnormality of language performance that could be seen to implicate semantic memory and the processes of access to semantic memory is that of abnormal word association performance. As reviewed above and noted since Kraepelin (1919) and Bleuler (1911), schizophrenic patients often make statements that are poorly or completely unrelated to their own prior communication or to the questions of a listener. This process of generation of disconnected speech could be explained partially by abnormalities of the connections between linguistic representations in semantics or abnormalities in the structure of the representations themselves. The classic word association study by Kent and Rosanoff (1910) demonstrated that patients with schizophrenia were quite likely to generate 'novel' responses to single word stimuli. These data provided the initial basis for the years of research into this topic since that time.

Later research has demonstrated that the characteristics of the linguistic representations themselves are unlikely to be abnormal, in that patients with schizophrenia have essentially normal performance on tests of their ability to recognize words and to define them lexicographically (O'Carroll et al., 1992). What appears to be clearly abnormal are those processes of connection between the linguistic representations in long-term semantic storage. There is an extensive literature in this area that was reviewed very well by Spitzer (1997). Elevag and Goldberg (1997) have also provided a specific theoretical formulation of the importance of these abnormalities. What follows here is a selective review of the major points of importance in this area of research.

Patients with schizophrenia have been shown in several studies to perform abnormally in tests that examine the rate and accuracy with which they access semantic information (e.g. Manschreck et al., 1988; Spitzer, 1997). The typical test used to examine the ability to access semantic structure is the lexical decision test. In this test, a subject views a briefly presented letter string and is requested to determine if the string was a word or not (Meyer and Schvaneveldt, 1971). If a highly related word is presented immediately before the letter string (e.g. 'Cat' followed by the stimulus DOG), the reaction time for lexical decision of the second string is facilitated. Unrelated words ('Table' followed by DOG) have no more effect than a flash of light on the reaction time for lexical decision. Patients with schizophrenia who manifest formal thought disorder have been found to manifest 'overpriming', in that their reaction time is markedly reduced for lexical decision compared with normal individuals. This finding may provide information about one of the potential mechanisms through which intrusions occur in speech. For example, rapid, wide-ranging and non-specific activation of a large number of semantic representations on an ongoing basis could lead to impairments in the ability to select the correct semantic/lexical item for production.

A complementary perspective is that of impoverishment or abnormality in the structure of the semantic structure itself. Patients with schizophrenia generate reduced and poorly connected verbal output in structured situations designed to elicit language (Gourovitch *et al.*, 1996). For example, the verbal fluency test requires patients to produce as many examples as they can from a variety of different semantic (e.g. Animals) or phonological (e.g. F–A–S) categories. When the output of patients with schizophrenia is examined with multi-dimensional scaling procedures, the structure of their representations is grossly different from that seen in normal individuals (Aloia *et al.*, 1996). This finding is complemented by the results of other studies indicating that patients with schizophrenia are not aided in their semantic (i.e. category) fluency performance through the provision of prompts (Joyce *et al.*, 1996). In contrast, normal individuals have their performance augmented considerably when a prompt is provided (Randolph *et al.*, 1993). Thus, it may be difficult or impossible for patients with schizophrenia to access semantic information in an appropriate manner, because of poorly structured semantic representations or impaired ability to access these representations efficiently.

As noted by Spitzer (1997), deficits in working memory and excessive priming activation can have a complementary effect, contributing to impaired communication in patients with schizophrenia. If such a patient has a working memory-based deficit in the ability to maintain and integrate newly presented information with their discourse plan, these deficits would only be compounded by an overactivated semantic system. If an individual had a deficit in correctly discriminating the status of information truly in their short-term memory, then the management of overactivated semantic nodes generating irrelevant information would be even more difficult. The input into working memory from overactivated semantic representations would provide multiple extraneous sources of input that would require discrimination. Thus, a patient with schizophrenia would not only have to discriminate whether they had yet uttered information that they planned to say and discriminate from information that was placed later in their discourse plan, but they would also have to determine if they had actually uttered information that was semantically related to, but not a part of, the information that they planned to say. Thus, for a schizophrenic patient, monitoring the discourse plan would require discriminations that normal individuals would never have to consider: determining if they had said irrelevant things that were never part of their plan in the first place. Thus, when the results of Aloia *et al.* (1996). are also considered, a third stratum of difficulty emerges: that of an abnormal underlying semantic structure which is activated abnormally and difficult to monitor. In this case, the information intruding into working memory might not even be directly relevant to the planned speech, arising from abnormal activations of essentially unrelated information.

The results of these studies highlight the fact that semantic memory is a dynamic process, with aspects of its structure and its patterns of access important. Also important, however, is what happens to the information that is entered into and retrieved from this system. Cognitive capacity and monitoring processes may be important for the understanding of the role of the semantic memory system and its role in language, in that if information is not entered into the system accurately, the structure and function of the system may not be important.

Summary

The language of schizophrenia has been a puzzle for the last century to listeners and to scientists trying to understand the reason for these communication problems. While the specific descriptive aspects of language problems in schizophrenia may be fully understood, the reasons for these abnormalities are still unclear. Cognitive capacity, attentional processes, working memory, source monitoring, and semantic structure and access have all been implicated. Yet, from the results of the studies correlating abnormalities in these processes and discrete language abnormalities, there is still no consensus about the specific interaction of these processes. That will be the goal of the next decade's research.

Developments in cognitive neuroscience and neuroimaging may provide some assistance in the immediate future, in that examination of brain functions in patients with schizophrenia when they are producing language or performing relevant cognitive tests may tell us a considerable amount about the biological substrates of these language abnormalities. It is somewhat ironic that the structural aspects of the brain that are important for language were discovered in the 19th century and yet we are still trying to understand their very complicated functions and interactions with other parts of the brain. An integrated clinical, cognitive and neuroscience approach will be most likely to reveal the actual parameters of the basic processes that cause formal thought disorder in schizophrenia. In the interim, several strong leads are being pursued, any one of which could provide the basis for interventions and any one of which could prove to be the crucial factor that causes formal thought disorder in schizophrenia.

References

Aloia, M.S., Gourovitch, M.L., Weinberger, D.R. and Goldberg, T.E. (1996) An investigation of semantic space in patients with schizophrenia. *Journal of the International Neuropsychological Society*, **2**, 267–273.

Andreasen, N.C. (1979a) Thought, language, and communication disorders: I. Clinical assessment, definition of terms, and assessment of their reliability. *Archives of General Psychiatry*, **36**, 1315–1321.

Andreasen, N.C. (1979b) Thought, language, and communication disorders: II. Diagnostic significance. *Archives of General Psychiatry*, **36**, 1325–1330.

Andreasen, N.C. and Grove, W.M. (1986) Thought, language, and communication in schizophrenia: diagnosis and prognosis. *Schizophrenia Bulletin*, **12**, 348–359.

Andreasen, N.C, Arndt, S., Alliger, R., Miller, D. and Flaum, M. (1995) Symptoms of schizophrenia: methods, meanings, mechanisms. *Archives of General Psychiatry*, **52**, 341–351.

Arndt, S., Allinger, R.J. and Andreasen, N.C. (1991) The distinction of positive and negative symptoms: a failure of a two-factor model. *British Journal of Psychiatry*, **158**, 317–322.

Barch, D. and Berenbaum, H. (1994) The relationship between information processing and language production. *Journal of Abnormal Psychology*, **103**, 241–250.

Barch, D.M. and Berenbaum, H. (1997) The effect of language production manipulations on negative thought disorder and discourse coherence disturbances in schizophrenia. *Psychiatry Research*, **71**, 115–127.

Berenbaum, H., Oltmanns, T.F. and Gottesman, I.I. (1985) Formal thought disorder in schizophrenic patients and their twins. *Journal of Abnormal Psychology*, **94**, 3–16.

Bleuler, E. (1911/950) *Dementia Praecox or the Group of Schizophrenias*. International Universities Press, New York.

Brebion, G., Smith, M.J., Gorman, J.M. and Amador, X. (1996) Reality monitoring failure in schizophrenia: the role of selective attention. *Schizophrenia Research*, **22**, 173–180.

Brebion, G., Smith, M.J., Gorman, J.M. and Amador, X. (1997) Discrimination accuracy and decision biases in different types of reality monitoring in schizophrenia. *Journal of Nervous and Mental Disease*, **185**, 247–253.

Callaway, E. and Naghdi, S. (1982) An information processing model for schizophrenia. *Archives of General Psychiatry*, **39**, 339–347.

Chaika, E.O. (1990) *Understanding Psychotic Speech*. Charles Thomas, Springfield, IL.

Chapman, L.J. and Chapman, J.M. (1973) *Disordered Thought in Schizophrenia*. Appleton, Century, Crofts, New York.

Cohen, J.D. and Servan-Schreiber, D. (1992) Context, cortex, and dopamine: a connectionist approach to behavior and biology in schizophrenia. *Psychological Review*, **99**, 45–77.

Cohen, J.D., Braver, T.S. and O'Reilly, R.C. (1996) A computational approach to prefrontal cortex, cognitive control and schizophrenia: recent developments and current challenges. *Philosophical Transactions of the Royal Society of London*, **351**, 1515–1527.

Cuesta, M.J. and Peralta V. (1993) Does formal thought disorder differ among patients with schizophrenic, schizophreniform, and manic schizoaffective disorders? *Schizophrenia Research*, **10**, 151–158.

Davidson, M., Harvey, P.D., Powchik, P., Parrella, M., White, L., Knobler, H.Y., Losonczy, M., Keefe, R.S.E., Katz, S. and Frecksa, E. (1995) Severity of symptoms in geriatric chronic schizophrenic patients. *American Journal of Psychiatry*, **152**, 197–207.

Docherty, N.M. (1993) Communication deviance, attention, and schizotypy in the parents of schizophrenic patients. *Journal of Nervous and Mental Disease*, **181**, 750–756.

Docherty, N.M. (1995) Linguistic reference patterns in the parents of schizophrenic patients. *Psychiatry*, **58**, 20–27.

Docherty, N.M., Schnur, M and Harvey, P.D. (1989) Reference performance and positive and negative thought disorder: a followup study of manics and schizophrenics. *Journal of Abnormal Psychology*, **97**, 437–442.

Docherty, N.M., DeRosa, M. and Andreasen, N.C. (1996a) Communication disturbances in schizophrenia and mania. *Archives of General Psychiatry*, **53**, 358–364.

Docherty, N.M., Hawkins, K.A., Hoffman, R.E., Quinlan, D.M., Rakfeldt, J. and Sledge, W.H. (1996b) Working memory, attention, and communication disturbances in schizophrenia. *Journal of Abnormal Psychology*, **105**, 212–219.

Docherty, N.M., Hall, M.J. and Gordinier, S.W. (1998) Affective reactivity of speech in schizophrenia patients and their nonschizophrenic relatives. *Journal of Abnormal Psychology*, **107**, 461–467.

Earle-Boyer, E.A., Levinson, J.C., Grant, R. and Harvey, P.D. (1986) The consistency of thought disorder in mania and schizophrenia: II. Stability across consecutive episodes. *Journal of Nervous and Mental Disease*, **174**, 443–447.

Elevag, B. and Goldberg, T.E. (1997) Formal thought disorder and semantic memory in schizophrenia. *CNS Spectrums*, **2**, 15–25.

Gold, J.M., Carpenter, C., Randolph, C., Goldberg, T.E. and Weinberger, D.R. (1997) Auditory working memory and Wisconsin Card Sorting Test performance in schizophrenia. *Archives of General Psychiatry*, **54**, 159–168.

Gourovitch, M.L., Goldberg, T.E. and Weinberger, D.R. (1996) Verbal fluency deficits in patients with schizophrenia: semantic fluency is differentially impaired as compared to phonological fluency. *Neuropsychology*, **10**, 573–577.

Granholm, E., Asarnow, R.F. and Marder, S. (1991) Controlled information resources and the development of automatic detection responses in schizophrenia. *Journal of Abnormal Psychology*, **100**, 22–30.

Granholm, E., Asarnow, R.F. and Marder, S.R. (1996) Dual task performance operating characteristics, resource limitations, and automatic processing in schizophrenia. *Neuropsychology*, **10**, 3–11.

Halladay, M.A.K and Hasan, R. (1976) *Cohesion in English*. Longman, London.

Harvey, P.D. (1983) Speech competence in manic and schizophrenic psychoses: the association between clinically rated thought disorder and cohesion and reference performance. *Journal of Abnormal Psychology*, **92**, 368–377.

Harvey, P.D. (1985) Reality monitoring in mania and schizophrenia: the association between thought disorder and performance. *Journal of Nervous and Mental Disease*, **173**, 67–73.

Harvey P.D. and Brault, J. (1986) Speech performance in mania and schizophrenia: the association of positive and negative thought disorder and reference failures. *Journal of Communication Disorders*, **16**, 161–173.

Harvey, P.D. and Pedley, M. (1989) Auditory and visual distractibility in schizophrenics: clinical and medication status correlations. *Schizophrenia Research*, **2**, 295–300.

Harvey, P.D., Weintraub, S. and Neale, J.M. (1982) Speech competence of children vulnerable to psychopathology. *Journal of Abnormal Child Psychology*, **10**, 373–388.

Harvey, P.D., Earle-Boyer, E.A. and Wielgus, M. (1984) The consistency of thought disorder in mania and schizophrenia: an assessment of acute psychotics. *Journal of Nervous and Mental Disease*, **172**, 458–463.

Harvey P.D., Earle-Boyer, E.A. and Levinson, J.C. (1988) Cognitive deficits and thought disorder: a retest study. *Schizophrenia Bulletin*, **14**, 57–66.

Harvey P.D., Docherty, N.M., Serper, M.R. and Rasmussen, M. (1990) Cognitive deficits and thought disorder: II. An eight month follow-up study. *Schizophrenia Bulletin*, **16**, 147–156.

Harvey, P.D., Lenzenweger, M.F., Keefe, R,S.E., Pogge, D.L., Serper, M.R. and Mohs, R.C. (1992) Empirical evaluation of the factorial structure of clinical symptoms in schizophrenia: formal thought disorder. *Psychiatry Research*, **44**, 141–151.

Harvey, P.D., Lombardi, J., Leibman, M., Parrella, M., White, L., Powchik, P., Mohs, R.C., Davidson, M. and Davis, K.L. (1997) Age-related differences in formal thought disorder in chronically hospitalized patients with schizophrenia: a cross-sectional study across nine decades. *American Journal of Psychiatry*, **154**, 205–210.

Heaton, R.K., Chelune, G.J., Talley, J.L., Kay, G.C. and Curtiss, G. (1993) *Wisconsin Card Sorting Test (WCST) Manual—Revised and Expanded*. Psychological Assessment Resources, Odessa, Florida.

Hoffman, R.S., Stopek, S. and Andreasen, N.C. (1986) A comparative study of manic versus schizophrenic speech disorganization. *Archives of General Psychiatry*, **43**, 831–838.

Hotchkiss, A.P. and Harvey, P.D. (1990) Effect of concurrent distraction on thought disorder in schizophrenia. *American Journal of Psychiatry*, **147**, 153–156.

Joyce, E.M. , Collinson, S.L. and Crichton, P. (1996) Verbal fluence in schizophrenia: relationship with executive function, semantic memory, and clinical alogia. *Psychological Medicine*, **26**, 39–49.

Keefe, R.S.E., Mohs, R.C., Losonczy, M., Davidson, M., Silverman, J.M., Kendler, K.S., Horvath, T.B., Nora, R. and Davis, K.L. (1987) Characteristics of very poor outcome schizophrenia. *American Journal of Psychiatry*, **144**, 889–895.

Keefe, R.S., Frescka, E., Apter, S.H., Davidson, M., Macaluso, J.M., Hirschowitz, J. and Davis, K.L. (1996) Clinical characteristics of Kraepelinian schizophrenia: replication and extension of previous findings. *American Journal of Psychiatry*, **153**, 806–811.

Kent, G.H. and Rosanaoff, A.J. (1910) A study of associations in insanity. *American Journal of Insanity*, 66, 37–47.

Kraepelin, E. (1919) *Dementia Praecox and Paraphrenia*. E. and S. Livingstone, Edinburgh.

Kraepelin, E. (1921) *Manic Depressive Insanity and Paranoia*. E. and S. Livingstone, Edinburgh.

Lanin-Kettering, I. and Harrow, M. (1985) The thought behind the words: a view of schizophrenic speech and thinking disorders. *Schizophrenia Bulletin*, **11**, 1–15.

Liddle, P.F. (1987) The symptoms of chronic schizophrenia: a re-examination of the positive–negative dichotomy. *British Journal of Psychiatry*, **151**, 145–151.

Manschreck, T.C., Maher, B.A., Milavetz, J.J., Ames, D., Weisstein, C.C. and Schneyer, M.L. (1988) Semantic priming in thought disordered schizophrenic patients. *Schizophrenia Research*, **1**, 61–68.

McGrath, J. (1991) Ordering thoughts on thought disorder. *British Journal of Psychiatry*, **158**, 307–316.

McPherson, L. and Harvey, P.D. (1996) Discourse connectedness in manic and schizophrenic psychoses: associations with derailment and other clinical thought disorders. *Cognitive Neuropsychiatry*, **1**, 41–54.

Meehl, P.E. (1989) Schizotaxia revisited. *Archives of General Psychiatry*, **46**, 935–944

Meyer, D.E. and Schvaneveldt, R.E. (1971) Facilitation in recognizing pairs of words: evidence of dependence between retrieval operations. *Journal of Experimental Psychology*, **20**, 227–234.

Moskowitz, J., Davidson, M. and Harvey, P.D. (1991) Effect of concurrent distraction on communication failures in schizophrenic patients: II. Medication effects. *Schizophrenia Research*, **5**, 153–159.

Neale, J.M. and Oltmanns, T.F. (1980) *Schizophrenia*. Wiley, New York.

O'Carroll, R.E., Walker, M. and Duncan, J. (1992) Selecting controls for schizophrenia research studies: the use of the National Adult Reading Test (NART) as a measure of premorbid ability. *Schizophrenia Research*, **8**, 137–141

Oltmanns, T.F., Ohayon, J. and Neale, J.M. (1979) The effect of medication and diagnostic criteria on distractibility in schizophrenia. *Journal of Psychiatric Research*, **14**, 81–91.

Oltmanns, T.F., Murphy, R., Berenbaum, H. and Dunlop, S.R. (1985) Rating verbal communication impairment in schizophrenia and affective disorders. *Schizophrenia Bulletin*, **11**, 292–299.

Peralta, V., Cuesta, M.J. and deLeon, J. (1992) Formal thought disorder in schizophrenia: a factor analytic study. *Comprehensive Psychiatry*, **33**, 105–110.

Randolph, C., Braun, A.R., Goldberg, T.E. and Chase, T.N. (1993) Semantic fluency in Alzheimer's, Parkinson's, and Huntington's disease: dissociation of storage and retrieval failures. *Neuropsychology*, **7**, 82–88.

Rochester, S.R. and Martin, J.R. (1979) *Crazy Talk: A Study of the Discourse of Schizophrenic Speakers*. Plenum, New York.

Serper, M.R. (1993) Visual controlled processing resources and formal thought disorder in schizophrenia and mania. *Schizophrenia Research*, **9**, 59–66.

Serper, M.R., Bergman, R.L. and Harvey, P.D. (1990) Medication may be required for the development of automatic information processing in schizophrenia. *Psychiatry Research*, **32**, 281–288.

Servan-Schreiber, D., Cohen, J.D. and Steingard, S. (1996) Schizophrenic deficits in the processing of context. A test of a theoretical model. *Archives of General Psychiatry*, **53**, 1105–1112.

Spitzer, M. (1997) A cognitive neuroscience view of schizophrenic thought disorder. *Schizophrenia Bulletin*, **23**, 29–50.

Vinogradov, S., Willis-Shore, J., Poole, J.H., Marten, E., Ober, B.A. and Shenaut, G.K. (1997) Clinical and neurocognitive aspects of source monitoring errors in schizophrenia. *American Journal of Psychiatry*, **154**, 1530–1537.

Walker, E and Harvey, P.D. (1986) Positive and negative symptoms in psychosis: attentional performance correlates. *Psychopathology*, **19**, 294–302.

Wykes, T. and Leff, J. (1982) Disordered speech: differences between schizophrenics and manics. *Brain and Language*, **15**, 117–124.

7 Glutamatergic contributions to cognitive dysfunction in schizophrenia

John H. Krystal, Aysenil Belger, Walid Abi-Saab, Bita Moghaddam, Dennis S. Charney, Amit Anand, Steven Madonick and Cyril D'Souza

Introduction

Both cognitive neuroscience and schizophrenia research have moved beyond the study of single regions and single neurotransmitters toward an appreciation of the importance of networks and neurotransmitter interactions (Krystal *et al.*, 1998b). One factor driving these shifts in schizophrenia research has been the appreciation that dopamine (DA) is one of many neurotransmitter systems implicated in the symptoms and cognitive dysfunction associated with schizophrenia (Carlsson and Carlsson, 1990). Rapid growth in the molecular neuroscience and psychopharmacology of glutamate systems has provided a number of potential insights into the pathophysiology of schizophrenia related to the N-methyl-D-aspartate (NMDA) antagonist model psychosis (Krystal *et al.*, 1998b). As a result, there is increasing interest in reviewing this progress in order to integrate this body of research more fully into the schizophrenia literature.

This review will attempt to provide a brief introduction into glutamatergic psychopharmacology. In particular, it will focus on NMDA antagonist models for psychoses, including schizophrenia. It will then briefly consider evidence of disturbances in glutamatergic systems based on post-mortem studies. It will conclude by taking stock of the current state of progress in glutamatergic studies and consider future directions of this research.

Introduction to glutamate receptors and glutamate drugs

The last 10 years have marked rapid advances in insights into the diversity of glutamate receptors (Table 7.1). These receptors are grouped, by prototypal ligands, into three families of inotropic receptors, i.e. receptors that are coupled to ion channels, including the NMDA receptors, α-amino-3-hydroxy-5-methyl-4-isoxazoleproprionate (AMPA) receptors and kainate receptors. Glutamate receptors also include a class of metabotropic receptors, i.e. receptors that are coupled to cellular second messenger systems via G-proteins.

The NMDA receptor subclass controls a calcium channel (Javitt and Zukin, 1991). The function of this receptor is dependent on the neuronal membrane potential. Under basal conditions, the calcium channel is blocked by magnesium. When the membrane is partially depolarized, the magnesium block is displaced and the binding of glutamate and glycine to their sites on the NMDA receptor complex opens the channel, allowing calcium to enter the neuron. When it enters the neuron, calcium is excitatory and, in sufficient quantities, toxic (Olney and Farber, 1995). NMDA receptors have other modulatory binding sites, depicted in Figure 7.1. NMDA receptors are composed of two subunits, NR1 and NR2. The NR1 subunit is common to most adult receptors, although post-translational splicing gives rise to functional diversity of the NR1 subunit (Hollmann *et al.*, 1993). There are four variants of the NR2 subunits (NR2A–2D) that have different regional localization and sensitivity to modulatory substances (Sucher *et al.*, 1996). In addition, a recently characterized NMDA receptor subunit that does not facilitate calcium entry appears to be expressed primarily *in utero* (Ciabarra *et al.*, 1995).

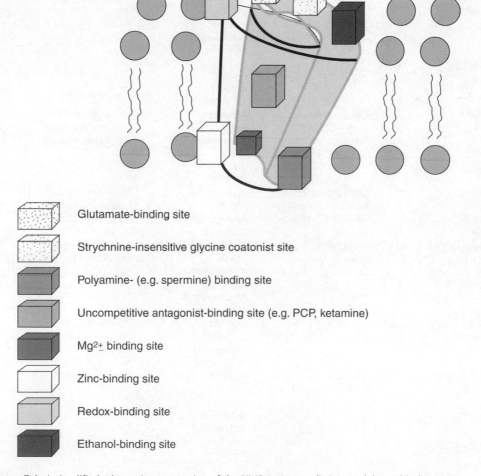

Glutamate-binding site

Strychnine-insensitive glycine coatonist site

Polyamine- (e.g. spermine) binding site

Uncompetitive antagonist-binding site (e.g. PCP, ketamine)

$Mg^{2\pm}$ binding site

Zinc-binding site

Redox-binding site

Ethanol-binding site

Figure 7.1 A simplified schematic presentation of the NMDA receptor listing modulatory binding sites.

Table 7.1 Glutamate receptors, glutamate agonists and glutamate antagonists

Receptor	Subunits	Agonists and antagonists	Function
NMDA	NR1 + NR2A–NR2D	**Agonist** NMDA **Competitive antagonist** CPP CGS19755 **Uncompetitive antagonist** D-AP5 Dizocilpine (MK-801) Phencyclidine (PCP) Ketamine Memantine Amantidine	Voltage-dependent calcium channel
GlycineB		**Agonist** Glycine D-Serine **Partial agonist** D-Cycloserine ACPC HA-966 Antagonist 5,7-DCKA	Required for NMDA receptor function
AMPA	Combination of GluR1–GluR4	**Agonist** AMPA **Antagonist** NBQX CNQX LY215490	Subtypes contain sodium, potassium, or calcium channels
Kainate	Combination of GluR5–GluR7 or KA1–KA2 subunits	**Agonist** AMPA **Antagonist** LY294486	Subtypes contain sodium, potassium, or calcium channels
Metabotropic group I	mGlu1 and mGlu5	**Agonist** DHPG **Antagonist-1** AIDA **Antagonist-5** 4CPG	Coupled to second messenger systems via $G_{q/11}$
Metabotropic group II	mGlu2 and mGlu3	**Agonist** LY354740 **Antagonist** LY307452	Coupled via $G_{i/o}$ Inhibit glutamate release
Metabotropic group III	mGlu4, mGlu6–mGlu8	**Agonist** L-AP4 Homo-AMPA (for mGlu6) **Antagonist** MAP4 MPPG (for mGlu8)	Coupled via $G_{i/o}$

Modified from Alexander and Peters (1998).
Abbreviations: ACPC, 1-aminocyclopropanecarboxylic acid; L-AP4, S-2-amino-4-phosphonobutyrate; D-AP5, D(–)-2-amino-5-phosphonopentanoate; AIDA, 1-aminocyclopentane-1S,3R-dicarboxylate; AMPA, α-amino-3-hydroxy-5-methyl-4-isoxazole propionic acid; CGS19755, 4-phosphonomethyl-2-piperidine carboxylic acid; CNQX, 6-cyano-7-nitroquinoxaline-2,3-dione; 4CPG, 4-carboxyphenylglycine; CPP: 3-(2-carboxypiperazin-4-yl)propyl-1-phosphonate; 5,7-DCKA, 5,7-dichlorokynurinate; DHPG, S-3,5-dihydroxyphenylglycine; (+)HA-966, (+)-3-amino-1-hydroxypyrrolid-2-one; LY215490, (3SR, 4αRS, 6RS, 8αPS)-6-[2-(1H-tetrazole-5yl)ethyl]decahydroisoquinoline-3-carboxylic acid; LY294486, (3SR, 4αRS, 6SR, 8RS)-6-((((1H-tetrazol-5yl)methyl)oxy)methyl)-1,2,3,4a,5,6,7,8,8a-decahydroisoquinolone-3-carboxylic acid; LY307452, 2S,4S-2-amino-4-(4,4-diphenylbut-1-yl)pentan-1,5-dioc acid; LY354740, (+)-2-aminobicyclic[3.1.0]hexane-2,6-dicarboxylate; MAP4, 2-methyl-2-amino-4-phosphonobutyrate; NBQX, 6-nitro-7-sulfamoyl-benz(f)quinoxaline-2,3-dione; NMDA. N-methyl-D-aspartate.

Several classes of drugs modulate NMDA receptor function (see Table 7.1). Uncompetitive NMDA antagonists, such as dizocilpine (MK-801), phencyclidine (PCP), ketamine and memantine bind to the open channel and obstruct calcium influx. Other antagonists, such as CGS19755 and D-CCP-ene, compete with glutamate for binding to the NMDA receptor. Ethanol, desipramine and nitroglycerine appear to antagonize NMDA receptor function via other sites of this receptor (Reynolds and Miller, 1988; Sucher *et al.*, 1996). There is growing interest in both agonists and antagonists of the strychnine-insensitive glycine (glycine-B) modulatory site of the NMDA receptor, including D-cycloserine, serine and ACPC (D'Souza, *et al.*, 1995).

AMPA receptors mediate fast excitatory neurotransmission. Kainate receptors contribute to fast excitatory neurotransmission, although they perform a wide diversity of excitatory and inhibitory functions. Metabotropic receptor subclasses also have excitatory, inhibitory and autoreceptor functions (Schoepp and Conn, 1993; Conn and Pin, 1997). Building on the inhibitory actions of the group 2 metabotropic glutamate receptor (mGluR2) agonists at this site are being developed to attenuate glutamate release (Schoepp *et al.*, 1997). A growing number of other drugs are being developed as anticonvulsants due, in part, to their capacity to attenuate glutamate release, including lamotrigine, topiramate, remacemide, felbamate and riluzole (Kanda *et al.*, 1996; Waldmeier *et al.*, 1996; Wang *et al.*, 1996; Davies, 1997; Johannessen, 1997; Stefani *et al.*, 1997). Many of these drugs block voltage-dependent sodium channels, an action held in common with more traditional anticonvulsants such as phenytoin and carbamazepine.

Introduction to human glutamatergic psychopharmacology: healthy humans

Studies in healthy humans suggest that NMDA receptor antagonists may model an abnormality in glutamatergic function in schizophrenic patients that contributes to the symptoms and cognitive deficits associated with this disorder.

Similarity to symptoms of schizophrenia

The signal observation in this field of research was that PCP produced cognitive, perceptual and emotional changes that impressed the initial investigative team as being 'schizophrenomimetic' (Luby *et al.*, 1959). Observations made during PCP administration or in individuals presenting with PCP intoxication essentially were replicated with subsequent studies of ketamine (Corssen and Domino, 1966; Ghoneim *et al.*, 1985; Oye *et al.*, 1992; Krystal *et al.*, 1994; Malhotra *et al.*, 1996). These increases are illustrated in Figure 7.2. Both drugs produced positive symptoms, such as hallucinations or delusions, negative symptoms, such as blunted affect and emotional withdrawal, and disorganization symptoms, such as disorganized thought and behavior. PCP intoxication was sufficiently similar to schizophrenia that these diagnoses were often confused in emergency rooms (Allen and Young, 1978). Similarly, ketamine acutely makes thought processes concrete, loosely organized and overpersonalized (Krystal *et al.*, 1998e). These changes were rated as quite similar to thought disorder measured in schizophrenic patients (Adler *et al.*, 1998).

The strength of the NMDA antagonist 'model' for schizophrenia is its capacity to mimic many types of symptoms of schizophrenia. The psychoses associated with amphetamine and serotonergic hallucinogens produce cognitive and perceptual effects that most closely resemble the positive symptoms of schizophrenia (Rosse *et al.*, 1994; Krystal *et al.*, 1998b) Their failure to produce negative, disorganization and other cognitive impairments seems to limit their relevance to paranoid psychoses, such as the paranoid subtype of schizophrenia, distinguished primarily by positive symptoms. In contrast, the range of symptoms and cognitive deficits produced by NMDA antagonists appear to resemble the breadth of

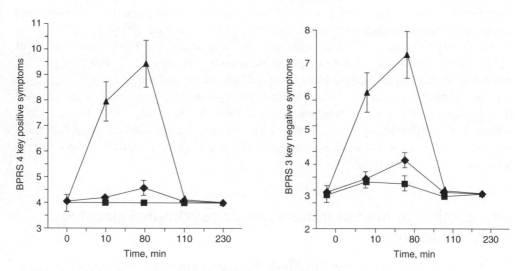

Figure 7.2 Left: ketamine hydrochloride effects on four key positive symptoms on the Brief Psychiatric Rating Scale (BPRS) in healthy subjects (*n* = 18). Cluster scores (mean ± SEM) are presented for placebo (■), ketamine hydrochloride (0.1 mg/kg, ●) and ketamine hydrochloride (0.5 mg/kg, ▲) test days. Repeated measures ANOVA performed on four key positive symptoms of the BPRS, ketamine dose?time interaction was highly significant [*F*(8,136) = 22.9, *P* = 0.0001]. Right: ketamine effects on three key negative symptoms of the BPRS in healthy subjects (*n* = 18). Repeated measures ANOVA performed on three key negative symptoms of the BPRS, ketamine dose?time interaction was highly significant [*F*(8,1360 = 18.0, *P* = 0.0001]. From Krystal *et al.* (1994).

symptoms seen in the disorganized or undifferentiated subtypes of schizophrenia. This breadth, however, may limit the relevance of the NMDA antagonist model for the paranoid subtype of schizophrenia.

The production of psychosis and perceptual change by ketamine is related to the degree of occupancy of DA receptors (Hartvig *et al.*, 1995) and the degree to which they modulate cerebral metabolism (Breier *et al.*, 1997; Vollenweider *et al.*, 1997). Among the uncompetitive DA antagonists, high affinity agents, such as PCP and ketamine, have relatively greater potential to produce psychosis at the same predicted level of receptor occupancy than do lower affinity drugs, such as memantine and amantidine (Kornhuber and Weller, 1997). Further, the schizophrenia-like symptoms produced by DA antagonists emerge within a narrow dose window. With ketamine, for example, anxiolytic effects are the most prominent effects observed at 0.1 mg/kg, while psychotigenic and anxiogenic effects occur at 0.5 mg/kg (Krystal *et al.*, 1994). Clouding of consciousness and anesthesia emerge at doses of 1.0 mg/kg or higher (Corssen and Domino, 1966).

GlycineB antagonists would be predicted to produce psychosis due to the dependence of DA receptor function upon the stimulation of this site. Although production or exacerbation of psychosis has been reported in association with chronic administration of high dose D-cycloserine and felbamate (Simeon *et al.*, 1970; Cascella *et al.*, 1994; Knable and Rickler, 1995; Theodore *et al.*, 1995), psychosis was not observed in healthy subjects during the acute administration of D-cycloserine at doses of 500 mg ($n = 45$) or 1000 mg ($n = 10$) (J. Krystal, unpublished observation). Overall, there has been relatively little published describing the dose-related cognitive and behavioral effects of full antagonists at the glycineB site in healthy subjects. Data reported to date suggest that the glycineB partial agonists have a low potential to produce psychosis.

Other glutamatergic drugs have been studied as potential antipsychotic treatments for the DA antagonist model psychosis. Two pilot studies have examined glutamatergic strategies for reducing psychosis produced by ketamine. The first study found that intravenous glycine (0.1 and 0.2 g/kg) attenuated psychoses produced by ketamine in healthy subjects (D'Souza *et al.*, 1997). This study supported a hypothesis growing from preclinical data that suggested that glycine reduces uncompetitive DA antagonist effects (D'Souza *et al.*, 1995). The second pilot study found a trend for lamotrigine pretreatment to attenuate the ketamine psychosis (Anand *et al.*, 1997). Lamotrigine more robustly reduced other perceptual changes produced by ketamine in healthy subjects. These data support a view growing from other basic studies that suggests that DA antagonists stimulate cortical and limbic glutamate release (Moghaddam *et al.*, 1997). The glutamate released by DA antagonists stimulates non-DA glutamate receptors (Krystal *et al.*, 1994). LY354740, an mGluR2 agonist that inhibits glutamate release, also prevents the DA antagonist stimulation of glutamate release in rats (Moghaddam and Adams, 1998). Similarly, there is increasing evidence that 5-hydroxytryptamine (5-HT$_{2A}$) antagonists might attenuate DA antagonist effects, perhaps via reductions in cortical glutamate release (Svensson *et al.*, 1995; Aghajanian and Marek, 1997).

The interaction of DA antagonists and drugs blocking kainate receptors has not yet been characterized. Overall, these studies suggest that AMPA antagonists, mGluR2 agonists and other glutamate release-inhibiting drugs might have therapeutic potential for treating hyperglutamatergic disorders, particularly those associated with deficits in DA receptor function.

The ketamine psychosis has been resistant to other pharmacological interventions. Positive symptoms produced in healthy subjects by ketamine, as measured by the Brief Psychiatric Rating Scale, were not reduced by pretreatment with lorazepam 2 mg ($n = 20$), haloperidol 5 mg ($n = 23$) or clozapine 25 mg ($n = 7$) (Krystal *et al.*, 1998b). In addition, psychosis was not increased by pretreatment with amphetamine 0.3 mg/kg i.v. ($n = 7$) (Krystal *et al.*, 1998f). These data suggest that the ketamine psychosis is not mediated by acute changes in dopaminergic systems or by global deficits in γ-aminobutyric acid (GABA)-A receptor stimulation.

Attention and working memory

Early reports suggested that PCP dose-dependently impaired these functions. For example, it reduced performance on the digit span test, digit–symbol substitution test, mental arithmetic, reaction time and the Stroop color word test (Rosenbaum *et al.*, 1959; Bakker and Amini, 1961; Cohen *et al.*, 1962). DA antagonist effects on attention have received closer evaluation in studies employing ketamine. This drug produces small, but consistent, reductions in vigilance as assessed by continuous performance tests. In general, ketamine impairments on vigilance and general orientation, as assessed by the Mini-Mental State Examination, are quite modest relative to impairments in executive functions and learning (Krystal *et al.*, 1994). Ketamine produced more pronounced increases in distractibility than reductions in vigilance (Krystal *et al.*, 1998e). The increase in distractibility produced by ketamine may be related to impairments in sensorimotor gating, as suggested by reductions in prepulse inhibition of the startle response (Krystal *et al.*, 1998b). This physiological measure has been associated with distractibility in schizophrenic patients (Karper *et al.*, 1996). This test encompasses elements of divided attention and response inhibition. Sedating medications such as lorazepam (Krystal *et al.*, 1998e), haloperidol (Krystal *et al.*, 1998d) and clozapine (Krystal *et al.*, 1998b) potentiate the impairment of attention produced by ketamine. In contrast, amphetamine pretreatment significantly attenuates the increase in distractibility produced by ketamine (Krystal *et al.*, 1998f). The current studies do not permit clear distinctions between attention and level of arousal.

DA antagonists also dose-dependently impair working memory. This construct has received a great deal of study in relation to growing insight into the functions of the prefrontal cortex (Goldman-Rakic, 1987). Working memory has been described as having three principal components (Baddeley, 1992): (i) a 'central executive' that guides the allocation of attention; (ii) a transient memory buffer described as a visuospatial sketchpad'; and (iii) a mechanism for verbal rehearsal called the 'phonological loop.' In rodents, non-human primates and humans, these functions appear to be subserved by networks including the frontal cortex (Baddeley, 1996; Goldman-Rakic, 1996). In both non-human primates (Wilson *et al.*, 1993) and humans (Belger *et al.*, 1998), different modalities of working memory, i.e. memory for shape, faces or location, are mediated by distinct cortical networks. PCP reduced verbal fluency and performance on a word association task (Bakker and Amini, 1961). In rodents, ketamine impairments of working memory are associated with increased glutamate and dopamine release (Verma and Moghaddam, 1996). Consistent with these findings, the dopamine-2 receptor antagonist, haloperidol, and the mGluR2 agonist, LY354740, reduced the cortical release of glutamate and working memory deficit produced by ketamine (Verma and Moghaddam, 1996; Moghaddam and Adams, 1998).

NMDA antagonist disruption of working memory has been demonstrated in humans. Ketamine reduced verbal fluency and immediate recall of suprasapan word lists (Ghoneim *et al.*, 1985; Krystal *et al.*, 1994). Similarly, ketamine increases the number and percentage of perseverative errors and decreases the number of criteria achieved on the Wisconsin Card Sorting Test (WCST) (Krystal *et al.*, 1994, 1998a). At subanesthetic doses, ketamine effects on the WCST are more prominent in WCST-naive subjects relative to WCST-experienced subjects. This difference suggests that ketamine has more detrimental effects on rule learning rather than on expression of learned rules (Krystal *et al.*, 1998a). Ketamine effects on WCST performance in healthy subjects are reduced by pretreatment with haloperidol, but not lorazepam (Krystal *et al.*, 1998de).

Ketamine also attenuated the frontal and cingulate, but not the parietal, component of the cortical activation on the odd-ball task as assessed using functional magnetic resonance imaging (fMRI; Krystal *et al.*, 1998c). This version of the odd-ball task, which evaluates the response to novel visual stimuli, has elements common to simple continuous performance and working memory tasks. As with healthy subjects administered ketamine, schizophrenic patients show deficits in the frontal, but not parietal, components of the cortical activation associated with the odd-ball task (Belger *et al.*, 1997).

Learning and memory

An extensive preclinical literature implicates NMDA receptors in a cellular model for the encoding of memory, long-term potentiation (Morris *et al.*, 1986; Maren and Baudry, 1995; Isaac *et al.*, 1996; Morris and Frey, 1997). Further, NMDA antagonists disrupt many types of learning in animals, ranging from fear conditioning to place learning (LeDoux, 1995). In several of these models, once a response is encoded, further expression of the learned behavior tends to be disrupted by non-NMDA antagonists (Miserendino *et al.*, 1990; Kim *et al.*, 1993).

The human literature implicates NMDA receptor function in many forms of learning. The interpretation of this literature is complicated by NMDA antagonist effects on attention, reviewed above. PCP impaired tests of declarative memory (Bakker and Amini, 1961). A converging body of evidence suggests that ketamine impairs the encoding of memory in humans. First, the recall impairment following administration of ketamine or other NMDA antagonists is dependent on dose and is evident when other behavioral effects are less prominent (Krystal *et al.*, 1994; Rockstroh *et al.*, 1996). Secondly, ketamine impairs memory when administered before, but not after, the presentation of stimuli (Oye *et al.*, 1992). Thirdly, free recall and recognition memory appear equally sensitive to ketamine effects (Malhotra *et al.*, 1996). Together, these data suggest that NMDA antagonists preferentially disrupt a relatively early stage of memory encoding. However, this effect was distinguished from the reduction of working memory in two studies where NMDA antagonists both spared working memory and had increasing effects with greater intervals between stimulus presentation and testing (Krystal *et al.*, 1994; Rockstroh *et al.*, 1996). Given the many cognitive effects of ketamine, it is likely that it effects many facets of memory function. Similarly, NMDA antagonists appear to disrupt many types of learning in humans, including fear conditioning (Hoehn-Saric *et al.*, 1991; Rockstroh *et al.*, 1996).

Glutamatergic abnormalities in schizophrenia

There is growing evidence of glutamatergic abnormalities in schizophrenia. However, the exact nature of these abnormalities is not clear currently. Despite the complexity of the current literature, a number of reviews have helped to organize current thinking on this topic (Kim *et al.*, 1980; Javitt and Zukin, 1991; Benes, 1995; Carlsson, 1995; Coyle, 1996; Deakin and Simpson, 1997; Hirsch *et al.*, 1997; Tamminga, 1998). The post-mortem studies are enormously difficult and expensive to conduct and they are complicated to interpret. They suffer from the fact that most studies evaluate elderly patients or younger patients who may not be representative due to factors that lead to their early death, including suicide (Nowak *et al.*, 1995). In these studies, the post-mortem interval often is highly variable between patients and there is very little control of factors that independently might alter glutamatergic function, such as alcohol consumption (Freund and Anderson, 1996). Most of these studies did not compare neuroleptic-treated and medication-free patients. Those that made these comparisons rarely studied sample sizes that were sufficiently large to be definitive. Further, those studies that compared patients with and without neuroleptic treatment did not account for differential effects of neuroleptic subclasses on glutamatergic regulation (Fitzgerald *et al.*, 1995). Despite these difficulties, post-mortem studies still provide the best detailed information available about glutamatergic pathology in schizophrenia.

A number of studies have described disturbances in glutamate receptors in schizophrenia, and these studies are summarized in Table 7.2. This table indicates that several studies described increases in NMDA receptor density based on ligand binding. While the increases in NMDA receptor binding are localized, the regions showing increased binding are not consistent between studies. To date, no studies have measured the level of NMDA subunit proteins in schizophrenic patients. Two published studies (see Table 7.2) report conflicting findings regarding mRNA levels for NMDA receptor subunits. One study reported decreased expression of the NR1 subunit in demented schizophrenic patients, but not cognitive preserved patients (Humphries *et al.*, 1996). A second study reported a relative enrichment of mRNA for the NR2D subunit in the prefrontal cortex of schizophrenic patients (Akbarian *et al.*, 1996b). A preliminary report from a third study suggested relative increases in mRNA levels for the NR1 and NR2A in the prefrontal cortex of schizophrenic patients, but not mRNA for the NR2B, NR2C or NR2D subunits (Meador-Woodruff *et al.*, 1998). Overall, the variability between studies suggests that the typical non-demented schizophrenic patient may demonstrate a regional increase in NMDA receptors.

The increase in NMDA receptors is perplexing. Increases in NMDA receptors are associated with tolerance to NMDA antagonists in animal models (Grant *et al.*, 1992; Follesa and Ticku, 1996). Other disorders, such as alcoholism, that are associated with increased NMDA receptor numbers show reduced sensitivity to NMDA antagonists (Krystal *et al.*,

Table 7.2 Reported abnormalities in glutamate receptor systems in post-mortem brain tissue from schizophrenic patients and controls

Target	Populations	No.[a]	Region	Measures	Comment
NMDA					
Binding	Schiz. Controls	6–13 3–12	Frontal Putamen Amygdala	[³H]MK-801	44% increase in B_{max} in putamen in patients (1)
Binding	Schiz. Control	9–13 10–14	Frontal (BA 10,11) Amygdala	[³H]TCP	B_{max} increased in orbital not effected by neuroleptic treatment (2)
Binding	Schiz., Undiff. Schiz., Paranoid Schizoaffective Suicide Control	17 27 9 7 112	Frontal, temporal, parietal, occipital, cingulate, putamen, cerebellum	[³H]TCP	Reduction in occipital B_{max} in all patient groups (3)
Binding	Schiz. Suicide Control, Neuroleptic Control	6 8 8 8	Striatum	[³H]MK801 (4)	No difference between groups
Binding	Schiz. Control	7 8	Hippocampus	[³H]MK-801	No group difference (5)
Glycine binding	Schiz., Drug-free Schiz., Medicated Control	5 6 10	13 regions	[³H]glycine binding	Increased frontal (premotor) B_{max} in treated patients Increased parietal B_{max} in both patient groups (6)
Glycine binding	Schiz., Medicated Controls	14 13	Nucleus accumbens, caudate, putamen	[³H]L-689,560	Increase in B_{max} in the putamen in patients (7)
mRNA	Schiz., Cog. Preserve Schiz., Cog. Impaired Controls	4 8 N.R.	Sup. temporal cortex (BA22)	NR1 mRNA level	Reduction only in patients with severe cognitive impairment (8)
mRNA	Schiz Controls, Neuroleptic Controls, Drug-free	15 8 15	Prefrontal, Cerebellum	NR1, NR2A–2D mRNA	Relative increase (53%) in prefrontal cortex NR2D in patients in relation to both control groups (9)
AMPA					
Binding	Schiz. Control	13 10	Frontal (6 regions), temporal (5 regions), parietal (4 regions), occipital (2 regions), piriform and cingulate	[³H]AMPA	No group differences (10)

Table 7.2 – *Continued*

Target	Populations	No.[a]	Region	Measures	Comment
Binding	Schiz. Suicide Control, Neuroleptic Control	6 8 8 8	Striatum	[³H]CNQX	Schizophrenics were higher than all groups, but suicides (4)
Binding	Schiz. Controls	7 8	Hippocampus	[³H]CNQX	B_{max} was lower in schizophrenics than controls (5)
Subunit protein levels	Schiz Control	10 11	Hippocampus	Antibodies to GluR1 and GluR2/3	GluR1 was reduced in parahippocampal gyrus while GluR2/3 was reduced in most hippocampal regions in patients (11)
Subunt protein levels	Schiz. Alcoholic Controls, Non-alc.	14 10 1	Hippocampus	Antibodies to GluR1–GluR3	Schizophrenics had reduced GluR2 and GluR3 relative to total controls, but not non-alcoholic controls. Alcoholics had elevated GluR2 and GluR3 levels (12)
Binding/ mRNA	Schiz., Medicated Schiz., Drug-free Control	10 6 9	Frontal, occipital cortex, nucleus accumbens, caudate, putamen	[³H]AMPA GluR1–GluR4 mRNA	No group differences and no impact of neuroleptics (13)
mRNA	Schiz Controls	6 8	Hippocampus	'non-NMDA' mRNA	Decrease in hippocampus mRNA levels (14)
mRNA	Schiz. Control	6 8	Hippocampus	'non-NMDA' mRNA	Decrease in hippocampal mRNA levels (15)
mRNA	Schiz Controls	9 14	Med. temporal, hippocampus	GluR1 and GluR2 mRNA levels	Both GluR1 and GluR2 mRNA levels were decreased in both regions in patients 25–70%. Reductions in GluR2 only in parahippocampal gyrus (16)
mRNA	Schiz. Control	11 11	Hippocampus	GluR2 (flip/flop)	Reduction in GluR2, especially the 'flop' isoform (17)
Kainate Binding	Schiz. Control	12 10	Prefrontal, putamen	[³H]kainate	Increase in medial prefrontal (48%) and eye movement area (25%) (18)
Binding	Schiz Control	14 14	Frontal (orbital, anterior), lateral temporal, amygdala, hippocampus	[³H]kainate	Increase in orbital frontal in patients bilaterally (19)

Measure	Group	n	Region	Ligand/Method	Findings
Binding	Schiz., Drug-free	6	4 Prefrontal regions	[3H]kainate	Increased B_{max} in both medicated and drug-free patients in medial and eye movement regions of prefrontal cortex. Increased B_{max} in three parietal regions only in medicated patients. There was a negative correlation between B_{max} and L-glutamate levels in many regions (20)
	Schiz., Medicated	6	4 Parietal regions		
	Control	10	2 Visual regions		
Binding	Schiz.	6	Striatum	[3H]kainate	No difference between groups(4)
	Suicide	8			
	Control, Neuroleptic	8			
	Control	8			
Subunit protein levels	Schiz.		Hippocampus	Antibodies to GluR5–GluR7	No group differences (12)
	Controls, Total				
	Controls, Non-alc.				
mRNA	Schiz	11	Hippocampus, Cerebellum (GluR6 only)	GluR6 and KA2 mRNA	Decrease in both measures in hippocampus in schizophrenics (21)
	Control	13			
Glutamate transporter					
Binding	Schiz	14	Frontal (orbital, anterior, lateral temporal, amygdala, hippocampus	D-[3H]aspartate	Increase in orbital frontal in patients bilaterally (19)
	Control	14			
Binding	Schiz	18	Caudate, putamen globus pallidus	D-[3H]aspartate	Reductions in putamen and ventral pallidum in schizophrenic patients (22)
	Control	20			
Binding	Schiz.	14	Frontal, temporal nucleus accumbens, caudate, putamen	D-[3H]aspartate	Reduced in nucleus accumbens caudate, and putamen in patients (23)
	Control	12			
Binding	Schiz.	6	Striatum	D-[3H]aspartate	No difference between groups(4)
	Suicide	8			
	Control, Neuroleptic	8			
	Control	8			

a In many studies, the number of brains studied varies by region.
N.R. = not reported.

[1]Kornhuber et al. (1989); [2]Simpson et al. (1991); [3]Weissman et al. (1991); [4]Noga et al. (1997); [5]Kerwin et al. (1990); [6]Ishimaru et al. (1994); [7]Aparicio-Legarza et al. (1998); [8]Humphries et al. (1996); [9]Akbarian et al. (1996b); [10]Kurumaji et al. (1992); [11]Eastwood et al. (1997b); [12]Breese et al. (1995); [13]Healy et al. (1998); [14]Collinge and Curtis (1991); [15]Harrison et al. (1991); [16]Eastwood et al. (1995); [17]Eastwood et al. (1997a); [18]Nishikawa et al. (1983); [19]Deakin et al. (1989); [20]Toru et al. (1994); [21]Porter et al. (1997); [22]Simpson et al. (1992); [23]Aparicio-Legarza et al. (1997).

1995). Yet, schizophrenic patients may show increased sensitivity to the hallucinatory and cognitive ketamine and other NMDA antagonists (Krystal *et al.*, 1995; Malhotra *et al.*, 1997). This paradox would be explained, for example, if there was an overabundant accumulation of an endogenous NMDA antagonist in schizophrenic patients. One candidate for this role is *N*-acetyl-aspartyl-glutamate (NAAG), a glutamate derivative that has NMDA antagonist and mGlu3 agonist actions (Coyle, 1997). Levels of this compound are elevated in post-mortem brain tissue from schizophrenic patients (Tsai *et al.*, 1995). Further research is needed in order to determine the precise involvement of NMDA receptors in schizophrenia.

Table 7.2 also reviews evidence of alterations in AMPA and kainate receptors in studies of post-mortem tissue from schizophrenic and comparison populations. As presented in this table, regional differences have been reported in AMPA receptor binding. In the striatum, levels were elevated or unchanged. In contrast, studies of the hippocampus generally reported reductions in AMPA receptor density. Overall, studies of AMPA receptor subunit protein levels and mRNA levels were consistent with the binding studies. Kainate receptor binding studies summarized in Table 7.2 suggested that the density of these receptors was elevated locally in several frontal cortical regions and unchanged in the striatum and hippocampus. In the hippocampus, the level of kainate receptor subunit protein was unchanged, but kainate receptor subunit mRNA levels were decreased (Table 7.2).

Alterations in the density of D-[^{3}H]aspartate binding to the glutamate transporter were also reported in schizophrenic patients (Table 7.2). Initial studies reported increased binding in the orbital frontal cortex, a non-significant trend for reductions in the left temporal cortex and significant reductions in the basal ganglia (reviewed in Table 7.2 and Deakin *et al.*, 1989). Deakin and Simpson (1997) suggested that increases in the density of binding to the glutamate transporter and glutamate receptors in the orbital frontal cortex reflected a hyperinnervation of this region that results in excessive activation of glutamatergic pathways terminating in target regions such as the anterior temporal cortex. They suggest that this glutamatergic hyper-activity is neurotoxic to these downstream sites, accounting for reductions in multiple glutamatergic indices in temporo-hippocampal structures. This model would also be consistent with neurotoxic hyperactivity in corticofugal pathways that might contribute to reductions in glutamatergic indices in the basal ganglia (Table 7.2). It also might fit with neuroanatomical data supporting the existence of increased glutamatergic innervation of the cingulate cortex (Benes *et al.*, 1992a) and reduced neuronal size in some cortical and hippocampal regions (Benes *et al.*, 1991b; Selemon *et al.*, 1995, 1998; Rajkowska *et al.*, 1998). However, one also could interpret the reductions in neuronal size and increased packing density to be in potential conflict with hyperinnervation of other regions arising from the prefrontal cortex. Thus, the exact pathological process that underlies these changes is open to multiple interpretations.

A growing body of data supports the existence of frontal cortical glutamatergic hyper-activity in schizophrenia. A recent study, for example, found evidence of increased glutamate cycling, i.e. elevation of cortical glutamine levels in the absence of other metabolic disturbances, in untreated schizophrenic patients in their first episode of illness (Bartha *et al.*, 1997). Similarly, the fact that NMDA receptor deficits activate glutamate systems and cause excitotoxicity was thought to support an excitotoxic model for the progression of neuro-pathology in some schizophrenic patients (Olney and Farber, 1995). These findings may conflict with an earlier positron emission tomography (PET) literature suggesting that frontal metabolism was reduced in schizophrenic patients (Wolkin *et al.*, 1992; Siegel *et al.*, 1993). However, variability in studies of the frontal cortex of schizophrenic patients at rest has shifted the current emphasis in research to evaluation of cognitive activation of the frontal cortex (Weinberger and Berman, 1996).

Frontal cortical glutamatergic hyperactivity may reflect inhibitory deficits arising from abnormalities in cortical GABA systems. Although no single finding regarding cortical GABA neurons has been replicated consistently, a number of reports point to deficits in this system. These findings include (i) reductions in the number of cortical GABA interneurons (Benes *et al.*, 1991a); (ii) migration deficits resulting in the inappropriate localization of interneurons (Akbarian *et al.*, 1993, 1996a); (iii) deficits in the GABA-synthetic enzyme (glutamic acid decarboxylase) by interneurons (Akbarian *et al.*, 1995); (iv) reductions in the number of inhibitory axon cartridges from a subset of interneurons, chandelier cells, that provide feedback inhibition to pyramidal neurons (Woo *et al.*, 1998); and (v) up-regulation of GABA-A receptor binding in some cortical layers (Benes *et al.*, 1992b, 1996).

Deficits in GABA systems may produce clinical consequences that are quite similar to those of NMDA antagonists. GABA systems may mediate the consequences of deficits in NMDA receptor function. Uncompetitive NMDA antagonists, such as ketamine, tend to block those receptors that are activated, i.e. where the neuronal membrane is partially depolarized. At rest, interneurons are partially depolarized while pyramidal neurons are partially hyperpolarized due to the tonic interneuronal activity. As a result, one would expect that uncompetitive NMDA antagonists would inhibit preferentially GABAergic inputs to pyramidal neurons. This hypothesis is consistent with a growing body of clinical and electrophysiologic data (reviewed in Krystal *et al.*, 1998e).

Therapeutic studies of NMDA receptor facilitation

A growing number of studies support the hypothesis that facilitation of NMDA receptor function in neuroleptic-treated patients reduces cognitive deficits and negative symptoms associated with schizophrenia (Deutsch *et al.*, 1989). However, the total number of patients treated with these agents are relatively small, and no large multicenter studies have yet been conducted. GlycineB receptor facilitation does not yet appear to substitute for typical or atypical antipsychotic treatment. As an adjunctive treatment to these medications, the magnitude of the therapeutic effect of glycineB agonists is modest but clinically significant (Krystal and D'Souza, 1998). After a series of initial ambiguous studies utilizing moderate doses of oral glycine, a relatively consistent literature is emerging involving the admin-istration of high dose oral glycine ($\geq$35 g/kg) (Javitt *et al.*, 1994; Heresco-Levy *et al.*, 1996a), D-serine (Tsai *et al.*, 1998) or D-cycloserine (Goff *et al.*, 1995). The initial placebo-controlled high-dose glycine study found that it reduced negative symptoms and had a trend to reduce performance deficits on the WCST (Javitt *et al.*, 1994). A subsequent study suggested that glycine had efficacy across a broader array of symptom classes (Heresco-Levy *et al.*, 1996b).

D-Cycloserine, as a partial glycineB agonist, produces a more complicated pattern of findings than glycine. When used as a stand-alone or as an adjunctive treatment, D-cycloserine doses of 250 mg per day or higher appear to worsen performance on the Stroop test and increase schizophrenia symptoms (Cascella *et al.*, 1994; Simeon *et al.*, 1970; Goff *et al.*, 1995). These effects of high dose D-cycloserine are similar to those reported for NMDA antagonists, reviewed earlier. NMDA antagonist-like effects of D-cycloserine most likely arise as a consequence of its capacity to displace endogenous glycine from glycineB sites, reducing NMDA receptor function by up to 50%. However, when D-cycloserine is administered under conditions of low glycineB receptor occupancy by endogenous glycine, it produces up to 50–60% of the maximal effects of glycine (Henderson *et al.*, 1990; Emmett *et al.*, 1991). Low dose (50–100 mg) (Goff *et al.*, 1995), but not lower (Rosse *et al.*, 1996) or higher (Cascella *et al.*, 1994) dose D-cycloserine has been reported to improve performance on the Stroop test and to reduce negative symptoms in schizophrenic patients. Two important controversial findings have been reported regarding D-cycloserine. One study found that D-cycloserine was ineffective as a supplement to atypical neuroleptics at doses that were effective for typical neuroleptics (Goff *et al.*, 1996). The second finding is that the therapeutic effects of D-cycloserine are approximately half of those associated with glycine (Heresco-Levy *et al.*, 1998). While this finding is attractive in light of evidence that D-cycloserine has half of the efficacy of glycine at the glycineB site, it has yet to be replicated.

Recent basic and clinical research suggests that superior pharmacological strategies are being developed to facilitate NMDA receptor function. The dosing and potential efficacy limitations of D-cycloserine as a partial agonist of glycineB receptors limit the potential utility of this agent. The poor central nervous system (CNS) penetration of oral glycine requires that massive amounts of glycine are administered relatively frequently, limiting the utility of this approach (D'Souza *et al.*, 1995). Two alternative strategies have been proposed. The first, is to use D-serine to stimulate glycineB receptors directly (Tsai *et al.*, 1998). This drug appears of equal, if not superior, efficacy to other strategies. Further, the fact that it is actively transported into the CNS reduces the amount needed with oral administration. Further, D-serine is more potent than glycine (Matsui *et al.*, 1995) and it may function more like a traditional neurotransmitter than glycine (Schell *et al.*, 1997). An alternative strategy is to facilitate NMDA receptor function by blocking the high-affinity glycine transporter (Supplisson and Bergman, 1997). Preclinical evaluations of this strategy appear quite promising (Javitt *et al.*, 1997). With all strategies that produce long-term enhancement of glycineB receptors, careful study will be needed to determine whether these strategies have neurotoxic consequences (Newell *et al.*, 1997).

Glutamate and the genetics of schizophrenia

To date, there is no strong evidence linking glutamate receptors to schizophrenia. Reported negative studies have included the NMDA receptor (NR1), the kainate receptor (GluR5, GluR6) and the glutamate transporter (Pariseau *et al.*, 1994; Chen *et al.*, 1996, 1997a,b). However, a recent report suggested that the number of repeats of the gene coding for the inward rectifying potassium channel might be related to the vulnerability for both schizophrenia and bipolar disorder (Chandy *et al.*, 1998). This channel is activated by calcium that enters the neuron when NMDA receptors and other calcium channels are activated. It, in turn, acts to terminate the neuronal response to NMDA receptor activation. Disturbances in the function of this channel could both enhance and reduce the efficacy of NMDA receptors.

Toward integration

Glutamatergic hypotheses regarding the etiology, pathophysiology and treatment of schizophrenia are not yet sufficiently mature to provide clarity regarding their long-term impact on the field of schizophrenia research. This field of research began on the foundation of the face validity of the similarity between NMDA antagonist effects and the signs and symptoms of schizophrenia. This is an imperfect foundation because NMDA antagonists produce some effects not typically associated with schizophrenia, and schizophrenia is a heterogeneous disorder, only some components of which are similar to NMDA antagonist effects. However, it remains the pharmacological model with the greatest degree of similarity to the types of schizophrenia that are most resistant to our currently available treatments. Thus, it is possible that NMDA antagonist models may serve to guide medication development for this subpopulation of schizophrenic patients.

The NMDA antagonist model has many implications for cognitive dysfunction in schizophrenic patients. This model produces many of the cognitive impairments associated with schizophrenia: impairments in the control of attention, executive cognitive dysfunction, deficits in sensory gating, disruption of smooth pursuit eye movements and impairments in memory encoding, among other perturbations of cognitive function. As a result, it provides one of the few human laboratory-based approaches for studying the human circuitry and pharmacological modulation of these functions. To this end, this model may help to generate new treatments even if glutamatergic systems turn out to be a secondary factor contributing to the etiology of schizophrenia. If this were true, NMDA antagonists might play a role in schizophrenia research similar to the role that anticholinergic models played in the development and evaluation of nootropic agents for Alzheimer's disease (Sunderland *et al.*, 1997).

However, the NMDA antagonist model of schizophrenia would clearly be most important if it was related directly to the etiology and pathophysiology of the disorder. In the case of Alzheimer's disease, characterization of the etiology and pathophysiology has raised real hopes of prevention (Cummings and Mendez, 1997). Thus, linking the NMDA antagonist model of schizophrenia to the pathology of this disorder is a high priority if it is to have a role in the development of treatments that serve more than a palliative role.

The post-mortem literature does not yet provide clear guidance on the pathology of schizophrenia or the role of glutamate systems in altering cortical circuitry in ways that might give rise to schizophrenia. However, the progress made to date does provide a provocative basis for further study. Disturbances in many glutamatergic markers have been reported. Opposing changes in brain regions, should they turn out to contribute to the pathophysiology of schizophrenia, suggest a primary region of developmental abnormality and other areas of secondary or adaptive disturbance. These processes might provide targets for pharmacological intervention.

The glutamatergic treatments introduced to date, glycine, D-cycloserine and D-serine, hold some promise of clinical benefit for cognitive dysfunction in schizophrenic patients. These treatments all highlight one aspect of the NMDA antagonist model, deficits in the function of the receptor itself. Efforts to modulate the intracellular consequences of deficits in NMDA receptor function, such as alterations in nitric oxide synthase activity, are already being explored in patients (Deutsch *et al.*, 1997).

However, the NMDA antagonist model has other facets that should be explored as targets for development of medications, particularly the capacity of NMDA antagonists to stimulate the release of glutamate. Thus strategies for reducing the release of glutamate or blocking the postsynaptic consequences of excessive glutamate release are potential new strategies for treating cognitive dysfunction in schizophrenia that are extensions of NMDA antagonist models (Anand *et al.*, 1997; Moghaddam and Adams, 1998).

Based on the recent genetic studies, one might also consider modulating the inward rectifying potassium channel in order to alter glutamatergic function. Further, it is quite possible that the NMDA antagonist model mimics schizophrenia because it produces a dysfunction in a non-glutamatergic system that mimics a primary deficit in schizophrenic patients. For example, NMDA antagonists could mimic a GABA deficit or dopaminergic hyperactivity, as noted earlier.

Thus, the study of glutamatergic contributions to cognitive dysfunction in schizophrenic patients appears to be at a mid-way point. There is compelling data that will stimulate research for many years to come without a clear sense, yet, where these systems will fit in the pathophysiology and treatment of this disorder. The explosion of research in this area in the last 10 years has produced a firm basic science understanding of glutamate systems that was absent when the PCP model of schizophrenia was introduced 40 years ago (Luby *et al.*, 1959). Building on a firm molecular neuroscience base, this field of research is poised for its most rigorous evaluation.

Acknowledgements

The authors thank Mr David Ansonoff for his assistance with the preparation of this review. Work related to this review was supported by the Department of Veterans Affairs through the Merit Review Program (J.H.K.), Schizophrenia Biological Research Center (all authors) and the VA-Yale Alcoholism Research Center (J.H.K.). It was also supported by NIMH grants MH-30929 (D.S.C. and J. Leckman), MH44866 (P. Goldman-Rakic), MH48404 (B.M.) and an NARSAD Independent Investigator Award (J.H.K.).

References

Adler, C.M., Malhotra, A.K., Goldberg, T., Elman, I., Pickar, D. and Breier, A. (1998) A comparison of ketamine-induced and schizophrenic thought disorder. *Society of Biological Psychiatry, Fifty-third Annual Convention*, pp. 83S–84S.

Aghajanian, G.K. and Marek, G.J. (1997) Serotonin induces excitatory postsynaptic potentials in apical dendrites of neocortical pyramidal cells. *Neuropharmacology*, **36**, 589–599.

Akbarian, S., Vinuela, A., Kim, J.J., Potkin, S.G., Bunney, W.E., Jr and Jones, E.G. (1993) Distorted distribution of nicotinamide-adenine dinucleotide phosphate-diaphorase neurons in temporal lobe of schizophrenics implies anomalous cortical development. *Archives of General Psychiatry*, **50**, 178–187.

Akbarian, S., Kim, J.J., Potkin, S.G., Hagman, J.O., Tafazzoli, A., Bunney, W.E., Jr and Jones, E.G. (1995) Gene expression for glutamic acid decarboxylase is reduced without loss of neurons in prefrontal cortex of schizophrenics [see comments]. *Archives of General Psychiatry*, **52**, 258–266, discussion 267–278.

Akbarian, S., Kim, J.J., Potkin, S.G., Hetrick, W.P., Bunney, W.E., Jr and Jones, E.G. (1996a) Maldistribution of interstitial neurons in prefrontal white matter of the brains of schizophrenic patients. *Archives of General Psychiatry*, **53**, 425–436.

Akbarian, S., Sucher, N.J., Bradley, D., Tafazzoli, A., Trinh, D., Hetrick, W.P., Potkin, S.G., Sandman, C.A., Bunney, W.E., Jr and Jones, E.G. (1996b) Selective alterations in gene expression for NMDA receptor subunits in prefrontal cortex of schizophrenics. *Journal of Neuroscience*, **16**, 19–30.

Alexander, S.P.H. and Peters, J.A. (1998) 1998 Receptor and Ion Channel Nomenclature Supplement. In *Trends in Pharmacological Sciences*, vol. 9th Edition.

Allen, R.M. and Young, S.J. (1978) Phencyclidine-induced psychosis. *American Journal of Psychiatry*, **135**, 1081–1084.

Anand, A., Charney, D.S., Cappiello, A., Berman, R.M., Oren, D.A. and Krystal, J.H. (1997) Lamotrigine reduces the psychotomimetic—but not the mood elevating—effects of ketamine in humans. *36th Annual Meeting, American College of Neuropsychopharmacology*, p. 251.

Aparicio-Legarza, M.I., Cutts, A.J., Davis, B. and Reynolds, G.P. (1997) Deficits of [^{3}H]D-aspartate binding to glutamate uptake sites in striatal and accumbens tissue in patients with schizophrenia. *Neuroscience Letters*, 232, 13–16.

Aparicio-Legarza, M.I., Davis, B., Hutson, P.H. and Reynolds, G.P. (1998) Increased density of glutamate/N-methyl-D-aspartate receptors in putamen from schizophrenic patients. *Neuroscience Letters*, **241**, 143–146.

Baddeley, A. (1992) Working memory. *Science*, **255**, 556–559.

Baddeley, A. (1996) The fractionation of working memory. *Proceedings of the National Academy of Sciences of the United States of America*, **93**, 13468–13472.

Bakker, C.B. and Amini, F.B. (1961) Observations on the psychotomimetic effects of serynyl. *Comprehensive Psychiatry*, **2**, 269–280.

Bartha, R., Williamson, P.C., Drost, D.J., Malla, A., Carr, T.J., Cortese, L., Canaran, G., Rylett, R.J. and Neufeld, R.W. (1997) Measurement of glutamate and glutamine in the medial prefrontal cortex of never-treated schizophrenic patients and healthy controls by proton magnetic resonance spectroscopy. *Archives of General Psychiatry*, **54**, 959–965.

Belger, A., Kirino, E., McCarthy, G., Gore, J.C. and Krystal, J.H. (1997) Assessment of prefrontal activation by infrequent visual targets and non-target novel stimuli in schizophrenia: a functional MRI study. *36th Annual Meeting, American College of Neuropsychopharmacology*, p 190.

Belger, A., Puce, A., Krystal, J., Gore, J., Goldman-Rakic, P. and McCarthy, G. (1998)

Dissociation of mnemonic and perceptual processes during spatial and non-spatial working memory using fMRI. *Human Brain Mapping*, **6**, 14–32.

Benes, F.M. (1995) Development of the glutamate, GABA, and dopamine systems in relation to NRH-induced neurotoxicity [editorial; comment]. *Biological Psychiatry*, **38**, 783–787.

Benes, F.M., McSparren, J., Bird, E.D., SanGiovanni, J.P. and Vincent, S.L. (1991a) Deficits in small interneurons in prefrontal and cingulate cortices of schizophrenic and schizoaffective patients. *Archives of General Psychiatry*, **48**, 996–1001.

Benes, F.M., Sorensen, I. and Bird, E.D. (1991b) Reduced neuronal size in posterior hippocampus of schizophrenic patients. *Schizophrenia Bulletin*, **17**, 597–608.

Benes, F.M., Sorensen, I., Vincent, S.L., Bird, E.D. and Sathi, M. (1992a) Increased density of glutamate-immunoreactive vertical processes in superficial laminae in cingulate cortex of schizophrenic brain. *Cerebral Cortex*, **2**, 503–512.

Benes, F.M., Vincent, S.L., Alsterberg, G., Bird, E.D. and SanGiovanni, J.P. (1992b) Increased GABA$_A$ receptor binding in superficial layers of cingulate cortex in schizophrenics. *Journal of Neuroscience*, **12**, 924–929.

Benes, F.M., Vincent, S.L., Marie, A. and Khan, Y. (1996) Up-regulation of GABA$_A$ receptor binding on neurons of the prefrontal cortex in schizophrenic subjects. *Neuroscience*, **75**, 1021–1031.

Breese, C.R., Freedman, R. and Leonard, S.S. (1995) Glutamate receptor subtype expression in human postmortem brain tissue from schizophrenics and alcohol abusers. *Brain Research*, **674**, 82–90.

Breier, A., Malhotra, A.K., Pinals, D.A., Weisenfeld, N.I. and Pickar, D. (1997) Association of ketamine-induced psychosis with focal activation of the prefrontal cortex in healthy volunteers. *American Journal of Psychiatry*, **154**, 805–811.

Carlsson, A. (1995) Neurocircuitries and neurotransmitter interactions in schizophrenia. *International Clinical Psychopharmacology*, **10**, 21–28.

Carlsson, M. and Carlsson, A. (1990) Interactions between glutamatergic and monoaminergic systems within the basal ganglia—implications for schizophrenia and Parkinson's disease. *Trends in Neuroscience*, **13**, 272–276.

Cascella, N.G., Macciardi, F., Cavallini, C. and Smeraldi, E. (1994) D-Cycloserine adjuvant therapy to conventional neuroleptic treatment in schizophrenia: an open-label study. *Journal of Neural Transmission—General Section*, **95**, 105–111.

Chandy, K.G., Fantino, E., Wittekindt, O., Kalman, K., Tong, L.L., Ho, T.H., Gutman, G.A., Crocq, M.A., Ganguli, R., Nimgaonkar, V., Morris-Rosendahl, D.J. and Gargus, J.J. (1998) Isolation of a novel potassium channel gene hSKCa3 containing a polymorphic CAG repeat: a candidate for schizophrenia and bipolar disorder? *Molecular Psychiatry*, **3**, 32–37.

Chen, A.C., Kalsi, G., Brynjolfsson, J., Sigmundsson, T., Curtis, D., Butler, R., Read, T., Murphy, P., Petursson, H., Barnard, E.A. and Gurling, H.M. (1996) Lack of evidence for close linkage of the glutamate GluR6 receptor gene with schizophrenia. *American Journal of Psychiatry*, **153**, 1634–1636.

Chen, A.C., Kalsi, G., Brynjolfsson, J., Sigmundsson, T., Curtis, D., Butler, R., Read, T., Murphy, P., Barnard, E.A., Petursson, H. and Gurling, H.M. (1997a) Exclusion of linkage between schizophrenia and the gene encoding a neutral amino acid glutamate/aspartate transporter, SLC1A5. *American Journal of Medical Genetics*, **74**, 50–52.

Chen, A.C., Kalsi, G., Brynjolfsson, J., Sigmundsson, T., Curtis, D., Butler, R., Read, T., Murphy, P., Petursson, H., Barnard, E.A. and Gurling, H.M. (1997b) Exclusion of linkage of schizophrenia to the gene for the glutamate GluR5 receptor. *Biological Psychiatry*, **41**, 243–245.

Ciabarra, A.M., Sullivan, J.M., Gahn, L.G., Pecht, G., Heinemann, S. and Sevarino, K.A. (1995) Cloning and characterization of chi-1: a developmentally regulated member of a novel class of the ionotropic glutamate receptor family. *Journal of Neuroscience*, **15**, 6498–6508.

Cohen, B.D., Rosenbaum, G., Luby, E.D. and Gottlieb, J.S. (1962) Comparison of phencyclidine hydrochloride (sernyl) with other drugs: simulation of schizophrenic performance with phencyclidine hydrochloride (sernyl), lysergic acid diethylamide (LSD-25), amobarbital (amytal) sodium; II. Symbolic and sequential thinking. *Archives of General Psychiatry*, **6**, 79–85.

Collinge, J. and Curtis, D. (1991) Decreased hippocampal expression of a glutamate receptor gene in schizophrenia. *British Journal of Psychiatry*, **159**, 857–859.

Conn, P.J. and Pin, J.P. (1997) Pharmacology and functions of metabotropic glutamate receptors. *Annual Review of Pharmacology and Toxicology*, **37**, 205–237.

Corssen, G. and Domino, E.F. (1966) Dissociative anesthesia: further pharmacologic studies and first clinical experience with the phencyclidine derivative CI-581. *Anesthesia and Analgesia*, **45**, 29–40.

Coyle, J.T. (1996) The glutamatergic dysfunction hypothesis for schizophrenia. *Harvard Review of Psychiatry*, **3**, 241–253.

Coyle, J.T. (1997) The nagging question of the function of *N*-acetylaspartylglutamate. *Neurobiology of Disease*, **4**, 231–238.

Cummings, J.L. and Mendez, M.F. (1997) Alzheimer's disease: cognitive and behavioral pharmacotherapy. *Connecticut Medicine*, **61**, 543–552.

Davies, J.A. (1997) Remacemide hydrochloride: a novel antiepileptic agent. *General Pharmacology*, **28**, 499–502.

Deakin, J.F. and Simpson, M.D. (1997) A two-process theory of schizophrenia: evidence from studies in post-mortem brain. *Journal of Psychiatric Research*, **31**, 277–295.

Deakin, J.F., Slater, P., Simpson, M.D., Gilchrist,A.C., Skan, W.J., Royston, M.C., Reynolds, G.P. and Cross, A.J. (1989) Frontal cortical and left temporal glutamatergic dysfunction in schizophrenia. *Journal of Neurochemistry*, **52**, 1781–1786.

Deutsch, S.I., Mastropaolo, J., Schwartz, B.L., Rosse, R.B. and Morihisa, J.M. (1989) A 'glutamatergic hypothesis' of schizophrenia. Rationale for pharmacotherapy with glycine. *Clinical Neuropharmacology*, **12**, 1–13.

Deutsch S.I., Rosse R.B., Schwartz B.L., Fay-McCarthy M., Rosenberg P.B. and Fearing K. (1997) Methylene blue adjuvant therapy of schizophrenia. *Clinical Neuropharmacology*, **20**, 357–363.

D'Souza, D.C., Charney, D.S. and Krystal, J.H. (1995) Glycine site agonists of the NMDA receptor: a review. *CNS Drug Reviews*, **1**, 227–260.

D'Souza, D.C., Gil, R., Belger, A., Zimmerman, L., Tracy, L., Larvey, K. and Cassello, K. and Krystal, J. (1997) Glycine–ketamine interactions in healthy humans. *36th Annual Meeting, American College of Neuropsychopharmacology*, p. 286.

Eastwood, S.L., McDonald, B., Burnet, P.W., Beckwith, J.P., Kerwin, R.W. and Harrison, P.J. (1995) Decreased expression of mRNAs encoding non-NMDA glutamate receptors GluR1 and GluR2 in medial temporal lobe neurons in schizophrenia. *Brain Research. Molecular Brain Research*, **29**, 211–223.

Eastwood, S.L., Burnet, P.W. and Harrison, P.J. (1997a) GluR2 glutamate receptor subunit flip and flop isoforms are decreased in the hippocampal formation in schizophrenia: a reverse transcriptase–polymerase chain reaction (RT–PCR) study. *Brain Research. Molecular Brain Research*, **44**, 92–98.

Eastwood, S.L., Kerwin, R.W. and Harrison, P.J. (1997b) Immunoautoradiographic evidence for a loss of alpha-amino-3-hydroxy-5-methyl-4-isoxazole propionate-preferring non-*N*-methyl-D-aspartate glutamate receptors within the medial temporal lobe in schizophrenia. *Biological Psychiatry*, **41**, 636–643.

Emmett, M.R., Mick, S.J., Cler, J.A., Rao, T.S., Iyengar, S. and Wood P.L. (1991) Actions of D-cycloserine at the *N*-methyl-D-aspartate-associated glycine receptor site *in vivo*. *Neuropharmacology*, 30, 1167–1171.

Fitzgerald, L.W., Deutch, A.Y., Gasic, G., Heinemann, S.F. and Nestler, E.J. (1995) Regulation of cortical and subcortical glutamate receptor subunit expression by antipsychotic drugs. *Journal of Neuroscience*, **15**, 2453–2461.

Follesa, P. and Ticku, M.K. (1996) NMDA receptor upregulation: molecular studies in cultured mouse cortical neurons after chronic antagonist exposure. *Journal of Neuroscience*, **16**, 2172–2178.

Freund, G. and Anderson, K.J. (1996) Glutamate receptors in the frontal cortex of alcoholics. *Alcoholism, Clinical and Experimental Research*, **20**, 1165–1172.

Ghoneim, M.M., Hinrichs, J.V., Mewaldt, S.P. and Petersen, R.C. (1985) Ketamine: behavioral effects of subanesthetic doses. *Journal of Clinical Psychopharmacology*, **5**, 70–77.

Goff, D.C., Tsai, G., Manoach, D.S. and Coyle, J.T. (1995) Dose-finding trial of D-cycloserine added to neuroleptics for negative symptoms in schizophrenia. *American Journal of Psychiatry*, **152**, 1213–1215.

Goff, D.C., Tsai, G., Manoach, D.S., Flood, J., Darby, D.G. and Coyle, J.T. (1996) D-Cycloserine added to clozapine for patients with schizophrenia. *American Journal of Psychiatry*, **153**, 1628–1630.

Goldman-Rakic, P.S. (1987) Circuitry of primate prefrontal cortex and regulation of behavior by representational memory. In: Plum, F. (ed.), *Handbook of Physiology, Section I. Higher Functions of the Brain*. Oxford University Press, New York, NY, pp. 373–417.

Goldman-Rakic, P.S. (1996) Regional and cellular fractionation of working memory. *Proceedings of the National Academy of Sciences of the United States of America*, **93**, 13473–13480.

Grant, K.A., Snell, L.D., Rogawski, M.A., Thurkauf, A. and Tabakoff, B. (1992) Comparison of the effects of the uncompetitive *N*-methyl-D-aspartate antagonist (+)-5-aminocarbonyl-10,11-dihydro-5H-dibenzo[a,d] cyclohepten-5,10-imine (ADCI) with its structural analogs dizocilpine (MK-801) and carbamazepine on ethanol withdrawal seizures. *Journal of Pharmacology and Experimental Therapeutics*, **260**, 1017–1022.

Harrison, P.J., McLaughlin, D. and Kerwin, R.W. (1991) Decreased hippocampal expression of a glutamate receptor gene in schizophrenia. *Lancet*, **337**, 450–452.

Hartvig, P., Valtysson, J., Lindner, K.J., Kristensen, J., Karlsten, R., Gustafsson, L.L., Persson, J., Svensson, J.O., Oye, I., Antoni, G. *et al.* (1995) Central nervous system effects of subdissociative doses of (S)-ketamine are related to plasma and brain concentrations measured with positron emission tomography in healthy volunteers. *Clinical Pharmacology and Therapeutics*, **58**, 165–173.

Healy, D.J., Haroutunian, V., Powchik, P., Davidson, M., Davis, K.L., Watson, S.J. and Meador-Woodruff, J.H. (1998) AMPA receptor binding and subunit mRNA expression in prefrontal cortex and striatum of elderly schizophrenics. *Neuropsychopharmacology*, **19**, 278–286.

Henderson, G., Johnson, J.W. and Ascher, P. (1990) Competitive antagonists and partial agonists at the glycine modulatory site of the mouse *N*-methyl-D-aspartate receptor. *Journal of Physiology*, **430**, 189–212.

Heresco-Levy, U., Javitt, D.C., Ermilov, M., Mordel, C., Horowitz, A. and Kelly, D. (1996a) Double-blind, placebo-controlled, crossover trial of glycine adjuvant therapy for treatment-resistant schizophrenia. *British Journal of Psychiatry*, **169**, 610–617.

Heresco-Levy, U., Javitt, D.C., Ermilov, M., Mordel, C., Horowitz, A. and Kelly, D. (1996b) Double-blind, placebo-controlled, crossover trial of glycine adjuvant therapy for treatment-resistant schizophrenia. *British Journal of Psychiatry*, **169**, 610–617.

Heresco-Levy, U., Javitt, D.C., Ermilov, M., Mordel, C., Silipo, G. and Lichtenstein, M. (1998) Double-blind, placebo-controlled, crossover trial of D-cycloserine adjuvant therapy for treatment-resistant schizophrenia. (in press).

Hirsch, S.R., Das, I., Garey, L.J. and de Belleroche, J. (1997) A pivotal role for glutamate in the pathogenesis of schizophrenia, and its cognitive dysfunction. *Pharmacology, Biochemistry and Behavior*, **56**, 797–802.

Hoehn-Saric, R., McLeod, D.R. and Glowa, J.R. (1991) The effects of NMDA receptor blockade on the acquisition of a conditioned emotional response. *Biological Psychiatry*, **30**, 170–176.

Hollmann, M., Boulter, J., Maron, C., Beasley, L., Sullivan, J., Pecht, G. and Heinemann, S. (1993) Zinc potentiates agonist-induced currents at certain splice variants of the NMDA receptor. *Neuron*, **10**, 943–954.

Humphries, C., Mortimer, A., Hirsch, S. and de Belleroche, J. (1996) NMDA receptor mRNA correlation with antemortem cognitive impairment in schizophrenia. *Neuroreport*, **7**, 2051–2055.

Isaac, J.T., Oliet, S.H., Hjelmstad, G.O., Nicoll, R.A. and Malenka, R.C. (1996) Expression mechanisms of long-term potentiation in the hippocampus. *Journal of Physiology, Paris*, **90**, 299–303.

Ishimaru, M., Kurumaji, A. and Toru, M. (1994) Increases in strychnine-insensitive glycine binding sites in cerebral cortex of chronic schizophrenics: evidence for glutamate hypothesis. *Biological Psychiatry*, **35**, 84–95.

Javitt, D.C. and Zukin, S.R. (1991) Recent advances in the phencyclidine model of schizophrenia [see comments]. *American Journal of Psychiatry*, **148**, 1301–1308

Javitt, D.C., Zylberman, I., Zukin, S.R., Heresco-Levy, U. and Lindenmayer, J.P. (1994) Amelioration of negative symptoms in schizophrenia by glycine. *American Journal of Psychiatry*, **151**, 1234–1236.

Javitt, D.C., Sershen, H., Hashim, A. and Lajtha, A. (1997) Reversal of phencyclidine-induced hyperactivity by glycine and the glycine uptake inhibitor glycyldodecylamide. *Neuropsychopharmacology*, **17**, 202–204.

Johannessen, S.I. (1997) Pharmacokinetics and interaction profile of topiramate: review and comparison with other newer antiepileptic drugs. *Epilepsia*, **38**, S18–S23.

Kanda, T., Kurokawa, M., Tamura, S., Nakamura, J., Ishii, A., Kuwana, Y., Serikawa, T., Yamada, J., Ishihara, K. and Sasa, M. (1996) Topiramate reduces abnormally high extracellular levels of glutamate and aspartate in the hippocampus of spontaneously epileptic rats (SER). *Life Sciences*, **59**, 1607–1616.

Karper, L.P., Freeman, G.K., Grillon, C., Morgan, C.A., 3rd, Charney, D.S. and Krystal, J.H. (1996) Preliminary evidence of an association between sensorimotor gating and distractibility in psychosis. *Journal of Neuropsychiatry and Clinical Neurosciences*, **8**, 60–66.

Kerwin, R., Patel, S. and Meldrum, B. (1990) Quantitative autoradiographic analysis of glutamate binding sites in the hippocampal formation in normal and schizophrenic brain post mortem. *Neuroscience*, **39**, 25–32.

Kim, J.S., Kornhuber, H.H., Schmid-Burgk, W. and Holzmuller, B. (1980) Low cerebrospinal fluid glutamate in schizophrenic patients and a new hypothesis on schizophrenia. *Neuroscience Letters*, **20**, 379–382.

Kim, M., Campeau, S., Falls, W.A. and Davis, M. (1993) Infusion of the non-NMDA receptor antagonist CNQX into the amygdala blocks the expression of fear-potentiated startle. *Behavioral and Neural Biology*, **59**, 5–8.

Knable, M.B. and Rickler, K. (1995) Psychosis associated with felbamate treatment [letter]. *Journal of Clinical Psychopharmacology*, **15**, 292–293.

Kornhuber, J. and Weller, M. (1997) Psychotogenicity and *N*-methyl-D-aspartate receptor antagonism: implications for neuroprotective pharmacotherapy. *Biological Psychiatry*, **41**, 135–144.

Kornhuber, J., Mack-Burkhardt, F., Riederer, P., Hebenstreit, G.F., Reynolds, G.P., Andrews, H.B. and Beckmann, H. (1989) [^{3}H]MK-801 binding sites in postmortem brain regions of schizophrenic patients. *Journal of Neural Transmission*, **77**, 231–236.

Krystal, J. and D'Souza, D.C. (1998) D-Serine and the therapeutic challenge posed by the NMDA antagonist model of schizophrenia. *Biological Psychiatry*, **44**, 1075–1076.

Krystal, J.H., Karper, L.P., Seibyl, J.P., Freeman, G.K., Delaney, R., Bremner, J.D., Heninger, G.R., Bowers, M.B., Jr and Charney, D.S. (1994) Subanesthetic effects of the noncompetitive NMDA antagonist, ketamine, in humans. Psychotomimetic, perceptual, cognitive, and neuroendocrine responses. *Archives of General Psychiatry*, **51**, 199–214.

Krystal, J., Karper, L., D'Souza, D.C., Webb, E., Bennett, A., Abi-Dargham, A., Petrakis, I.L., Brenner, L., Morrissey, K., Abi-Saab, D. and Charney, D.S. (1995) Differentiating NMDA dysregulation in schizophrenia and alcoholism using ketamine. *Schizophrenia Research*, **15**, 156.

Krystal, J., Bennett, A., Abi-Saab, D., Belger, A., Karper, L.P., D'Souza, D.C., Lipschitz, D., Abi-Dargham, A. and Charney, D.S. (2000) Dissociation of ketamine effects on rule acquisition and rule implementation: possible relevance to NMDA receptor contributions to executive cognitive functions. *Biological Psychiatry*, **47**, 137–143.

Krystal, J.H., Abi-Dargham, A., Laruelle, M. and Moghaddam, B. (1999) Pharmacologic model psychoses. In: Charney, D.S., Nestler, E. and Bunney, B.S. (eds), *Neurobiology of Mental Illness*. Oxford University Press, New York, pp. 214–224.

Krystal, J.H., Belger, A., Kirino, E., Gore, J. and McCarthy, G. (1998c) Ketamine effects on the cortical processing of novelty in humans assessed with fMRI. *Society for Neuroscience Abstracts*, **24** (in press).

Krystal, J.H., D'Souza, D.C., Karper, L.P., Bennett, A., Abi-Dargham, A., Abi-Saab, D., Bowers, M.B., Jr, Jatlow, P., Heninger, G.R. and Charney, D.S. (1999) Interactive effects of subanesthetic ketamine and haloperidol in healthy humans. *Psychopharmacology*, **145(2)**, 193–204.

Krystal, J.H., Karper, L.P., Bennett, A., D'Souza, D.C., Abi-Dargham, A., Morrissey, K., Abi-Saab, D., Bremner, J.D., Bowers, M.B., Jr, Suckow, R.F., Stetson, P., Heninger, G.R. and Charney, D.S. (1998e) Interactive effects of subanesthetic ketamine and subhypnotic lorazepam in humans. *Psychopharmacology*, **135**, 213–229.

Krystal, J.H., Moghaddam, B., Breier, A., Goldman-Rakic, P. and McElvey, J. (1998f) Glutamate, dopamine, the frontal cortex, and schizophrenia. *Biological Psychiatry*, 43, 60S.

Kurumaji, A., Ishimaru, M. and Toru, M. (1992) α-[^{3}H]Amino-3-hydroxy-5-methylisoxazole-4-propionic acid binding to human cerebral cortical membranes: minimal changes in postmortem brains of chronic schizophrenics. *Journal of Neurochemistry*, **59**, 829–837.

LeDoux, J.E. (1995) Emotion: clues from the brain. *Annual Review of Psychology*, **46**, 209–235.

Luby, E.D., Cohen, B.D., Rosenbaum, G., Gottlieb, J.S. and Kelley, R. (1959) Study of a new schizophrenomimetic drug—sernyl. *Archives of Neurological Psychiatry*, **81**, 363–369.

Malhotra, A.K., Pinals, D.A., Weingartner, H., Sirocco, K., Missar, C.D., Pickar, D. and Breier, A. (1996) NMDA receptor function and human cognition: the effects of ketamine in healthy volunteers. *Neuropsychopharmacology*, **14**, 301–307.

Malhotra, A.K., Pinals, D.A., Adler, C.M., Elman, I., Clifton, A., Pickar, D. and Breier, A. (1997) Ketamine-induced exacerbation of psychotic symptoms and cognitive impairment in neuroleptic-free schizophrenics. *Neuropsychopharmacology*, **17**, 141–150.

Maren, S. and Baudry, M. (1995) Properties and mechanisms of long-term synaptic plasticity in the mammalian brain: relationships to learning and memory. *Neurobiology of Learning and Memory*, **63**, 1–18.

Matsui, T., Sekiguchi, M., Hashimoto, A., Tomita, U., Nishikawa, T. and Wada, K. (1995) Functional comparison of D-serine and glycine in rodents: the effect on cloned NMDA receptors and the extracellular concentration. *Journal of Neurochemistry*, **65**, 454–458.

Meador-Woodruff, J.H., Haroutunian, V., Davis, K.L. and Watson, S.J. (1998) NMDA receptor dysregulation in schizophrenic prefrontal cortex. *Biological Psychiatry*, **43**, 83S.

Miserendino, M.J., Sananes, C.B., Melia, K.R. and Davis, M. (1990) Blocking of acquisition but not expression of conditioned fear-potentiated startle by NMDA antagonists in the amygdala. *Nature*, **345**, 716–718.

Moghaddam, B. and Adams, B.W. (1998) Reversal of phencyclidine effects by a group II metabotropic glutamate receptor agonist in rats. *Science*, **281**, 1349–1352.

Moghaddam, B., Adams, B., Verma, A. and Daly, D. (1997) Activation of glutamatergic neurotransmission by ketamine: a novel step in the pathway from NMDA receptor blockade to dopaminergic and cognitive disruptions associated with the prefrontal cortex. *Journal of Neuroscience*, **17**, 2921–2927.

Morris, R.G. and Frey, U. (1997) Hippocampal synaptic plasticity: role in spatial learning or the automatic recording of attended experience? *Philosophical Transactions of the Royal Society of London, Series B*, **352**, 1489–1503.

Morris, R.G., Anderson, E., Lynch, G.S. and Baudry, M. (1986) Selective impairment of learning and blockade of long-term potentiation by an N-methyl-D-aspartate receptor antagonist, AP5. *Nature*, **319**, 774–776.

Newell, D.W., Barth, A., Ricciardi, T.N. and Malouf, A.T. (1997) Glycine causes increased excitability and neurotoxicity by activation of NMDA receptors in the hippocampus. *Experimental Neurology*, **145**, 235–244.

Nishikawa, T., Takashima, M. and Toru, M. (1983) Increased [^{3}H]kainic acid binding in the prefrontal cortex in schizophrenia. *Neuroscience Letters*, **40**, 245–250.

Noga, J.T., Hyde, T.M., Herman, M.M., Spurney, C.F., Bigelow, L.B., Weinberger, D.R. and Kleinman, J.E. (1997) Glutamate receptors in the postmortem striatum of schizophrenic, suicide, and control brains. *Synapse*, **27**, 168–176.

Nowak, G., Ordway, G.A. and Paul, I.A. (1995) Alterations in the N-methyl-D-aspartate (NMDA) receptor complex in the frontal cortex of suicide victims. *Brain Research*, **675**, 157–164.

Olney, J.W. and Farber, N.B. (1995) Glutamate receptor dysfunction and schizophrenia [see comments]. *Archives of General Psychiatry*, **52**, 998–1007.

Oye, I., Paulsen, O. and Maurset, A. (1992) Effects of ketamine on sensory perception: evidence for a role of N-methyl-D-aspartate receptors. *Journal of Pharmacology and Experimental Therapeutics*, **260**,1209–1213.

Pariseau, C., Gregor, P., Myles-Worsley, M., Holik, J., Hoff, M., Waldo, M., Freedman R., Coon H. and Byerley W. (1994) Schizophrenia and glutamate receptor genes. *Psychiatric Genetics*, **4**, 161–165.

Porter, R.H., Eastwood, S.L. and Harrison, P.J. (1997) Distribution of kainate receptor subunit mRNAs in human hippocampus, neocortex and cerebellum, and bilateral reduction of hippocampal GluR6 and KA2 transcripts in schizophrenia. *Brain Research*, **751**, 217–231.

Rajkowska, G., Selemon, L.D. and Goldman-Rakic, P.S. (1998) Neuronal and glial somal size in the prefrontal cortex: a postmortem morphometric study of schizophrenia and Huntington disease. *Archives of General Psychiatry*, **55**, 215–224.

Reynolds, I.J. and Miller, R.J. (1988) Tricyclic antidepressants block N-methyl-D-aspartate receptors: similarities to the action of zinc. *British Journal of Pharmacology*, **95**, 95–102.

Rockstroh, S., Emre, M., Tarral, A. and Pokorny, R. (1996) Effects of the novel NMDA-receptor antagonist SDZ EAA 494 on memory and attention in humans. *Psychopharmacology*, **124**, 261–266.

Rosenbaum, G., Cohen, B.D., Luby, E.D., Gottlieb, J.S. and Yelen, D. (1959) Comparison of sernyl with other drugs: simulation of schizophrenic performance with sernyl, LSD-25, and amobarbital (amytal) sodium; I. Attention, motor function, and proprioception. *Archives of General Psychiatry*, **1**, 651–656.

Rosse, R.B., Collins, J.P., Jr, Fay-McCarthy, M., Alim, T.N., Wyatt, R.J. and Deutsch, S.I. (1994) Phenomenologic comparison of the idiopathic psychosis of schizophrenia and drug-induced cocaine and phencyclidine psychoses: a retrospective study. *Clinical Neuropharmacology*, **17**, 359–369.

Rosse, R.B., Fay-McCarthy, M., Kendrick, K., Davis, R.E. and Deutsch, S.I. (1996) D-Cycloserine adjuvant therapy to molindone in the treatment of schizophrenia. *Clinical Neuropharmacology*, **19**, 444–450.

Schell, M.J., Brady, R.O., Jr, Molliver, M.E. and Snyder, S.H. (1997) D-Serine as a neuromodulator: regional and developmental localizations in rat brain glia resemble NMDA receptors. *Journal of Neuroscience*, **17**, 1604–1615.

Schoepp, D.D. and Conn, P.J. (1993) Metabotropic glutamate receptors in brain function and pathology. *Trends in Pharmacological Sciences*, **14**, 13–20.

Schoepp, D.D., Johnson, B.G., Wright, R.A., Salhoff, C.R., Mayne, N.G., Wu, S., Cockerman, S.L., Burnett, J.P., Belegaje,R., Bleakman,D. and Monn, J.A. (1997) LY354740 is a potent and highly selective group II metabotropic glutamate receptor agonist in cells expressing human glutamate receptors. *Neuropharmacology*, **36**, 1–11.

Selemon, L.D., Rajkowska, G. and Goldman-Rakic, P.S. (1995) Abnormally high neuronal density in the schizophrenic cortex. A morphometric analysis of prefrontal area 9 and occipital area 17. *Archives of General Psychiatry*, **52**, 805–818, discussion 819–820.

Selemon, L.D., Rajkowska, G. and Goldman-Rakic, P.S. (1998) Elevated neuronal density in prefrontal area 46 in brains from schizophrenic patients: application of a three-dimensional, stereologic counting method. *Journal of Comparative Neurology*, 392, 402–412.

Siegel, B.V., Jr, Buchsbaum, M.S., Bunney, W.E., Jr, Gottschalk, L.A., Haier, R.J., Lohr, J.B., Lottenberg, S., Najafi, A., Nuechterlein, K.H., Potkin, S.G. *et al.* (1993) Cortical–striatal–thalamic circuits and brain glucose metabolic activity in 70 unmedicated male schizophrenic patients. *American Journal of Psychiatry*, 150, 1325–1336.

Simeon, J., Fink, M., Itil, T.M. and Ponce, D. (1970) D-Cycloserine therapy of psychosis by symptom provocation. *Comprehensive Psychiatry*, 11, 80–88.

Simpson, M.D., Slater, P., Royston, M.C. and Deakin, J.F. (1991) Alterations in phencyclidine and sigma binding sites in schizophrenic brains. Effects of disease process and neuroleptic medication. *Schizophrenia Research*, **6**, 41–48.

Simpson, M.D., Slater, P., Royston, M.C. and Deakin, J.F. (1992) Regionally selective deficits in uptake sites for glutamate and γ-aminobutyric acid in the basal ganglia in schizophrenia. *Psychiatry Research*, **42**, 273–282.

Stefani, A., Spadoni, F. and Bernardi, G. (1997) Differential inhibition by riluzole, lamotrigine, and phenytoin of sodium and calcium currents in cortical neurons: implications for neuroprotective strategies. *Experimental Neurology*, 147, 115–122.

Sucher, N.J., Awobuluyi, M., Choi, Y.B. and Lipton, S.A. (1996) NMDA receptors: from genes to channels. *Trends in Pharmacological Sciences*, **17**, 348–355.

Sunderland, T., Molchan, S.E., Little, J.T., Bahro, M., Putnam, K.T. and Weingartner, H. (1997) Pharmacologic challenges in Alzheimer disease and normal controls: cognitive modeling in humans. *Alzheimer Disease and Associated Disorders*, **11**, S23–S26.

Supplisson, S. and Bergman, C. (1997) Control of NMDA receptor activation by a glycine transporter co-expressed in *Xenopus* oocytes. *Journal of Neuroscience*, **17**, 4580–4590.

Svensson, T.H., Mathe, J.M., Andersson, J.L., Nomikos, G.G., Hildebrand, B.E. and Marcus, M. (1995) Mode of action of atypical neuroleptics in relation to the phencyclidine model of schizophrenia: role of 5-HT$_2$ receptor and α1-adrenoceptor antagonism [published erratum appears in *Journal of Clinical Psychopharmacology* 1995 Apr; **15**(2): 154]. *Journal of Clinical Psychopharmacology*, **15**, 11S–18S.

Tamminga, C.A. (1998) Schizophrenia and glutamatergic transmission. *Critical Reviews in Neurobiology*, **12**, 21–36

Theodore, W.H., Albert, P., Stertz, B., Malow, B., Ko, D., White, S., Flamini, R. and Ketter, T. (1995) Felbamate monotherapy: implications for antiepileptic drug development. *Epilepsia*, **36**, 1105–1110.

Toru, M., Kurumaji, A. and Ishimaru, M. (1994) Excitatory amino acids: implications for psychiatric disorders research. *Life Sciences*, **55**, 1683–1699.

Tsai, G., Passani, L.A., Slusher, B.S., Carter, R., Baer, L., Kleinman, J.E. and Coyle, J.T. (1995) Abnormal excitatory neurotransmitter metabolism in schizophrenic brains. *Archives of General Psychiatry*, **52**, 829–836.

Tsai, G., Yang, P., Chung, L.-C., Lange, N. and Coyle, J. (1998) D-Serine added to antipsychotics for the treatment of schizophrenia. *Biological Psychiatry*, **44**, 1081–1089.

Verma, A. and Moghaddam, B. (1996) NMDA receptor antagonists impair prefrontal cortex function as assessed via spatial delayed alternation performance in rats: modulation by dopamine. *Journal of Neuroscience*, **16**, 373–379.

Vollenweider, F.X., Leenders, K.L., Oye, I., Hell, D. and Angst, J. (1997) Differential psychopathology and patterns of cerebral glucose utilisation produced by (S)- and (R)-ketamine in healthy volunteers using positron emission tomography (PET). *European Neuropsychopharmacology*, **7**, 25–38.

Waldmeier, P.C., Martin, P., Stocklin, K., Portet, C. and Schmutz, M. (1996) Effect of carbamazepine, oxcarbazepine and lamotrigine on the increase in extracellular glutamate elicited by veratridine in rat cortex and striatum. *Naunyn-Schmiedeberg's Archives of Pharmacology*, **354**, 164–172.

Wang, S.J., Huang, C.C., Hsu, K.S., Tsai, J.J. and Gean, P.W. (1996) Presynaptic inhibition of excitatory neurotransmission by lamotrigine in the rat amygdalar neurons. *Synapse*, **24**, 248–255.

Weinberger, D.R. and Berman, K.F. (1996) Prefrontal function in schizophrenia: confounds and controversies. *Philosophical Transactions of the Royal Society of London, Series B*, **351**, 1495–1503.

Weissman, A.D., Casanova, M.F., Kleinman, J.E., London, E.D. and De Souza, E.B. (1991) Selective loss of cerebral cortical sigma, but not PCP binding sites in schizophrenia. *Biological Psychiatry*, **29**, 41–54.

Wilson, F.A., Scalaidhe, S.P. and Goldman-Rakic, P.S. (1993) Dissociation of object and spatial processing domains in primate prefrontal cortex [see comments]. *Science*, **260**, 1955–1958.

Wolkin A., Sanfilipo, M., Wolf, A.P., Angrist, B., Brodie, J.D. and Rotrosen J. (1992) Negative symptoms and hypofrontality in chronic schizophrenia. *Archives of General Psychiatry*, **49**, 959–965.

Woo, T.U., Whitehead, R.E., Melchitzky, D.S. and Lewis, D.A. (1998) A subclass of prefrontal γ-aminobutyric acid axon terminals are selectively altered in schizophrenia. *Proceedings of the National Academy of Sciences of the United States of America*, **95**, 5341–5346.

Section 2:
The importance of cognitive impairment and its correlates in schizophrenia

8 Cognitive functioning, social adjustment and long-term outcome in schizophrenia

Kim T. Mueser

Introduction

This review evaluates the evidence suggesting a link between cognitive functioning in schizophrenia and long-term outcome. In considering the course and outcome of schizophrenia, special emphasis is given to impairments in social (including vocational) functioning, which both characterize the illness and present the greatest challenge to treatment providers and families. While I review research on the association between cognitive functioning and outcome for patients who receive routine treatment (e.g. psychopharmacology and case management), I examine more closely the relationship between cognitive impairment and response to psychosocial rehabilitation. Understanding whether cognitive functioning limits (or precludes) the ability to benefit from psychosocial rehabilitation has important implications for the development, evaluation and modification of interventions designed to improve social functioning in schizophrenia.

I begin with a brief discussion of the importance of social functioning in schizophrenia. Then, I review contemporary theories of social adjustment which posit that cognitive functioning plays a pivitol role in mediating social competence and interpersonal effectiveness. Next, research on the relationship between cognitive functioning and outcome is reviewed, followed by consideration of the overlap between cognitive impairment, negative symptoms and outcome. Next, I review research on the prediction of response to psychosocial treatment from cognitive functioning. I conclude with a discussion of the theoretical and clinical implications of cognitive deficits for improving the long-term outcome of schizophrenia.

The importance of social functioning in schizophrenia

When considering the relationship between cognitive impairment and the course of schizophrenia, there are several reasons for focusing on social functioning as an especially important dimension of outcome. First, according to many modern diagnostic systems, impairment in social functioning, broadly construed as the ability to work, maintain interpersonal relationships or to care for oneself, is necessary to establish a diagnosis of schizophrenia (e.g. DSM-

IV; American Psychiatric Association, 1994). Thus, by definition, schizophrenia entails deficits in social functioning.

Second, not only does the diagnosis of schizophrenia require impairment in social functioning, but poor social functioning frequently precedes the onset of the disorder, and premorbid adjustment is predictive of a more severe course of illness (Langfeldt, 1937; Zigler and Glick, 1986; Stephens *et al.*, 1966, 1997; MacEwan and Athawe, 1997). Third, social functioning after the onset of schizophrenia continues to be a robust predictor of long-term outcome, including relapses, rehospitalizations and social functioning (Strauss and Carpenter, 1974, 1977; Tsuang, 1986; Rajkumar and Thara, 1989; Jonsson and Nyman, 1991; Perlick *et al.*, 1992; Harrison *et al.*, 1996). Fourth and last, social functioning tends to be improved only marginally by antipsychotic medication, mainly to the extent that it prevents or reduces the disruptive effects of relapses and rehospitalizations. In line with this, social functioning is correlated less strongly with positive symptoms than negative symptoms (Liddle, 1987; Bellack, 1990a; Glynn *et al.*, 1992; Brekke *et al.*, 1994).

Thus, poor social functioning is an integral feature of schizophrenia that defines the disorder, antedates its onset, predicts its outcome and is influenced minimally by available pharmacological interventions. Improvement in social functioning lies at the heart of psychosocial treatment, yet progress on this front has been slow. A more complete understanding of the interface between cognitive impairment and social functioning in schizophrenia may be useful in improving upon our existing treatment technology.

The role of cognition in social competence

Over the past several decades, as it became clear that deinstitutionalization offered little promise for improving the pervasive social deficits in schizophrenia, attention has turned to the development of theoretical models for understanding the nature and determinants of these deficits. Two interrelated models have been advanced that postulate the necessary components of effective social behavior, the tripartite model of social skills and the social skills model of social competence. Cognitive functioning is hypothesized to be a critical component of social skill, which is an important determinant of social competence and social functioning. These models, and the evidence supporting them, are reviewed briefly below.

The tripartite model of social skills proposes that effective social behavior requires three different types of skills, including social perception, cognition and behavioral skills (Trower *et al.*, 1978; Wallace *et al.*, 1980; Morrison and Bellack, 1981; McFall, 1982; Liberman *et al.*, 1986; Spaulding *et al.*, 1986). Significant impairments in any of these skill areas can interfere with social competence and the ability to fulfill social roles and responsibilities. First, in order to be effective in a social situation, the person must be able accurately to perceive relevant situational parameters, such as his or her relationship to the other person, whether the setting is public or private and the other person's affective response (i.e. *social perception skills*). Recognition of these situational features is crucial as they may determine the appropriateness of social behaviors. Extensive research has documented that patients with schizophrenia demonstrate impairments in their social perception skills, including their ability to perceive accurately the facial expressions of others (Morrison *et al.*, 1988; Gaebel and Wölwer, 1992;

Mueser *et al.*, 1997a), to extract relevant social cues (Corrigan *et al.*, 1992), to process contextual factors adequately (Servan-Schreiber *et al.*, 1996) and to identify problems in interpersonal situations (e.g. Donahoe *et al.*, 1990; Bellack *et al.*, 1994).

Second, after the relevant social information has been extracted from a situation, the individual must be able to formulate a goal, generate possible response alternatives for achieving the goal, weigh the benefits and disadvantages of each possible solution and choose the best solution (i.e. *problem-solving* or *cognitive skills*). Although these cognitive operations may occur implicitly, they have an important bearing on the success of any plan, and hence are of direct relevance to an individual's social competence. In addition to the cognitive skills generally subsumed under the rubric of 'problem-solving skills', other cognitive skills can also influence social competence. Abstract thinking is crucial for an individual to grasp a concept related to solving a particular problem or achieving a desired goal. Memory impairment may interfere with selecting appropriate social responses by rendering it more difficult for individuals to learn from past mistakes or to recall critical features of situations. Impairment in cognitive functioning is a core feature of schizophrenia which may limit the ability of patients to identify suitable response options in interpersonal situations (e.g. Bellack *et al.*, 1994).

Third, after social perception and cognitive skills have been used to appraise a situation and formulate a plan of action, behavioral skills or *social skills* are required to implement the plan. Social skills refer to the actual behaviors emitted in interpersonal situations that are necessary to achieve a particular goal, including non-verbal components (e.g. facial expression), paralinguistic skills (e.g. voice volume), verbal content (i.e. the appropriateness of what is said) and interactive balance (e.g. timing of turn-taking). Numerous studies have shown that patients with schizophrenia have poorer social skills than other clinical populations and non-patient controls, and that social skills in schizophrenia are correlated with social functioning (e.g. Argyle, 1981; Bellack *et al.*, 1990a, 1992).

Thus, the tripartite model of social skills proposes that perceptual, cognitive and behavioral skills are necessary for social competence. Considering the central role of cognition in this model, what is the evidence that cognitive impairment is correlated with social perception and social skill? As reviewed below, research provides strong support for the association between cognitive impairment and deficits in both social perception and social skill.

Several studies suggest that social perception is correlated with cognitive functioning in schizophrenia. The associations between cognitive performance and social perception probably reflect the bi-directional nature of their inter-relationship. Certain cognitive functions, such as vigilance, are needed to attend accurately to and perceive relevant situational information, whereas perception may contribute to more complex cognitive operations, such as executive functions. Social knowledge is correlated with a variety of parietal functions (McEvoy *et al.*, 1996). The ability to perceive intentions in indirect speech acts is correlated with IQ in patients with schizophrenia, but not normal controls (Corcoran *et al.*, 1995). Social cue recognition has been found to be correlated with verbal memory and vigilance (Corrigan *et al.*, 1992, 1994a). Deficits in emotion recognition are correlated with generalized perceptual (or neurocognitive) deficits in schizophrenia in numerous studies (e.g. Novic *et al.*, 1984; Feinberg *et al.*, 1986; Archer and Hay, 1992; Kerr and Neale, 1993; Mueser *et al.*, 1996; Salem *et al.*, 1996).

There continues to be debate as to whether cognitive impairment entirely accounts for social perception deficits in schizophrenia (e.g. Novic *et al.*, 1984; Heimberg *et al.*, 1992; Schneider *et al.*, 1995; Bryson *et al.*, 1997). For example, Penn *et al.* (1997) suggest that patients with schizophrenia demonstrate a unique impairment in cognitive operations performed on social stimuli (i.e. social cognition), as compared with other stimuli. Phillips and David (1995) suggested, based on a general cognitive model of Bruce and Young (1986), that delusional misidentification could mediate at least some of the impaired facial processing (and presumably the processing of other social stimuli) observed in schizophrenia. If this speculation is correct, deficits in social perception may be accounted for substantially, but not entirely, by cognitive factors.

Similarly to social perception, there is also abundant evidence that social skills are related to cognitive functioning (Mueser *et al.*, 1991, 1995; Brenner *et al.*, 1992; Bellack *et al.*, 1994; Bowen *et al.*, 1994; Corrigan and Toomey, 1995; Lysaker *et al.*, 1995; Penn *et al.*, 1995a; Ikebuchi *et al.*, 1996). The strength of the association between social skill and cognitive functioning varies considerably from one study to the next, as do the methods for assessing cognitive performance. Furthermore, other variables only partially related to cognitive performance also appear to contribute to social skill, such as negative symptoms (Jackson *et al.*, 1989; Bellack *et al.*, 1990a). Nevertheless, the consistent research showing an association between cognitive functioning and social skill provides ample support for the role of cognition as a mediator of social skill in the tripartite model.

The social skills model addresses the relationships between social skills, social competence and social adjustment (Bellack *et al.*, 1997). *Social competence* is defined as the ability to achieve desired goals. *Social adjustment* refers to an individual's actual attainment of those goals, including the ability to function in different social roles (e.g. worker, parent, spouse, student), to enjoy leisure and recreational activities and to care for oneself (Mueser *et al.*, 1990a). Central to the social skills model is the hypothesis that social competence requires the effective integration of a set of component behaviors or social skills, such as non-verbal behaviors, paralinguistic features and verbal content. A corollary to this hypothesis is that impairments in these component skills contribute to poor social competence, and hence poor social functioning. The social skills model does not assume that social skill is the only determinant of social functioning; a wide range of other factors may also influence social adjustment, such as psychotic symptoms, environmental conditions and mood. However, adequate social skills are postulated to be critical for interpersonal success.

The available research supports this hypothesis. For example, Bellack *et al.* (1990b) showed that social skills, assessed with a role play test, were correlated significantly with independent ratings of social adjustment in the community as well as ratings of social competence based on more naturalistic family problem-solving discussions. Other studies have also found associations between social skill and social functioning (Penn *et al.*, 1995a,b), even when psychopathology has been statistically controlled (Hoffman *et al.*, 1998).

To summarize, the social skills and tripartite models propose that social competence and social functioning require the smooth integration of a complex set of component behaviors. Effective performance of these behaviors (social skills), in turn, requires both accurate social perception and cognitive skills. Research provides strong support for each of these assumptions. In addition, cognitive functioning has been established to be related to both social perception and social skills. The implication of these models is that social functioning is expected to be correlated with cognitive impairment, which is also supported by extensive research (Spaulding, 1978; Allen, 1990; Breier *et al.*, 1991; Jaeger and Douglas, 1992; Dickerson *et al.*, 1996; Penn *et al.*, 1996; Bartels *et al.*, 1997; Brekke *et al.*, 1997; Spaulding *et al.*, 1997). The conclusion that cognitive deficits contribute to functional impairment in schizophrenia is generally supported by Green's (1996) review.

Prediction of outcome from cognitive functioning

Both neurocognitive and social impairments are often present long before the onset of schizophrenia. The strong associations between cognitive and social functioning in schizophrenia, reviewed in the previous section, suggest that these domains are mutually interactive. Research on premorbid adjustment and functioning after the onset of schizophrenia provides some support for this. For example, neurological symptoms during childhood and adolescence are related to poorer social functioning in adulthood in patients with schizophrenia (Jonsson and Nyman, 1991). Conversely, premorbid childhood social behaviors predict adult neurocognitive deficits (Baum and Walker, 1995).

The associations between cognitive and social functioning suggest that cognitive impairment may be an important predictor of outcome in schizophrenia. There are numerous studies reporting that cognitive impairment is prospectively predictive of a worse outcome (e.g. Cancro *et al.*, 1971; Zahn and Carpenter, 1978; Tsuang, 1986; Breier *et al.*, 1991; Goldman *et al.*, 1993; Silverstein *et al.*, 1994). For example, Jaeger and Douglas (1992) reported that performance on the Wisconsin Card Sorting Task (WCST) predicted social functioning 18 months later. Cognitive or neurocognitive impairment, measured in various ways, including disorganization on psychiatric rating scales, IQ, performance on the WCST and early information processing measures, is predictive of later vocational outcomes in schizophrenia, including work and work performance (Solinski *et al.*, 1992; Bryson *et al.*, 1998; Nuechterlein *et al.*, 1998; Mueser *et al.*, in press).

To the extent that cognitive functioning in schizophrenia is related to social and vocational disability, it may also be predictive of psychiatric service utilization. Limited research supports this hypothesis. Wykes *et al.* (Wykes *et al.*, 1990; Wykes and Dunn, 1992; Wykes, 1994) examined predictors of service utilization in patients 3–6 years following the closure of a partial hospital program. A simple response processing measure (reaction time) was a robust predictor of poorer functioning in less restrictive environments, lower capacity for independent living and need for higher levels of supervision.

The relationship between cognitive impairment, service utilization and need for supervision has also been examined in elderly patients with schizophrenia. Residential status (nursing home versus in the community) was found to be strongly related to cognitive impairment in the elderly (Bartels *et al.*, 1997). Furthermore, cognitive deficits in the elderly with schizophrenia was prospectively predictive of both service utilization and treatment costs (S.J.Bartels and K.T.Mueser, unpublished data). Harvey *et al.* (1998) has also reported that geriatric patients with schizophrenia and severe cognitive deficits are more likely to require nursing home care than similar patients with more intact cognitive functioning. Although the question of service utilization and cognitive impairment has not been studied extensively, it may have important implications for the planning and delivery of rehabilitation services for persons with schizophrenia.

Research on cognitive performance and the outcome of schizophrenia points to a significant relationship. Cognitive impairment, both premorbidly and after onset of the illness, is related to a more severe course of the disorder and higher utilization of more costly psychiatric services. However, caution must be exercised before concluding prematurely that cognitive impairment causes a worse outcome, and that some third factor, such as negative symptoms, is not responsible for the association between cognitive impairment and course of illness.

Cognitive functioning, negative symptoms and course of illness

There are several reasons for considering whether the prognostic significance of cognitive impairment in schizophrenia can be explained by negative symptoms such as anhedonia, apathy, social withdrawal, blunted affect, alogia and anergia. First, there is a conceptual overlap between the constructs, with certain symptoms or deficits considered both negative symptoms and cognitive impairment. For example, impairment in attention and slowness or paucity of cognitive processing (alogia) are included on the Scale for the Assessment of Negative Symptoms (SANS; Andreasen, 1984). Factor analysis of the SANS suggests that negative symptoms can be divided into three correlated dimensions, including apathy–anhedonia, blunting and alogia–inattention (Sayers et al., 1996). Furthermore, when considered together, only the apathy–anhedonia dimension was related to premorbid functioning, concurrent social functioning and future relapse in a dosage reduction study (Sayers et al., 1996). Thus, negative symptoms are not a unitary dimension of psychopathology; some dimensions overlap more clearly with cognitive functioning than others, and differential associations may be present between dimensions of negative symptoms and other domains of functioning.

Second, negative symptoms tend to be correlated moderately with the severity of cognitive deficits (McCreadie et al., 1994; Roy and DeVriendt, 1994; Davidson and McGlashan, 1997). Third, as for cognitive impairment, negative symptoms are relatively stable over time (McGlashan and Fenton, 1992; Eaton et al., 1995; Husted et al., 1995), are associated with a more severe psychopathology (Robins and Guze, 1970; Keefe et al., 1987; Salokangas et al., 1989; Bailer et al., 1996) and are associated with worse premorbid functioning and a worse outcome (Pogue-Geile, 1989; Mueser et al., 1990a; Gupta et al., 1995; Larsen et al., 1996).

Fourth, similarly to cognitive functioning, the severity of negative symptoms is correlated with both social perception performance (Gaebel and Wölwer, 1992; Schneider et al., 1995; Mueser et al., 1996) and social skill (Jackson et al., 1989; Bellack et al., 1990a), which, according to the social skill model, may contribute to poorer social competence and adjustment. Fifth, consistent with the social skill model, negative symptoms are associated with impairment in social functioning (Glynn et al., 1992; Brekke et al., 1994; Palacios-Araus et al., 1995). Thus, like poor cognitive functioning, negative symptoms are related to social dysfunction in schizophrenia and portend a worse course of illness. This raises the question of whether the importance of cognitive functioning in predicting outcome is due to its relationship with negative symptoms.

Despite the apparent overlap in constructs, it is unlikely that the associations between cognitive functioning, social adjustment and outcome are entirely accounted for by the severity of negative symptoms. Not all studies report that negative symptoms are more predictive of functioning than cognitive impairment; some studies find that cognitive impairment is more predictive of outcome than negative symptoms, while others report that both are independently predictive (e.g. Breier *et al.*, 1991; Goldman *et al.*, 1993; Palacios-Araus *et al.*, 1995; Penn *et al.*, 1995a; Hoffman *et al.*, 1998). Furthermore, cognitive impairment and negative symptoms may be associated differentially with dimensions of social functioning. For example, Liddle (1987) found that negative symptoms were related to poor social relationships and lack of recreational activities, whereas cognitive (disorganization) symptoms were related to poor hygiene and grooming, and impersistence at work.

The term 'cognitive functioning' subsumes a wide variety of different cognitive abilities and processes, ranging from general intellectual functioning and reaction time to arousal, early information processing, attention, memory and executive functions. Apart from evidence suggesting differential associations between negative symptoms and cognitive functioning, different areas of cognitive impairment appear to be related to different areas of social functioning. For example, Ikebuchi *et al.* (1996) reported that the amplitude and latency of N1 brain waves, which are related to sensory function and selective attention, are associated with social skills. On the other hand, Brekke *et al.* (1997) found that more traditional neuropsychological measures bore no relationship to social functioning, but were associated with employment and independent living which, in turn, showed no relationship to arousal and orienting responses. This evidence suggests that social interaction may depend more upon fundamental attentional processes, such as the capacity to orient and reorient to changing stimuli, whereas success in employment and independent living may rely more on the mastery of instrumental tasks requiring neurocognitive skills.

A final argument for the importance of cognitive functioning to social adjustment concerns evidence indicating that neurocognitive deficits, but not negative symptoms, are related to the acquisition of social skills in skills training (Green, 1996; see next section). To the extent that learning appropriate social behavior is more dependent upon intact cognitive processing abilities than the absence of negative symptoms, cognitive impairment would appear to be a determinant of social functioning in patients participating in skills training (and perhaps other?) programs. Thus, the available research suggests that cognitive deficits contribute to social functioning independently of negative symptoms. However, the failure to measure negative symptoms in some studies may result in an overestimate of the contribution of cognitive impairment to social adjustment and outcome.

The prediction of rehabilitation outcome

The prominence of cognitive impairment in schizophrenia and its associations with negative symptoms, social functioning and outcome of the illness suggest that it may play an important role in determining the success of psychosocial rehabilitation. Research has supported the efficacy of several different psychosocial treatment models for schizophrenia, including social skills training for social dysfunction, family psychoeducation for relapse prevention and support for obtaining competitive employment (Mueser *et al.*, 1997b). More recently, cognitive therapy for psychosis has also been found to improve the outcome of schizophrenia (Haddock *et al.*, 1998).

The possible role of cognitive factors in mediating response to rehabilitation may depend on the type of intervention in question. Social skills training is based on the assumption that systematically teaching the component skills necessary for socially competent behavior will result in improved social functioning (Bellack *et al.*, 1997). As the learning of social skills presumably is a prerequisite to improvements in social skills training, cognitive impairment may be hypothesized to limit either the rate of improvement or the final attainment of targeted behaviors (Green, 1996; Silverstein *et al.*, 1998). The role of cognitive impairment as a mediator of response to other rehabilitation methods is less clear. Family psychoeducation is aimed at lowering stressful levels of family tension (i.e. 'expressed emotion'), improving the ability of the family to monitor the course of the illness and achieve goals, and promoting adherence to recommended treatments (Mueser and Glynn, 1998). Cognitive impairment may limit the substantive contributions of the patient to family sessions, but it is uncertain whether this results in less benefit from family intervention.

Supported employment interventions de-emphasize traditional prevocational assessment and sheltered employment in favor of rapid job search and acquisition that is guided by patients' preferences, and the provision of ongoing job support after competitive work has been obtained in order to promote job retention or transition to another job (Bond *et al.*, 1997). As supported employment is not primarily a learning-oriented rehabilitation strategy (although learning may occur in an incidental fashion), the effect of cognitive impairment on program success is uncertain. It may be speculated, based on evidence that cognitive functioning contributes to vocational success in the general population (Herrnstein and Murray, 1994), that a minimal level of effective cognitive functioning is necessary in order to succeed in a supported employment program for schizophrenia.

Cognitive therapy focuses on helping patients to examine the evidence supporting the psychotic beliefs in order to determine whether alternative conceptualizations would be more suitable (Fowler *et al.*, 1995; Chadwick *et al.*, 1996). Although cognitive restructuring (i.e. teaching patients how to evaluate the support for their beliefs) can be taught as a skill for the management of negative emotions, such as in applications to depression (Beck *et al.* 1979), post-traumatic stress disorder (Foa and Rothbaum, 1997) and borderline personality disorder (Linehan, 1993), cognitive therapy in schizophrenia is used to help patients challenge the empirical basis for their delusions and hallucinations, with less effort focused on teaching a specific self-regulatory skill. Learning may be less critical to the success of cognitive therapy than social skills training, but other cognitive abilities may be even more important, such as reasoning, memory and capacity for flexible thinking.

Thus, cognitive impairment could interfere with the ability to benefit from psychosocial treatment, especially interventions based on learning such as social skills training. Despite the intuitive appeal of this hypothesis, only limited research has evaluated the relationship between cognitive functioning and response to rehabilitation in schizophrenia. We review research on cognitive impairment and the effects of vocational rehabilitation, cognitive therapy and social skills training below.

Mueser *et al.* (1997c) failed to find an association between disorganization on the Brief Psychiatric Rating Scale (Overall and Gorham, 1962; Woerner *et al.*, 1988) and competitive employment outcomes over 18 months in a mixed sample (40% schizophrenia spectrum) of patients participating in a study of supported employment compared with group skills training. In contrast, two other studies using different cognitive measures and studying different approaches to vocational rehabilitation reported significant associations. Hoffman and Kupper (1997) reported that conceptual disorganization on the Positive and Negative Syndrome Scale (Kay *et al.*, 1987) predicted work outcome in patients with schizophrenia over 18 months in a traditional vocational rehabilitation program including skills training, sheltered work, job coaches and competitive work. Lysaker (Lysaker and Bell, 1995; Lysaker *et al.*, 1995), in a study of a work program for schizophrenia including paid work and group support, reported that performance on the WCST at baseline predicted improvements in both social skill and work performance at 12 weeks.

Only one study has examined whether cognitive functioning is predictive of the success of cognitive therapy for schizophrenia. Garety *et al.* (1997) reported that better performance on the Cognitive Estimates Test (Shallice and Evans, 1978) predicted more improvement in psychotic symptoms after 9 months of cognitive therapy. However, improvement was unrelated to verbal fluency, intelligence or reasoning. Memory and executive functions were not assessed.

Several studies have evaluated whether cognitive deficits mediate the acquisition of social skills in social skills training. Two studies examined the associations between cognitive functioning and social skills following exposure to social skills training (Bowen *et al.*, 1994; Corrigan *et al.*, 1994b), with both studies reporting that vigilance and verbal memory correlated with post-training levels of social skill. These studies are consistent with the hypothesis that cognitive factors are related to social skills acquisition. However, neither study measured pretreatment social skills, so it remains unclear whether cognitive functioning actually predicted the learning of new skills, rather than just pretreatment levels of social skill.

Four studies have examined the relationship between cognitive functioning and the acquisition of social skills using pre- and post-treatment assessments of social skill. Mueser *et al.* (1991) reported that memory (especially verbal memory) predicted both the acquisition of social skills in 30 acute inpatients with schizophrenia or schizoaffective disorder over a 2 week training period and the retention of skills 1 month later. Kern *et al.* (1992), in a study of social skills training with 17 in-patients with chronic schizophrenia over 8 months, found that vigilance predicted skill acquisition; other cognitive measures, including early information processing (backward masking), memory, distractibility, executive functions (WCST performance), perceptual organization or intelligence, were not related to learning skills, although auditory memory and distraction were related to 'on-task behavior' during the social skills training.

Silverstein *et al.* (1998) examined the prediction of skill acquisition in 21 in-patients with chronic schizophrenia participating in UCLA social skills training modules using a comprehensive battery of cognitive assessments, including perceptual organization, reaction time, visual information processing, attention, memory, executive functions and intelligence.

Auditory attention and verbal memory skills were most predictive of learning new social skills. Finally, in 26 in-patients with chronic schizophrenia, Silverstein *et al.* (1998) evaluated whether cognitive functioning was predictive of social skills acquisition in a brief learning test designed to measure patients' responsiveness to social skills training procedures, the UCLA Micro-Module Learning Test (Wallace, 1997; cited by Silverstein *et al.*, 1998). Findings indicated that responsiveness to social skills training procedures was predicted by pretreatment verbal memory, verbal fluency and inferential reasoning ability.

In summary, relatively little research has evaluated the utility of cognitive functioning as a predictor of vocational rehabilitation (Lysaker and Bell, 1995; Hoffman and Kupper, 1997; Mueser *et al.*, 1997c) or cognitive therapy (Garety *et al.*, 1997), although the available evidence suggests that cognitive impairment may limit response to these interventions. More research has examined the associations between cognitive functioning and response to social skills training (Mueser *et al.*, 1991; Kern *et al.*, 1992; Silverstein *et al.*, 1998), with a convergence of findings indicating that verbal memory was related to skill acquisition in three of the four studies. These findings provide moderately strong evidence that memory deficits may act as a rate-limiting factor in social skills training. The evidence is especially compelling considering the different methods used to assess memory across the studies, the different characteristics of the patients included in the studies (acute versus chronic schizophrenia), the different skills training interventions examined and the different treatment and follow-up periods, ranging from less than a day to over 6 months. The role of specific cognitive abilities, such as vigilance and executive functions, in mediating response to skills training is less certain due to the variability of different cognitive measures employed across the studies.

Implications of cognitive deficits for social rehabilitation

Considering the progress that has been achieved in the development and validation of rehabilitation methods for persons with schizophrenia and other severe mental disorders (Mueser *et al.*, 1997b), and the prominence of cognitive deficits in schizophrenia, it is remarkable that so few studies have examined whether these deficits impede response to psychosocial treatment. Therefore, there is a need to include measures of cognitive functioning, both symptom-based measures and neuropsychological measures, in longitudinal studies of psychiatric rehabilitation. Analyses that focus on behavior *change*, rather than the prediction of outcome at the end of treatment irrespective of pretreatment level of functioning, are of primary interest in determining whether cognitive factors limit clinical response to an intervention. Furthermore, research is needed to evaluate both theoretical constructs hypothesized to mediate outcome, such as social skills, and the domains of functioning that are the target of intervention, such as social functioning, in order to understand how cognitive functioning interacts with the process of rehabilitation. To date, research on the relationship between cognitive impairment and response to social skills training has focused on the evaluation of social skill, but not on improvement in social functioning. Therefore, the evidence suggesting that cognitive impairment limits the rate of improvement in social skills training is indirect. There is a need for research that directly examines the relationship between cognitive functioning and improved social functioning during social skills training.

In addition to the evaluation of cognitive functioning as a predictor of response to rehabilitation, future research needs to consider the associations between cognitive impairment and service utilization and costs. If cognitive deficits are associated with a more severe course of illness, the utilization of more costly services would be expected in patients with greater impairments. The determination of how cognitive impairment influences the utilization of services could lead to the development or refinement of interventions designed to manage schizophrenia more cost-effectively in these patients and to make progress towards rehabilitation goals.

Another area in need of research is the issue of whether pharmacological interventions that improve cognitive impairment in schizophrenia (Green *et al.*, 1997; Andersson *et al.*, 1998) also confer benefits in social functioning. It is possible that improved cognitive functioning will result automatically in concomitant improvements in social and vocational adjustment. For example, increased ability to focus attention may permit patients to utilize skills already in their behavioral repertoires in order to attain psychosocial goals. Alternatively, decreased distractibility and improved memory may enable patients with both premorbid and morbid social skill deficits to acquire new skills spontaneously through observation of available role models. On the other hand, it is also possible that enhanced cognitive functioning will improve the *capacity* of patients to respond to psychosocial rehabilitation, but that spontaneous improvements in social outcomes will not occur in most patients without the benefit of systematic programing. For example, Rosenheck *et al.* (1998) has reported that clozapine augments response to psychosocial rehabilitation in persons with severe and persistent mental illness, although the mechanism of this effect is unknown.

Although more effective medications may ameliorate some of the cognitive deficits of schizophrenia, the association between premorbid cognitive impairment and subsequent development of schizophrenia (e.g. Mirsky *et al.*, 1995) suggests that at least some of these deficits are long-standing and are unlikely to remit completely, even with optimal pharmacotherapy. Furthermore, in the absence of even more effective neuroleptics, cognitive deficits will probably continue to be an important feature of schizophrenia for some time to come. Considering the evidence suggesting that cognitive impairment both contributes to poor social functioning and limits response to psychosocial treatment, clinical interventions are needed either to rehabilitate cognitive functions or to teach compensatory strategies for helping patients to achieve goals despite their deficits.

Cognitive rehabilitation for persons with schizophrenia has been a topic of much debate (e.g. Penn, 1991; Bellack, 1992; Brenner *et al.*, 1992; Hogarty and Flesher, 1992; Liberman and Green, 1992; Spaulding, 1992). Although progress has been slow, some positive findings have been reported (Olbrich and Lutz, 1990; Spaulding *et al.*, 1999; Wykes *et al.*, 1999). Less attention has been paid to the development of strategies to help patients manage cognitive deficits in areas such as attention and memory. Interestingly, both patients with schizophrenia and their relatives report successfully using coping strategies to manage problems with patients' inattention (Mueser *et al.*, 1997d). However, little research has attempted systematically to teach and evaluate self-management strategies for the management of cognitive problems in schizophrenia (Velligan *et al.*, 1996).

A final area in need of further investigation concerns gender differences. Data from three independent samples of patients with schizophrenia indicate that social skills are related to cognitive impairment in women but not men (Mueser *et al.*, 1995; Penn *et al.*, 1996). The reasons for this are unclear and the studies reporting these associations are limited to in-patient samples. However, it raises the question of whether the contribution of cognitive impairment to poor social functioning differs as a function of gender. Women with schizophrenia have a more benign course of illness, including better premorbid social functioning, fewer hospitalizations, and better social and occupational functioning than men (Haas and Garratt, 1998). Furthermore, men with schizophrenia tend to have worse negative symptoms (Goldstein and Link, 1988; Shtasel *et al.*, 1992), worse social skills (Mueser and Bellack, 1998) and are more likely to benefit from social skills training (Mueser *et al.*, 1990b; Smith *et al.*, 1997; Schaub *et al.*, 1998). In recent years, there has been debate as to whether impaired social functioning in schizophrenia (i.e. 'disorders of relating') is an independent (or semi-independent) dimension of psychopathology not fully explained by negative symptoms or cognitive impairment (Strauss and Carpenter, 1974; Dworkin, 1990; Peralta *et al.*, 1994). If the determinants of social functioning differ between men and women, different treatments may be necessary in order to improve long-term outcome. Future research examining the predictive utility of cognitive impairment in schizophrenia, and the interactions between cognitive functioning and response to rehabilitation, needs to explore whether the observed relationships vary by gender.

In summary, the role of cognitive impairment as a predictor of social functioning and outcome in schizophrenia has been well established. Cognitive impairment is associated with social perception, social skill, social functioning, the course of illness and response to psychosocial treatment. However, cognitive functioning is also correlated with the severity of negative symptoms, which is associated independently with social skill and social functioning. The weight of evidence supporting a critical role for cognitive impairment in determining the outcome of schizophrenia points to the need for work that addresses how to better treat these deficits, including either cognitive remediation or compensatory strategies. At the same time, research indicates that not all impairments in social functioning can be attributed to cognitive deficits, suggesting that improved cognitive functioning (resulting from either pharmacological or psychosocial treatment) will not obviate the need for other interventions aimed at improving social adjustment. The combination of treatments that target both cognitive and social dimensions of schizophrenia appears to have the greatest potential for improving the course of this illness.

References

Allen, H. (1990) Cognitive processing and its relationship to symptoms and social functioning in schizophrenia. *British Journal of Psychiatry*, **156**, 201–203.

American Psychiatric Association (1994) *Diagnostic and Statistical Manual of Mental Disorders (Fourth Edition) (DSM-IV)*. American Psychiatric Association, Washington, DC.

Andersson, C., Chakos, M., Mailman, R. and Lieberman, J. (1998) Emerging roles for novel antipsychotic medications in the treatment of schizophrenia. *The Psychiatric Clinics of North America*, **21**, 151–179.

Andreasen, N.C. (1984) *Scale for the Assessment of Negative Symptoms (SANS)*. University of Iowa, Iowa City.

Archer, J. and Hay, D.C. (1992) Face processing in psychiatric conditions. *British Journal of Clinical Psychology*, **31**, 45–61.

Argyle, M.F. (1981) The contribution of social interaction research to social skills training. In: Wine, J.D. and Srnnye, M.D. (eds), *Social Competence*. Guilford, New York, pp. 261–286.

Bailer, J., Brauer, W. and Rey, E.R. (1996) Premorbid adjustment as predictor of outcome in schizophrenia: results of a prospective study. *Acta Psychiatrica Scandinavica*, **93**, 368–377.

Bartels, S.J., Mueser, K.T. and Miles, K.M. (1997) A comparative study of elderly patients with schizophrenia and bipolar disorder in nursing homes and the community. *Schizophrenia Research*, **27**, 181–190.

Baum, K.M. and Walker E.F. (1995) Childhood behavioral precursors of adult symptom dimensions in schizophrenia. *Schizophrenia Research*, **16**, 111–120.

Beck, A.T., Rush, A.J,. Shaw, B.F. and Emery G. (1979) *Cognitive Therapy of Depression*. Guilford, New York.

Bellack, A.S. (1992) Cognitive rehabilitation for schizophrenia: is it possible? Is it necessary? *Schizophrenia Bulletin*, **18**, 43–50.

Bellack, A.S., Morrison, R.L., Wixted, J.T. and Mueser, K.T. (1990a) An analysis of social competence in schizophrenia. *British Journal of Psychiatry*, **156**, 809–818.

Bellack, A.S., Morrison, R.L., Mueser, K.T., Wade, J.H. and Sayers, S.L. (1990b) Role play for assessing the social competence of psychiatric patients. *Psychological Assessment*, **2**, 248–255.

Bellack, A.S., Mueser, K.T., Wade, J.H., Sayers, S.L. and Morrison, R.L. (1992) The ability of schizophrenics to perceive and cope with negative affect. *British Journal of Psychiatry*, **160**, 473–480.

Bellack, A.S., Sayers, M., Mueser, K.T. and Bennett, M. (1994) An evaluation of social problem solving in schizophrenia. *Journal of Abnormal Psychology*, **103**, 371–378.

Bellack, A.S., Mueser, K.T., Gingerich, S. and Agresta, J. (1997) *Social Skills Training for Schizophrenia: A Step-by-Step Guide*. Guilford, New York.

Bond, G.R., Drake, R.E., Mueser, K.T. and Becker, D.R. (1997) An update on supported employment for people with severe mental illness. *Psychiatric Services*, **48**, 335–346.

Bowen, L., Wallace, C.J., Glynn, S.M., Nuechterlein, K.H., Lutzker, J.R. and Kuehnel, T.G. (1994) Schizophrenic individuals' cognitive functioning and performance in interpersonal interactions and skills training procedures. *Journal of Psychiatric Research*, **28**, 289–301.

Breier, A., Schreiber, J.L., Dyer, J. and Pickar, D. (1991) National Institute of Mental Health longitudinal study of chronic schizophrenia: prognosis and predictors of outcome. *Archives of General Psychiatry*, **48**, 239–246.

Brekke, J.S., Debonis, J.A. and Graham, J.W. (1994) A latent structure analysis of the positive and negative symptoms in schizophrenia. *Comprehensive Psychiatry*, **35**, 252–259.

Brekke, J.S., Raine, A., Ansel, M., Lencz, T. and Bird, L. (1997) Neuropsychological and psychophysiological correlates of psychosocial functioning in schizophrenia. *Schizophrenia Bulletin*, **23**, 19–28.

Brenner, H.D., Hodel, B., Roder, V. and Corrigan, P. (1992) Treatment of cognitive dysfunctions and behavioral deficits in schizophrenia. *Schizophrenia Bulletin*, **18**, 21–26.

Bruce, V. and Young, A.W. (1986) Understanding face recognition. *British Journal of Psychology*, **77**, 305–327.

Bryson, G., Bell, M. and Lysaker, P. (1997) Affect recognition in schizophrenia: a function of global impairment or a specific cognitive deficit? *Psychiatric Research*, **71**, 105–114.

Bryson, G., Bell, M.D., Kaplan, E. and Greig, T. (1998) The functional consequences of memory impairments on initial work performance in people with schizophrenia. *Journal of Nervous and Mental Disease*, **186**, 610–615.

Cancro, R., Sutton, S., Kerr, J. and Sugarman, A. (1971) Reaction time and prognosis in acute schizophrenia. *Journal of Nervous and Mental Disease*, **151**, 351–359.

Chadwick, P., Birchwood, M. and Trower, P. (1996) *Cognitive Therapy for Delusions, Voices and Paranoia*. John Wiley & Sons, Chichester, UK.

Corcoran, R., Mercer, G. and Frith, C.D. (1995) Schizophrenia, symptomatology and social inference: investigating 'theory of mind' in people with schizophrenia. *Schizophrenia Research*, **17**, 5–13.

Corrigan, P.W. and Toomey, R. (1995) Interpersonal problem-solving and information-processing in schizophrenia. *Schizophrenia Bulletin*, **21**, 395–403.

Corrigan, P.W., Wallace, C.J. and Green, M.F. (1992) Deficits in social schemata in schizophrenia. *Schizophrenia Research*, **8**, 129–135.

Corrigan, P.W., Green, M.F. and Toomey, R. (1994a) Cognitive correlates to social cue perception in schizophrenia. *Psychiatry Research*, **53**, 141–151.

Corrigan, P.W., Wallace, C.J., Schade, M.L. and Green, M.F. (1994b) Learning medication self-management skills in schizophrenia: relationships with cognitive deficits and psychiatric symptoms. *Behavior Therapy*, **25**, 5–15.

Davidson, L. and McGlashan, T.H. (1997) The varied outcomes of schizophrenia. *Canadian Journal of Psychiatry—Revue Canadienne de Psychiatrie*, **42**, 34–43.

Dickerson, F., Boronow, J.J., Tringel, N. and Parente, F. (1996) Neurocognitive deficits and social functioning in outpatients with schizophrenia. *Schizophrenia Research*, **21**, 75–83.

Donahoe, C.P., Carter, M.J., Bloem, W.D., Hirsch, G.L., Laasi, N. and Wallace, C.J. (1990) Assessment of interpersonal problem-solving skills. *Psychiatry*, **53**, 329–339.

Dworkin, R.H. (1990) Patterns of sex differences in negative symptoms and social functioning consistent with separate dimensions of schizophrenic psychopathology. *American Journal of Psychiatry*, **147**, 347–349.

Eaton, W.W., Thara, R., Federman, B., Melton, B. and Liang, K. (1995) Structure and course of positive and negative symptoms in schizophrenia. *Archives of General Psychiatry*, **52**, 127–134.

Feinberg, T.E., Rifkin, A., Schaffer, C. and Walker, E. (1986) Facial discrimination and emotional recognition in schizophrenia and affective disorders. *Archives of General Psychiatry*, **43**, 276–9.

Foa, E.B. and Rothbaum, B.O. (1997) *Treating the Trauma of Rape: Cognitive-Behavioral Therapy for PTSD*. Guilford, New York.

Fowler, D., Garety, P. and Kuipers, E. (1995) *Cognitive Behaviour Therapy for Psychosis: Theory and Practice*. John Wiley & Sons, Chichester, UK.

Gaebel, W. and Wölwer, W. (1992) Facial expression and emotional face recognition in schizophrenia and depression. *European Archives of Psychiatry and Clinical Neuroscience*, **242**, 46–52.

Garety, P., Fowler, D., Kuipers, E., Freeman, D., Dunn, G., Bebbington, P., Hadley, C. and Jones, S. (1997) London–East Anglia randomised controlled trial of cognitive–behavioral therapy for psychosis. *British Journal of Psychiatry*, **171**, 420–426.

Glynn, S.M., Randolph, E.M., Eth, S., Paz, G.G., Leong, G.B., Shaner, A.L. and VanVort, W. (1992) Schizophrenic symptoms, work adjustment, and behavioral family therapy. *Rehabilitation Psychology*, **37**, 323–338.

Goldman, R.S., Axelrod, B.N., Tandon, R., Ribeiro, S.C.M., Craig, K. and Berent, S. (1993) Neuropsychological prediction of treatment efficacy and one-year outcome in schizophrenia. *Psychopathology*, **26**, 122–126.

Goldstein, J.M. and Link, B.G. (1988) Gender and the expression of schizophrenia. *Journal of Psychiatric Research*, **22**, 141–155.

Green, M.F. (1996) What are the functional consequences of neurocognitive deficits in schizophrenia? *American Journal of Psychiatry*, **153**, 321–330.

Green, M.F., Marshall, B.D., Wirshing, W.C., Ames, Marder, S.R., McGurk, S., Kern, R.S. and Mintz, J. (1997) Does risperidone improve verbal working memory in treatment-resistant schizophrenia? *American Journal of Psychiatry*, **154**, 799–804.

Gupta, S., Rajaprabhakaran, R., Arndt, S., Flaum, M. and Andreasen, N.C. (1995) Premorbid adjustment as a predictor of phenomenological and neurobiological indices in schizophrenia. *Schizophrenia Research*, **16**, 189–197.

Haas, G.L. and Garrett, L.S. (1998) Gender differences in social functioning. In: Mueser, K.T. and Tarrier, N. (eds), *Handbook of Social Functioning in Schizophrenia*. Allyn & Bacon, Boston, pp. 149–180.

Haddock, G., Tarrier, N., Spaulding, W., Yusupoff, L., Kinney, C. and McCarthy, E. (1998) Individual cognitive-behavior therapy in the treatment of hallucinations and delusions: a review. *Clinical Psychology Review*, **18**, 821–838.

Harrison, G., Croudace, T., Mason, P., Glazebrook, C. and Medley, I. (1996) Predicting the long-term outcome of schizophrenia. *Psychological Medicine*, **26**, 697–705.

Harvey, P.D., Howanitz, E., Parrella, M., White, L., Davidson, M., Mohs, R.C., Hoblyn, J. and Davis, K.L. (1998) Symptoms, cognitive functioning, and adaptive skills in geriatric patients with lifelong schizophrenia: a comparison across treatment sites. *American Journal of Psychiatry*, **155**, 1080–1086.

Heimberg, C., Gur, R.E., Erwin, R.J., Shtasel, D.L. and Gur, R.C. (1992) Facial emotion discrimination: III. Behavioral findings in schizophrenia. *Psychiatry Research*, **42**, 253–265.

Herrnstein, R.J. and Murray, C. (1994) *The Bell Curve: Intelligence and Class Structure in American Life*. Free Press, New York.

Hoffman, H. and Kupper, Z. (1997) Relationships between social competence, psychopathology and work performance and their predictive value for vocational rehabilitation of schizophrenic outpatients. *Schizophrenia Research*, **23**, 69–79.

Hoffman, H., Kupper, Z. and Kunz, B. (1998) Predicting schizophrenic outpatients' behavior by symtomatology and social skills. *Journal of Nervous and Mental Disease*, **186**, 214–222.

Hogarty, G.E. and Flesher, S. (1992) Cognitive remediation in schizophrenia: proceed . . . with caution! *Schizophrenia Bulletin*, **18**, 51–57.

Husted, J.A., Beiser, M. and Iacono, W.G. (1995) Negative symptoms in the course of first-episode affective psychosis. *Psychiatry Research*, **56**, 145–154.

Ikebuchi, E., Nakagome, K., Tugawa, R., Asada, Y., Mori, K., Takahashi, N., Takazawa, S., Ichikawa, I. and Akaho, R. (1996) What influences social skills in patients with schizophrenia? Preliminary study using the role play test, WAIS-R and event-related potential. *Schizophrenia Research*, **22**, 143–150.

Jackson, H.J., Minas, I.H., Burgess, P.M., Joshua, S.D., Charisiou, J. and Campbell, I.M. (1989) Is social skills performance a correlate of schizophrenia subtypes? *Schizophrenia Research*, **2**, 301–309.

Jaeger, J. and Douglas, E. (1992) Neuropsychiatric rehabilitation for persistent mental illness. *Psychiatric Quarterly*, **63**, 71–94.

Jonsson, H. and Nyman, A.K. (1991) Predicting long-term outcome in schizophrenia. *Acta Psychiatrica Scandinavica*, **83**, 342–346.

Kay, S.R., Fiszbein, A. and Opler, L.A. (1987) The Positive and Negative Syndrome Scale (PANSS) for schizophrenia. *Schizophrenia Bulletin*, **13**, 261–276

Keefe, R.S., Mohs, R.C., Losonczy, M.F., Davidson, M., Silverman, J.M., Kendler, K.S., Horvath, T.B., Nora, R. and Davis, K.L. (1987) Characteristics of very poor outcome schizophrenia. *American Journal of Psychiatry*, **144**, 889–895.

Kern, R.S., Green, M.F. and Satz, P. (1992) Neuropsychological predictors of skills training for chronic psychiatric patients. *Psychiatry Research*, **43**, 223–230.

Kerr, S.L. and Neale, J.M. (1993) Emotion perception in schizophrenia: specific deficit or further evidence of generalized poor performance? *Journal of Abnormal Psychology*, **102**, 312–318.

Langfeldt, G. (1937) *The Prognosis in Schizophrenia and Factors Influencing the Course of the Disease*. Munksgaard, Copenhagen.

Larsen, T.K., McGlashan, T.H., Johannessen, J.O. and Vibe-Hansen, L. (1996) First-episode schizophrenia: II. Premorbid patterns by gender. *Schizophrenia Bulletin*, **22**, 257–269.

Liberman, R.P. and Green, M.F. (1992) Whither cognitive-behavioral therapy for schizophrenia? *Schizophrenia Bulletin*, **18**, 27–35.

Liberman, R.P., Mueser, K.T., Wallace, C.J., Jacobs, H.E., Eckman, T. and Massel, H.K. (1986) Training skills in the psychiatrically disabled: learning coping and competence. *Schizophrenia Bulletin*, **12**, 631–647.

Liddle, P.F. (1987) The symptoms of chronic schizophrenia: a re-examination of the positive–negative dichotomy. *British Journal of Psychiatry*, **151**, 145–151.

Linehan, M.M. (1993) *Cognitive-Behavioral Treatment of Borderline Personality Disorder*. Guilford Press, New York.

Lysaker, P. and Bell, M. (1995) Work rehabilitation and improvements in insight in schizophrenia. *Journal of Nervous and Mental Disease*, **183**, 103–107.

Lysaker, P.H., Bell, M.D., Zito, W.S. and Bioty, S.M. (1995) Social skills at work: deficits and predictors of improvement in schizophrenia. *Journal of Nervous and Mental Disease*, **183**, 688–692.

MacEwan, T.H. and Athawes, R.W.B. (1997) The Nithsdale Schizophrenia Surveys. XV.

Social adjustment in schizophrenia: associations with gender, symptoms and childhood antecedents. *Acta Psychiatrica Scandinavica*, **95**, 254–258.

McCreadie, R.G., Connolly, M.A., Williamson, D.J., Athawes, R.W. and Tilak-Singh, D. (1994) The Nithsdale Schizophrenia Surveys. XII. 'Neurodevelopmental' schizophrenia: a search for clinical correlates and putative aetiological factors. *British Journal of Psychiatry*, **165**, 340–346.

McEvoy, J.P., Hartman, M., Gottlieb, D., Godwin, S., Apperson, L.J. and Wilson, W. (1996) Common sense, insight, and neuropsychological test performance in schizophrenia patients. *Schizophrenia Bulletin*, **22**, 635–641.

McFall, R.M. (1982) A review and reformulation of the concept of social skills. *Behavioral Assessment*, **4**, 1–33.

McGlashan, T.H. and Fenton, W.S. (1992) The positive–negative distinction in schizophrenia. Review of natural history validators. *Archives of General Psychiatry*, **49**, 63–72.

Mirsky, A.F., Ingraham, L.J. and Kugelmass, S. (1995) Neuropsychological assessment of attention and its pathology in the Israeli cohort. *Schizophrenia Bulletin*, **21**, 193–204.

Morrison, R.L. and Bellack, A.S. (1981) The role of social perception in social skill. *Behavior Therapy*, **12**, 69–79.

Morrison, R.L., Bellack, A.S. and Mueser, K.T. (1988) Facial affect recognition deficits and schizophrenia. *Schizophrenia Bulletin*, **14**, 67–83.

Mueser, K.T. and Bellack, A.S. (1998) Social skills and social functioning. In: Mueser, K.T. and Tarrier, N. (eds), *Handbook of Social Functioning in Schizophrenia*. Allyn & Bacon, Needham Heights, MA, pp. 79–96.

Mueser, K.T. and Glynn, S.M. (1998) Family intervention for schizophrenia. In: Dobson, K.S. and Craig, K.D. (eds), *Empirically Supported Therapies: Best Practice in Professional Psychology*. Sage Publications, Thousand Oaks, CA, pp. 157–186.

Mueser, K.T., Bellack, A.S., Morrison, R.L. and Wixted, J.T. (1990a) Social competence in schizophrenia: premorbid adjustment, social skill, and domains of functioning. *Journal of Psychiatric Research*, **24**, 51–63.

Mueser, K.T., Levine, S., Bellack, A.S., Douglas, M.S. and Brady, E.U. (1990b) Social skills training for acute psychiatric patients. *Hospital and Community Psychiatry*, **41**, 1249–1251.

Mueser, K.T., Bellack, A.S., Douglas, M.S. and Wade, J.H. (1991) Prediction of social skill acquisition in schizophrenic and major affective disorder patients from memory and symptomatology. *Psychiatry Research*, **37**, 281–296.

Mueser, K.T., Blanchard, J.J. and Bellack, A.S. (1995) Memory and social skill in schizophrenia: the role of gender. *Psychiatry Research*, **57**, 141–153.

Mueser, K.T., Doonan, R., Penn, D.L., Blanchard, J.J., Bellack, A.S., Nishith, P. and deLeon, J. (1996) Emotion recognition and social competence in chronic schizophrenia. *Journal of Abnormal Psychology*, **105**, 271–275.

Mueser, K.T., Penn, D.L., Blanchard, J.J. and Bellack, A.S. (1997a) Affect recognition in schizophrenia: a synthesis of findings across three studies. *Psychiatry: Interpersonal and Biological Processes*, **60**, 301–308.

Mueser, K.T., Drake, R.E. and Bond, G.R. (1997b) Recent advances in psychiatric rehabilitation for patients with severe mental illness. *Harvard Review of Psychiatry*, **5**, 123–137.

Mueser, K.T., Becker, D.R., Torrey, W.C., Xie, H., Bond, G.R., Drake, R.E. and Dain, B.J. (1997c) Work and nonvocational domains of functioning in persons with severe mental illness: a longitudinal analysis. *Journal of Nervous and Mental Disease*, **185**, 418–428.

Mueser, K.T., Valentiner, D.P. and Agresta, J. (1997d) Coping with negative symptoms of schizophrenia: patient and family perspectives. *Schizophrenia Bulletin*, **23**, 329–339.

Mueser, K.T., Salyers, M. and Mueser, P.R. A prospective analysis of work in schizophrenia. (in press). *Schizophrenia Bulletin*.

Novic, J., Luchins, D.J. and Perline, R. (1984) Facial affect recognition in schizophrenia: is there a differential deficit? *British Journal of Psychiatry*, **144**, 533–537.

Nuechterlein, K., Ventura, J., Snyder, K., Gitlin, M., Subotnik, K., Dawson, M. and Mintz, J. (1998) The role of stressors in schizophrenic relapse: longitudinal evidence and implication for psychosocial interventions. Presented at: *IV World Congress: World Association for Psychosocial Rehabilitation*. Hamburg, Germany.

Olbrich, R. and Lutz, M. (1990) Reduction of schizophrenic deficits by cognitive training: an evaluative study. *European Archives of Psychiatric and Neurological Sciences*, **239**, 366–369.

Overall, J.E. and Gorham, D.R. (1962) The Brief Psychiatric Rating Scale. *Psychological Reports*, **10**, 799–812.

Palacios-Araus, L., Herran, A., Sandoya, M., Gonzalez, H.E., Vazquez-Barquero, J.L. and Diez-Manrique, J.F. (1995) Analysis of positive and negative symptoms in schizophrenia: a study from a population of long-term outpatients. *Acta Psychiatrica Scandinavica*, **92**, 178–182.

Penn, D. (1991) Cognitive rehabilitation of social deficits in schizophrenia: a direction of promise or following a primrose path? *Psychosocial Rehabilitation Journal*, **15**, 27–41.

Penn, D.L., Mueser, K.T., Spaulding, W., Hope, D.A. and Reed, D. (1995a) Information processing and social competence in chronic schizophrenia. *Schizophrenia Bulletin*, **21**, 269–281.

Penn, D.L., Mueser, K.T., Doonan, R. and Nishith, P. (1995b) Relations between social skills and ward behavior in chronic schizophrenia. *Schizophrenia Research*, **16**, 225–232.

Penn, D.L., Mueser, K.T. and Spaulding, W. (1996) Information processing, social skill, and gender in schizophrenia. *Psychiatry Research*, **59**, 213–220.

Penn, D.L., Corrigan, P.W., Bentall, R.P., Racenstein, J.M. and Newman, L. (1997) Social cognition in schizophrenia. *Psychological Bulletin*, **121**, 114–132.

Peralta, V., Cuesta, M.J. and deLeon, J. (1994) An empirical analysis of latent structures underlying schizophrenic symptoms: a four-syndrome model. *Biological Psychiatry*, **36**, 726–736.

Perlick, D., Stastny, P., Mattis, S. and Teresi, J. (1992) Contribution of family, cognitive, and clinical dimensions to long-term outcome in schizophrenia. *Schizophrenia Research*, **6**, 257–265.

Phillips, M.L. and David, A.S. (1995) Facial processing in schizophrenia and delusional misidentification: cognitive neuropsychiatric approaches. *Schizophrenia Research*, **17**, 109–114.

Pogue-Geile, M.F. (1989) The prognostic significance of negative symptoms in schizophrenia. *British Journal of Psychiatry*, **Suppl. 7**, 123–127.

Rajkumar, S. and Thara, R. (1989) Factors affecting relapse in schizophrenia. *Schizophrenia Research*, **2**, 403–409.

Robins, E. and Guze, S.B. (1970) Establishment of diagnostic validity in psychiatric illness: its application to schizophrenia. *American Journal of Psychiatry*, **126**, 983–987.

Rosenheck, R., Tekell, J., Peters, J., Cramer, J., Fontana, A., Xu, W., Thomas, J., Henderson, W. and Charney, D. (1998) Does participation in psychosocial treatment augment the benefit of clozapine? *Archives of General Psychiatry*, **55**, 618–625.

Roy, M.A. and DeVriendt, X. (1995) Positive and negative symptoms in schizophrenia: a current overview. *Canadian Journal of Psychiatry*, **39**, 407–414.

Salem, J.E., Kring, A.M. and Kerr, S.L. (1996) More evidence for generalized poor performance in facial emotion perception in schizophrenia. *Journal of Abnormal Psychology*, **105**, 480–483.

Salokangas, R.K., Rakkolainen, V. and Alanen, Y.O. (1989) Maintenance of grip on life and goals of life: a valuable criterion for evaluating outcome in schizophrenia. *Acta Psychiatrica Scandinavica*, **80**, 187–193.

Sayers, S.L., Curran, P.J. and Mueser, K.T. (1996) Factor structure and construct validity of the Scale for the Assessment of Negative Symptoms. *Psychological Assessment*, **8**, 269–280.

Schaub, A., Behrendt, B., Brenner, H.D., Mueser, K.T. and Liberman, R.P. (1998) Training schizophrenic patients to manage their symptoms: predictors of treatment response to the German version of the Symptom Management Module. *Schizophrenia Research*, **31**, 121–130.

Schneider, F., Gur, R.C., Gur, R.E. and Shtasel, D.L. (1995) Emotional processing in schizophrenia: neurobehavioral probes in relation to psychopathology. *Schizophrenia Research*, **17**, 67–75.

Servan-Schreiber, D., Cohen, J.D. and Steingard, S. (1996) Schizophrenic deficits in the processing of context: a test of theoretical model. *Archives of General Psychiatry*, **53**, 1105–1112.

Shallice, T. and Evans, M. (1978) The involvement of the frontal lobes in cognitive estimation. *Cortex*, **14**, 292–303.

Shtasel, D.L., Gur, R.E., Gallacher, F., Heimberg, C. and Gur, R.C. (1992) Gender differences in the clinical expression of schizophrenia. *Schizophrenia Research*, **7**, 225–231.

Silverstein, S.M., Maxey, J.T. and West, L.L. (1994) Cognitive and symptom factors related to treatment outcome in a partial hospitalization program. *Continuum*, **1**, 251–261.

Silverstein, S.M., Schenkel, L.S., Valone, C. and Nuernberger, S.W. (1998) Cognitive deficits and psychiatric rehabilitation outcomes in schizophrenia. *Psychiatric Quarterly*, **69**, 169–191.

Smith, T.E., Hull, J.W., Anthony, D.T., Goodman, M., Hedayat-Harris, A., Felger, T., Kentros, M.K., MacKain, S. and Romanelli, S. (1997) Post-hospitalization treatment adherence of schizophrenic patients: gender differences in skill acquisition. *Psychiatry Research*, **69**, 123–129.

Solinski, S., Jackson, H.J. and Bell, R.C. (1992) Prediction of employability in schizophrenic patients. *Schizophrenia Research*, **7**, 141–148.

Spaulding, W.D. (1978) The relationships of some information-processing factors to severely disturbed behavior. *Journal of Nervous and Mental Disease*, **166**, 417–428.

Spaulding, W.D. (1992) Design prerequisites for research on cognitive therapy for schizophrenia. *Schizophrenia Bulletin*, **18**, 39–42.

Spaulding, W.D., Storms, L., Goodrich, V. and Sullivan, M. (1986) Applications of experimental psychopathology in psychiatric rehabilitation. *Schizophrenia Bulletin*, **12**, 560–577.

Spaulding, W.D., Reed, D., Elting, D., Sullivan, M. and Penn, D.L. (1997) Cognitive changes in the course of rehabilitation. In: Brenner, H.D., Boeker, W. and Genner, R. (eds), *Towards a Comprehensive Therapy for Schizophrenia*. Hofgrefe-Huber, Seattle, pp. 106–117.

Spaulding, W.D., Reed, D., Sullivan, M., Richardson, C. and Weiler, M. (1999) Effects of cognitive treatment in psychiatric rehabilitation. *Schizophrenia Bulletin*, **25**, 657–676.

Stephens, J.H., Astrup, C. and Mangrum, J.C. (1966) Prognostic factors in recovered and deteriorated schizophrenia. *American Journal of Psychiatry*, **122**, 1116–1121.

Stephens, J.H., Richard, P. and McHugh, P.R. (1997) Long-term follow-up of patients hospitalized for schizophrenia, 1913–1940. *Journal of Nervous and Mental Disease*, **185**, 715–721.

Strauss, J.S. and Carpenter, W.T. (1974) The prediction of outcome in schizophrenia II. Relationships between predictor and outcome variables: a report from the WHO International Pilot Study of schizophrenia. *Archives of General Psychiatry*, **31**, 37–42.

Strauss, J.S. and Carpenter, W.T. (1977) Prediction of outcome in schizophrenia: III. Five-year outcome and its predictors. *Archives of General Psychiatry*, **34,** 159–163.

Trower, P., Bryant, B.M. and Argyle, M. (1978) *Social Skills and Mental Health*. Methuen, London.

Tsuang, M.T. (1986) Predictors of poor and good outcome in schizophrenia. In: Erlenmeyer-Kimling, L. and Miller, N.E. (eds), *Life-span Research on the Prediction of Psychopathology*. Lawrence Erlbaum, Hillsdale, NJ. pp. 195–203.

Velligan, D.I., Mahurin, R.K., True, J.E., Lefton, R.S. and Flores, C.V. (1996) Preliminary evaluation of cognitive adaptation training to compensate for cognitive deficits in schizophrenia. *Psychiatric Services*, **47**, 415–417.

Wallace, C.J. (1997) Psychometric properties of the Micro-module Learning Test. Unpublished data UCLA Clinical Research Center for Schizophrenia and Psychiatric Rehabilitation.

Wallace, C.J., Nelson, C.J., Liberman, R.P., Aitchison, R.A., Lukoff, D., Elder, J.P. and Ferris, C. (1980) A review and critique of social skills training with schizophrenic patients. *Schizophrenia Bulletin*, **6**, 42–63.

Woerner, M.G., Mannuzza, S. and Kane, J.M. (1988) Anchoring the BPRS: an aid to improved reliability. *Psychopharmacology Bulletin*, **24**, 112–117.

Wykes, T. (1994) Predicting symptomatic and behavioural outcomes of community care. *British Journal of Psychiatry*, **165**, 486–492.

Wykes, T. and Dunn, G. (1992) Cognitive deficit and the prediction of rehabilitation success in a chronic psychiatric group. *Psychological Medicine*, **22**, 389–398.

Wykes, T., Sturt, E. and Katz, R. (1990) The prediction of rehabilitative success after three years: the use of social, symptom, and cognitive variables. *British Journal of Psychiatry*, **157**, 865–877.

Wykes, T., Reeder, C., Corner, J., Williams, C. and Everitt, B. (1999) The effects of neurocognitive remediation on executive processing in patients with schizophrenia. *Schizophrenia Bulletin*, **25**, 291–307.

Zahn, T.P. and Carpenter, W.T. (1978) Effects of short term outcome and clinical improvement on RT in acute schizophrenia. *Journal of Psychiatric Research*, **14**, 59–68.

Zigler, E. and Glick, M. (1986) *A Developmental Approach to Adult Psychopathology.* Weiner, I.B. (Series ed.), *Wiley Series on Personality Processes*. John Wiley and Sons, New York.

9 Relevance of neurocognitive deficits for functional outcome in schizophrenia

Michael Foster Green, Robert S. Kern, Mary Jane Robertson, Mark J. Sergi and Kimmy S. Kee

Introduction

In a research area characterized by differences of opinion, there is remarkable agreement on the point that neurocognitive deficits are part and parcel of schizophrenia. In other words, they generally do not derive from the symptoms of the disorder, nor are they a result of medication nor are they induced by institutionalization. On the contrary, many (though not all) of the neurocognitive deficits seem to reflect predisposition to the illness as opposed to the presence of illness. Hence, the neurocognitive deficits of schizophrenia can be considered central to the disorder.

Evidence for this centrality comes from several sources. Some neurocognitive deficits are present in children who are at 'high risk' for schizophrenia, with risk for illness usually defined as having a schizophrenic parent (Nuechterlein, 1983; Cornblatt and Erlenmeyer-Kimling, 1985; Rutschmann et al., 1986; Cornblatt et al., 1989; Asarnow et al., 1977). These studies indicate that neurocognitive deficits are apparent long before the onset of overt, psychotic symptoms. Further support for the centrality of the deficits is that they endure after a psychotic episode when symptoms have subsided and patients are in remission (Asarnow and MacCrimmon, 1978; Miller et al., 1979; Nuechterlein et al., 1992). Neurocognitive deficits are also found in first-degree relatives of patients, who do not have a schizophrenic disorder (Grove et al., 1991; Steinhauer et al., 1991; Mirsky et al., 1992; Green et al., 1997; Keefe et al., 1997). Moreover, these deficits can be observed in non-psychotic individuals who are considered to be in the schizophrenia spectrum because they have clinical symptoms of schizotypal personality disorder or high scores on tests of psychosis proneness (Braff, 1981; Asarnow et al., 1983; Balogh and Merritt, 1985; Lenzenweger et al., 1991).

Awareness of the centrality of neurocognitive deficits is not new. Bleuler made a similar observation when he labeled attentional deficits as a 'fundamental' symptom of schizophrenia (Bleuler, 1950). Much of the research over the past century has been directed toward understanding the nature of neurocognitive deficits in schizophrenia. However, only relatively recently has a concerted effort been made to understand the functional implications of these deficits. The literature in this area has grown rapidly; in fact this literature doubled between

1996 and 1998. Because of this recent surge in interest in functional consequences, we now have a sufficient database on which to make inferences.

In this chapter, we have three goals. First, we want to provide a brief orientation to some terminology in this area. This area tends to become jargon filled, and our intention is to make this chapter relatively non-technical and reader friendly. We include one section for neurocognitive constructs and one for categories of functional outcome. Second, we will survey the literature in this area in a selective, not comprehensive, fashion. We will focus on studies that have been published after 1995. Finally, we will discuss a question that has received little attention: if neurocognitive deficits are related to functional outcome, what are critical mediators for these relationships? Two candidate mediators will be evaluated.

What is meant by neurocognition

Although assessments of neurocognition in schizophrenia run the gamut from standardized clinical neuropsychological tests to specialized measures from experimental psychology, a wide-ranging review of assessment methods is not needed for the purposes of this chapter. In general, research in this area has centered on a few key neurocognitive constructs.

(i) Global or composite measures of neurocognitive functioning. Some studies use a brief global measure, such as a mental status exam, to provide a rough estimate of neurocognitive ability. Other studies have used prorated IQ scores for the same reason. These are examples of global indices. In some instances, a variety of rather specific neurocognitive measures are summed into an overall score called a composite neurocognitive index. These global and composite measures are useful for many questions, but they do not provide information on the relationships between particular neurocognitive abilities and functional outcome.

(ii) Types of memory. There are many ways to subtype memory and a large variety of assessment methods. Two types of memory are especially relevant to the current topic, namely immediate/working memory and secondary memory. Immediate or working memory refers to the ability to hold information 'on-line' for a brief period of time (usually a few seconds). Repeating a telephone number is an example of immediate or working memory. Many measures of working memory assess not only the ability to store information on-line, but also the ability to manipulate or process the information that is being held. If you needed to remember a list of numbers and then repeat them backwards, that would involve a manipulation of the information.

Secondary memory refers to the ability to acquire and store information over a longer period of time (usually lasting for several minutes and longer). This type of memory is usually assessed with lists of words or passages of text. The stimuli that are to be remembered exceed the immediate memory span, meaning that they contain too much information to be held on-line at any one time.

(iii) Vigilance (also sometimes called sustained attention) refers to the ability to maintain a readiness to respond to target stimuli and not respond to non-targets. In signal detection terms, this involves an ability to distinguish signal from noise. Vigilance typically is measured with the Continuous Performance Test in which subjects are presented with a series of briefly presented stimuli and instructed to respond only to selected target stimuli and ignore all others.

(iv) Executive functioning refers to volition, planning, purposive action and self-monitoring of behavior (Lezak, 1995). With such a broad range of abilities, it is not surprising that few measures of executive functioning assess all of them. Frequently, executive functioning in schizophrenia is measured with card sorting measures that assess the subject's ability to attain, maintain and shift a cognitive set. Card sorting tests are used commonly in the studies reviewed here.

(v) Verbal fluency tests involve measures of the ability to generate words. Subjects may be asked to produce words that begin with a certain letter, or to produce words from a certain category (e.g. animals). The term verbal fluency potentially is misleading because the subject never speaks fluently, but only generates one-word responses that fall within the specified category.

(vi) Early visual processing refers to the basic stages of visual processing such as the visual scanning of a display and the early detection and identification of visual stimuli. Assessments of these processes involve the very brief presentation of visual stimuli, either alone or in the presence of competing stimuli.

What is meant by functional outcome in schizophrenia

Outcomes in schizophrenia can be divided into several categories that are largely independent: clinical or symptomatic outcome, subjective variables and functional (social and vocational) outcome (Brekke *et al.*, 1993). Clinical outcome frequently includes measures related to psychiatric symptoms such as time to positive symptom remission. Subjective variables include subjective satisfaction and self-esteem. Functional outcome, which is the focus of this chapter, includes a variety of domains involved with the acquisition and retention of skills that are needed for social, vocational and community functioning.

There is wide variability in the outcome measures for studies of neurocognition and functional outcome in schizophrenia. The outcome measures fit into three general categories: (i) success on psychosocial rehabilitation programs; (ii) studies of laboratory assessment of instrumental skills and social problem-solving ability; and (iii) studies that have considered broader aspects of behavior in community outcome and activities of daily living. The first two categories are highly interconnected because performance of skills in the laboratory obviously is dependent on the acquisition of those skills. We suggest that these outcome areas can be considered as running along a proximal to distal dimension (see Figure 9.1). The dimension is offered as a heuristic, and is not meant to be taken too literally. We view as 'proximal' aspects of outcome that involve acquisition and performance of isolated skills, as well as laboratory analogs of social and work functioning. We view as 'distal' behaviors that involve the integration of multiple skill areas, and community-based outcomes that are actual, not simulated.

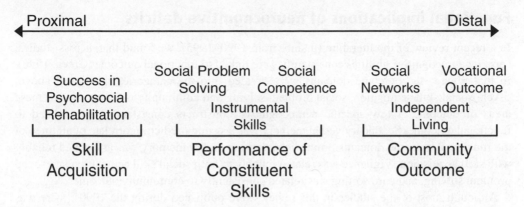

Figure 9.1. Key domains of functional outcome in schizophrenia. The outcome domains are depicted along a hypothetical proximal to distal dimension.

Psychosocial skill acquisition

Psychosocial skills training is perhaps the most widely used psychosocial treatment for schizophrenic patients. These programs are designed to teach patients basic skills that enable them to attain greater functional independence (e.g. programs in basic conversation skills, symptom and medication management, and leisure skills). Because these training programs tend to be highly structured and closely monitored, it is possible to track the amount of success in a skills training program and the degree to which a patient acquires component skills.

Laboratory assessments of instrumental skills and social problem-solving ability

Studies in this category examine performance within the laboratory, often using analog measures of social competence and problem solving. For example, in a typical assessment for this category, subjects may watch a series of videotaped vignettes which depict a social interaction with a problem. Subjects may be asked to identify the problem, suggest solutions to the problem and then demonstrate how they would act out the solution through a role play.

Community outcome/daily activities

This is the broadest category of functional outcome and includes such outcomes as occupational and social attainment. Because of its breadth, this outcome area is sometimes difficult to measure and would include aspects such as the ability to carry out activities of daily living, amount or level of work or school, or type and quality of social support that one has.

Functional implications of neurocognitive deficits

In a recent review of the literature (mainly from 1990–1995), we found that, across studies, certain neurocognitive abilities consistently were linked to functional outcome (Green, 1996). In that review, the outcome domains were divided into the categories mentioned above: psychosocial skill acquisition, social problem solving and community outcome. Across these areas of outcome, a few specific neurocognitive constructs consistently were related to functional outcome. Secondary verbal memory was a strong predictor/correlate of all three of the functional outcome domains. Immediate/working verbal memory was associated reliably with skill acquisition. Vigilance was related reliably to both social skill acquisition and social problem solving, and card sorting was related consistently to community outcome.

Although most of the studies in this review were published during the 1990s, there was precedence for these studies. Heaton and colleagues (Heaton et al., 1978; Heaton and Pendelton, 1981) previously had examined the role of neuropsychological variables in outcome for mixed patient groups. Further, neurocognitive abilities are related to functional (i.e. occupational) outcome in other disorders such as multiple sclerosis and human immunodeficiency virus (HIV) infection (Heaton et al., 1994), so it should not be surprising that similar relationships also exist in schizophrenia.

In the 4 years since our published review, the literature in this area has doubled, and over 20 additional articles have been published that have examined the relationships between neurocognition and aspects of functional outcome. These studies are reviewed in more detail in Green et al. (2000). We will review selectively some of the articles to illustrate key points. Studies are divided into three outcome domains that are similar, but not identical to, the outcome domains discussed in Green (1996): community outcome and daily activities; laboratory assessments of social problem solving and instrumental skills; and psychosocial skill acquisition.

Psychosocial skill acquisition

Relatively few studies have been published in the past few years that examined the relationship between neurocognition and skill acquisition in psychosocial rehabilitation. One reason for the paucity of studies is that, depending on the design, they can be rather time-consuming. It is unfortunate that this area is somewhat understudied because the neuro-cognitive connections to psychosocial rehabilitation may provide one of the most practical implications for this line of inquiry.

One study (Silverstein et al., 1998) used a measure of within-session learning as an index of skill acquisition. This is essentially a measure of brief learning capacity for social skill training material. Some of the measures (e.g. verbal memory, verbal fluency and inferential thinking) were correlated with skill acquisition on this method. However, other areas, such as vigilance, were not related. In a small sample of patients ($n = 19$), McKee et al. (1997) observed patients during a long-term rehabilitation program. Patients were observed for program attendance and level of participation during the sessions. Executive functioning (measured with an interference task, the Stroop) was significantly related to participation in psychosocial rehabilitation, but secondary verbal memory was not.

Across all studies published to date, the most consistent predictors and correlates of skill acquisition in rehabilitation programs include secondary verbal memory, immediate/working memory, vigilance and psychomotor speed. This pattern suggests that memory and vigilance are needed for success in skill acquisition programs, and the findings have good face validity (i.e. they make sense). Because rehabilitation programs are similar in format to interactive classes, it makes sense that recall and vigilance would be needed to keep track of the session and to encode new material.

Social problem solving and instrumental skills

Among the outcome areas, studies in this domain may have the most consistency in assessment. Laboratory analogs of social problem solving tend to follow similar formats in which a subject is shown an interpersonal problem and then asked to identify the problem and generate solutions. Frequently, subjects are asked to demonstrate in a role play how they would solve social problems. Also included in this outcome area are studies in which subjects demonstrate competence on certain instrumental life skills, perhaps by simulating daily activities. Across published studies in this area, secondary verbal memory and vigilance have both been shown to be highly consistent correlates of laboratory assessments of social problem solving and performance of instrumental skills.

One of the innovative aspects of recent studies in this area has been an extension of the types of predictors and correlates. Some studies have included measures that lie at the interface of basic neurocognition and social functioning, an area known as social cognition. For example, Corrigan and Toomey (1995) used a measure of social perception in which subjects identified cues in a series of interpersonal situations. Social perception was significantly related to a measure of social problem solving. Notably, this relationship generally was stronger than relationships between basic neurocognitive measures (i.e. without a social component) and social problem solving. This differential relationship suggests that social cognition, including social perception, may be more closely related to social competence than is basic neurocognition because of its proximity to social competence (see Figure 9.1).

Another aspect of social cognition is affect perception (e.g. identifying the emotion in facial expression). Mueser *et al.* (1996) examined emotion recognition in a sample of schizophrenic inpatients. Affect perception was associated with social competence assessed through an unstructured role play. We will discuss affect perception in more detail below.

Community and activities of daily living

Across studies, neurocognitive measures have been reported to be reliable predictors and correlates of community outcome. Some of the most consistent neurocognitive constructs associated with this aspect of functional outcome include secondary verbal memory, card sorting and verbal fluency.

One of the recent developments for these studies has been the inclusion of older schizophrenic patients (Bartels *et al.*, 1997; Harvey *et al.*, 1997, 1998). These studies have used rather general measures of neurocognition, such as the Mini-Mental State Examination

(MMSE) or a composite score from the Consortium to Establish a Registry for Alzheimer's Disease (CERAD) battery, and have shown strong relationships between composite neurocognitive indicators and adaptive living skills. The study by Harvey *et al.* (1998) is notable in that it included three separate groups of elderly patients who differed substantially in their level of adaptive functioning. One group was from a nursing home and had low levels of adaptive functioning. Another group of elderly acute patients had relatively high adaptive functioning, and a group of chronic hospitalized patients was intermediate. The key point is that differences in overall level of adaptive functioning did not affect the patterns of correlations. For each group, a composite cognitive measure correlated most strongly with adaptive functioning, explaining in the neighborhood of 40–50% of the variance. Negative symptoms correlated slightly less than cognition, and positive symptoms correlated almost not at all.

Similarly, Klapow *et al.* (1997) reported that a global measure of neurocognition from the MMSE was related to an assessment of simulated daily activities in older schizophrenic patients. This relationship held even after controlling for the effects of symptoms and subject demographics.

One study in this area has included a measure of social cognition. Penn *et al.* (1996) reported relationships between affect recognition and adaptive unit behavior, and, not surprisingly, these relationships were stronger than those between basic neurocognition and adaptive unit behavior.

Although the results across studies are generally consistent in showing relationships, some of the studies (Heslegrave *et al.*, 1997; Addington *et al.*, 1998; Addington and Addington, 1999) had results, that while not entirely negative, were not as robust as other studies in this area. How can we explain this? Addington and Addington (1999) assessed aspects of social outcome that included social competence and social problem solving. The relationships between neurocognitive measures and social competence were fairly weak; however, the relationships with social problem solving were much stronger. Perhaps neurocognitive abilities are related more closely to social problem solving than they are to social competence because social problem solving (a component of social cognition) is closer to basic neuro-cognition than is social outcome (see Figure 9.1).

In the article by Heslegrave *et al.* (1997), the largely negative results involved a quality of life assessment that was based, at least partially, on subjective satisfaction. As mentioned above, subjective variables constitute a separate domain of outcome, and it may be one that is not strongly related to neurocognition.

Candidate mediators

At this point, we should ask what has been learned from this literature so far. The simplest and the safest conclusion is that relationships exist between aspects of neurocognition and domains of functional outcome. These relationships are best documented for secondary verbal memory, immediate/working verbal memory, vigilance and card sorting. However, the literature has taught us relatively little about the *mechanisms* that can account for these relationships. In other words, the question shifts from *whether* a particular neurocognitive deficit is related to functional outcome to *how* a particular neurocognitive deficit is related to functional outcome. To understand the mechanisms of these interactions, we need to consider possible mediators, i.e. variables that are intermediate between the basic neurocognitive abilities measured in the laboratory and the specific outcome areas.

In a recent article (Green and Nuechterlein, 1999), we proposed several candidate variables that may be mediators between neurocognition and functional outcome. Two of these candidate mediators, affect perception and awareness of illness, will be considered in this section. Based on the current literature, it is difficult to demonstrate with certainty that a particular variable serves as a mediator. Instead it is possible to say that a certain variable *may* serve as a mediator (i.e. we cannot rule out this possibility). At a minimum, a mediator between basic neurocognition and functional outcome in schizophrenia should have reasonably strong associations with both of these types of variables.

Affect perception

Affect perception is the ability to accurately perceive, interpret and process emotional expression in others. Dating back to the mid-1800s, Darwin proposed that the ability to perceive affect is a universal human accomplishment. Almost a century later, his theory was tested empirically across different cultures in a series of studies by Ekman and colleagues. For example, in one study (Ekman *et al.*, 1969), college students in the USA, Brazil, Chile, Argentina and Japan were asked to identify one of six emotions displayed in various photographs of facial expressions. Results showed considerable agreement among individuals from different cultures in perceiving affect. A follow-up study (Ekman and Friesen, 1971) found similar results comparing affect recognition among college students from the five countries and preliterate tribesmen in New Guinea. More recently, in the psychopathology literature, several investigators have examined perception of affect in samples of schizophrenia patients, and the majority have reported that schizophrenia patients are less accurate than normals in their ability to recognize facial and vocal emotion (Turner, 1964; Walker *et al.*, 1984; Feinberg *et al.*, 1986; Borod *et al.*, 1993; Kerr and Neale, 1993; Bellack *et al.*, 1996).

Perception of affect can be considered a complex social cognitive ability, which relies on the integrity of a select set of more basic neurocognitive processes (Schneider *et al.*, 1995; Bryson *et al.*, 1997; Addington and Addington, 1998). As such, it is possible that deficits in a certain group, such as schizophrenic patients, could be attributed to deficits in a more basic neurocognitive ability. In a recent study from our laboratory, 28 treatment-resistant schizophrenia patients received a battery of facial and vocal affect perception measures and assessments of a discrete set of neurocognitive abilities (Kee *et al.*, 1998). Measures of affect perception included a visual emotion identification test (still photographs presented on videotape; Kerr and Neale, 1993), an auditory emotion identification test (audiotape; Kerr and Neale, 1993) and a combined visual and auditory affect perception test (brief interpersonal vignettes presented on videotape; Bellack *et al.*, 1996). Measures of neurocognitive functioning included a measure of early visual processing and visual scanning, a measure of visual vigilance and a measure of immediate/working memory. Among these measures, performance on the measure of early visual processing (The Span of Apprehension) strongly correlated with performance on all affect perception tasks, regardless of the modality of the stimulus presentation. Associations between perception of affect and the other two types of measures were in the same direction, but were significantly smaller. These findings indicate that affect perception in schizophrenia is related to basic neurocognition and that associations are particularly strong for early perceptual processing and visual scanning.

The next question concerns the relationships between affect perception and an aspect of social competence, social perception. Two studies mentioned above are relevant here. Penn *et al.* (1996) examined the relationship between affect perception and adaptive behavior in a sample of 27 chronic in-patients with diagnoses of schizophrenia or schizoaffective disorder. They reported that perception of affect was related to social competence, social interest and neatness, as measured by the Nurse's Observation Scale for Inpatient Evaluation (NOSIE-30). Similarly, Mueser *et al.* (1996) found that perception of affect was related to social adjustment on the ward, such as social mixing, personal appearance and hygiene, in a sample of 28 long-term schizophrenia in-patients.

Putting the findings together, we can generate a simple diagram such as Figure 9.2. Although it is diagramed as a single model, it has not been tested as such. Instead, we have support for the individual arrows, but the components could be configured in another way. Nonetheless, at this point, we can consider affect perception to be a possible mediator between basic neurocognition and social competence in schizophrenia (i.e. we cannot rule out this possibility).

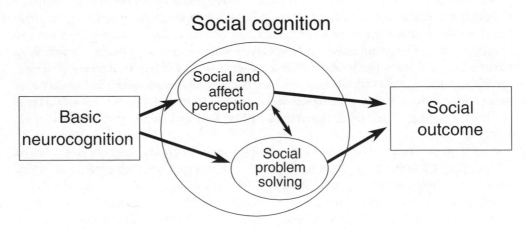

Figure 9.2. Social cognition is represented as a possible mediator between basic neurocognition and social outcome.

Insight

Insight is a multidimensional construct that includes awareness of the symptoms and consequences of one's disorder, as well as awareness of one's need for treatment (Amador *et al.*, 1991). Most studies examining the association between insight and functional outcome in schizophrenia have found significant relationships (Schwartz, 1998). One study found that insight was related to the quality of social skills displayed in a psychosocial rehabilitation program (Lysaker *et al.*, 1994). Another study found that insight in schizophrenia was associated with the frequency and quality of social relationships and the quantity and quality of useful work (McGlashan and Carpenter, 1981). Also, two studies found that better insight was related to reduced re-hospitalization (McGlashan and Carpenter, 1981; McEvoy *et al.*, 1989).

Many studies have examined the relationship between neurocognition and insight in schizophrenia, and the results have been entirely mixed. We found 13 studies that examined this question, and six found support for an association between neurocognition and insight. Among the neurocognitive measures, insight has been examined most frequently in relation to tests that presumably assess frontal lobe functioning (e.g. Lysaker and Bell, 1994, 1995; Young *et al.*, 1993). For example, several studies examined whether insight is related to performance on a card sorting test (the Wisconsin Card Sorting Test, WCST). Two studies found that patients' responses on the insight item of a clinical symptom assessment (the Positive and Negative Syndrome Scale) correlated with their performance on the WCST (Voruganti *et al.*, 1997; Lysaker *et al.*, 1998). Likewise, Young *et al.* (1998) found that poor awareness of symptoms, misattribution of symptoms and denial of minor character flaws were all correlated with performance on the WCST.

However, the majority of published studies have failed to find a clear relationship between neurocognition and insight in schizophrenia (e.g. David *et al.*, 1995; Kemp and David, 1996). Sometimes, insight appears to be related to clinical factors such as psychosis and depression (Collins *et al.*, 1997; Dickerson *et al.*, 1997). Curiously, one study reported a paradoxical finding; that impaired insight was associated with better verbal and visual memory (Cuesta and Peralta, 1994).

The inconsistency of the findings suggests that insight and neurocognition do not have a linear relationship; however, an intriguing possibility is that they have a non-linear relationship. In a recent study, Startup (1996) found a curvilinear relationship between neurocognition and insight such that patients with relatively intact neurocognition were characterized by both relatively good and relatively poor insight. In other words, two forces may be at work. One influence is neurocognitive: insight requires a certain neurocognitive foundation. The second influence is psychological: patients have a motivation for positive self-evaluation that might lead to reduced awareness of illness. Hence, depending on which factor is predominant, a patient with good neurocognitive abilities might have either high insight (because they have a good neurocognitive foundation) or low insight (because they are actively maintaining a positive self-evaluation).

Overall, insight does not appear to be a likely mediator between basic neurocognition and functional outcome. The literature is inconsistent and, to the extent that relationships exist between neurocognition and insight, they may be complex and non-linear. Hence, at this time, insight or awareness of illness does not seem to account (at least not in any simple way) for the observed associations between neurocognition and functional outcome in schizophrenia.

A multilevel view of functional outcome

At this point, there is highly convincing support for relationships between neurocognition and functional outcome across three types of functional outcome domains. The most consistent relationships have included the neurocognitive domains of secondary memory, immediate/working memory, vigilance and card sorting as predictors of functional outcome.

Still unknown are the ways in which these relationships are mediated. In other words, what are the steps running from basic neurocognition at one end to functional outcome at the other? We discussed two possible mediators in the previous section. By considering the mediating steps, we can understand the determinants of disturbances in social and occupational functioning at multiple levels. Much like an illness in the human body can be viewed as a disruption at multiple levels (e.g. individual, organ, cell or molecule), so too can a disturbance in functional outcome be viewed at multiple levels. Consider a first person account.

> "Having a major mental illness has had a devastating effect on all aspects of my life. My relationships with others are, at best, very loose. I recently read in a brochure that people with schizophrenia have difficulty making and keeping friends, which has definitely been true in my case. I have given up on the idea of getting married and having children someday. Instead, I have decided to devote my life to writing. Above all else, I want my life to have meaning apart from my diagnosis." Dykstra (1997, p. 698).

The poignant difficulties in establishing and maintaining friendships described in this personal narrative could be understood as the end product of a host of determinants. Clearly, we can view the problems at the social level. In addition, we can view the difficulties one level lower as problems in mediators such as social cognition (perhaps difficulties in perception of emotion in others). Lower still, we may conceptualize the social difficulties as the final product of problems in basic neurocognition (perhaps visual scanning or secondary memory). Viewing the problem in this descending fashion illustrates a type of 'psychosocial reductivism' in which relatively complex aspects of social dysfunction can be understood in terms of more basic disturbances.

References

Addington, J. and Addington, D. (1998) Facial affect recognition and information processing in schizophrenia and bipolar disorder. *Schizophrenia Research*, **32**, 171–181.

Addington, J. and Addington, D. (1999) Neurocognitive and social functioning in schizophrenia. *Schizophrenia Bulletin*, **25**, 173–182.

Addington, J., McCleary, L. and Munroe-Blum, H. (1998) Relationship between cognitive and social dysfunction in schizophrenia. *Schizophrenia Research*, **34**, 59–66.

Amador, X.F., Strauss, D.H., Yale, S.A. and Gorman, J.M. (1991) Awareness of illness in schizophrenia. *Schizophrenia Bulletin*, **17**, 113–132.

Asarnow, R.F. and MacCrimmon, D.J. (1978) Residual performance deficit in clinically remitted schizophrenics: a marker of schizophrenia? *Journal of Abnormal Psychology*, **87**, 597–608.

Asarnow, R.F., Nuechterlein, K.H. and Marder, S.R. (1983) Span of apprehension performance, neuropsychological functioning, and indices of psychosis-proneness. *Journal of Nervous and Mental Disease*, **171**, 662–669.

Asarnow, R.F., Steffy, R.A., MacCrimmon, D.J. and Cleghorn, J.M. (1977) An attentional assessment of foster children at risk for schizophrenia. *Journal of Abnormal Psychology*, **86**, 267–275.

Balogh, D.W. and Merritt, R.D. (1985) Susceptibility to type A backward pattern masking among hypothetically psychosis-prone college students. *Journal of Abnormal Psychology*, **94**, 377–383.

Bartels, S.J., Mueser, K.T. and Miles, K.M. (1997) A comparative study of elderly patients with schizophrenia and bipolar disorder in nursing homes and the community. *Schizophrenia Research*, **27**, 181–190.

Bellack, A.S., Blanchard, J.J. and Mueser, K.T. (1996) Cue availability and affect perception in schizophrenia. *Schizophrenia Bulletin*, **22**, 535–544.

Bleuler, E. (1950) *Dementia Praecox or the Group of Schizophrenias*. International Universities Press, New York.

Borod, J.C., Martin, C.C., Alpert, M., Brozgold, A. and Welkowitz, J. (1993) Perception of facial emotion in schizophrenic and right brain-damaged patients. *Journal of Nervous and Mental Disease*, **181**, 494–502.

Braff, D.L. (1981) Impaired speed of information processing in nonmedicated schizotypal patients. *Schizophrenia Bulletin*, **7**, 499–508.

Brekke, J.S., Levin, S., Wolkon, G., Sobel, G. and Slade, B. (1993) Psychosocial functioning and subjective experience in schizophrenia. *Schizophrenia Bulletin*, **19**, 599–608.

Bryson, G., Bell, M. and Lysaker, P. (1997) Affect recognition in schizophrenia: a function of global impairment or a specific cognitive deficit? *Psychiatric Research*, **71**, 105–114.

Collins, A.A., Remington, G.J., Coulter, K. and Birkett, K. (1997) Insight, neurocognitive function and symptom clusters in chronic schizophrenia. *Schizophrenia Research*, **27**, 37–44.

Cornblatt, B.A. and Erlenmeyer-Kimling, L. (1985) Global attentional deviance as a marker of risk for schizophrenia: specificity and predictive validity. *Journal of Abnormal Psychology*, **94**, 470–486.

Cornblatt, B.A., Lenzenweger, M.F. and Erlenmeyer-Kimling, L. (1989) The continuous performance test, identical pairs version: II. Contrasting attentional profiles in schizophrenic and depressed patients. *Psychiatric Research*, **29**, 65.

Corrigan, P.W. and Toomey, R. (1995) Interpersonal problem-solving and information-processing in schizophrenia. *Schizophrenia Bulletin*, **21**, 395–403.

Cuesta, M.J. and Peralta, V. (1994) Lack of insight in schizophrenia. *Schizophrenia Bulletin*, **20**, 359–366.

David, A., Van Os, J., Jones, P., Harvey, I., Forester, A. and Fahy, T. (1995) Insight and psychotic illness: cross-sectional and longitudinal associations. *British Journal of Psychiatry*, **167**, 621–628.

Dickerson, F.B., Boronow, J.J., Ringel, N. and Parente, F. (1997) Lack of insight among outpatients with schizophrenia. *Psychiatric Services*, **48**, 195–199.

Dykstra, T. (1997) First person account: how I cope. *Schizophrenia Bulletin*, **23**, 697–699.

Ekman, P. and Friesen, W. (1971) Constants across cultures in the face and emotion. *Journal of Personality and Social Psychology*, **17**, 124–129.

Ekman, P., Sorenson, E.R. and Friesen, W.V. (1969) Pan-cultural elements in facial displays of emotion. *Science*, **164**, 86–88.

Feinberg, T.E., Rifkin, A., Schaffer, C. and Walker, E. (1986) Facial discrimination and emotional recognition in schizophrenia and affective disorders. *Archives of General Psychiatry*, **43**, 276–279.

Green, M.F. (1996) What are the functional consequences of neurocognitive deficits in schizophrenia? *American Journal of Psychiatry*, **153**, 321–330.

Green, M.F. and Nuechterlein, K.H. (1999) Should schizophrenia be treated as a neurocognitive disorder? *Schizophrenia Bulletin*, **25**, 309–319.

Green, M.F., Nuechterlein, K.H. and Breitmeyer, B. (1997) Backward masking performance in unaffected siblings of schizophrenia patients: evidence for a vulnerability indicator. *Archives of General Psychiatry*, **54**, 465–472.

Green, M.F., Kern, R.S., Braff, D. and Mintz, J. (2000) Neurocognition and functional outcome in schizophrenia: are we measuring the right stuff? *Schizophrenia Bulletin*, **26**, 119–136.

Grove, W.M., Lebow, B.S., Clementz, B.A., Cerri, A., Medus, C. and Iacono, W.G. (1991) Familial prevalence and coaggregation of schizotypy indicators: a multitrait family study. *Journal of Abnormal Psychology*, **100**, 115–121.

Harvey, P.D., Sukhodolsky, D., Parrella, M., White, L. and Davidson, M. (1997) The association between adaptive and cognitive deficits in geriatric chronic schizophrenic patients. *Schizophrenia Research*, **27**, 211–218.

Harvey, P.D., Howanitz, E., Parrella, M., White, L., Davidson, M., Mohs, R.C., Hoblyn, J. and Davis, K.L. (1998) Symptoms, cognitive functioning, and adaptive skills in geriatric patients with lifelong schizophrenia: a comparison across treatment sites. *American Journal of Psychiatry*, **155**, 1080–1086.

Heaton, R.K. and Pendelton, M.G. (1981) Use of neuropsychological tests to predict adult patients' everyday functioning. *Journal of Consulting and Clinical Psychology*, **49**, 807–821.

Heaton, R.K., Baade, L.E. and Johnson, K.L. (1978) Neuropsychological test results associated with psychiatric disorders in adults. *Psychology Bulletin*, **85**, 141–162.

Heaton, R.K., Velin, R.A., McCutchan, J.A., Gulevich, S.J., Atkinson, J.H., Wallace, M.R. *et al.* (1994) Neuropsychological impairment in human immunodeficiency virus-infection: implications for employment. *Psychosomatic Medicine*, **56**, 8–17.

Heslegrave, R.J., Awad, A.G. and Voruganti, L.N.P. (1997) The influence of neurocognitive deficits and symptoms on quality of life in schizophrenia. *Journal of Psychiatry and Neuroscience*, **22**, 235–243.

Kee, K.S., Kern, R.S. and Green, M.F. (1998) Perception of emotion and neurocognitive functioning in schizophrenia: what's the link? *Psychiatry Research*, **81**, 57–65.

Keefe, R.S.E., Silverman, J., Mohs, R.C., Siever, L.J, Harvey, P.D., Friedman, L. *et al.* (1997) Eye tracking, attention, and schizotypal personality symptoms in nonpsychotic relatives of patients with schizophrenia. *Archives of General Psychiatry*, **54**, 169–177.

Kemp, R. and David, A. (1996) Psychological predictors of insight and compliance in psychotic patients. *British Journal of Psychiatry*, **169**, 444–450.

Kerr, S.L. and Neale, J.M. (1993) Emotion perception in schizophrenia: specific deficit or further evidence of generalized poor performance? *Journal of Abnormal Psychology*, **102**, 312–318.

Klapow, J.C., Evans, J., Patterson, T.L., Heaton, R.K., Koch, W.L. and Jeste, D.V. (1997) Direct assessment of functional status in older patients with schizophrenia. *American Journal of Psychiatry*, **154**, 1022–1024.

Lenzenweger, M.F., Cornblatt, B.A. and Putnick, M. (1991) Schizotypy and sustained attention. *Journal of Abnormal Psychology*, **100**, 84–89.

Lezak, M.D. (1995) *Neuropsychological Assessment*. Oxford University Press, New York.

Lysaker, P. and Bell, M. (1994) Insight and cognitive impairments in schizophrenia: performance on repeated administrations of the Wisconsin Card Sorting Test. *Journal of Nervous and Mental Disease*, **182**, 656–660.

Lysaker, P. and Bell, M. (1995) Work rehabilitation and improvements in insight in schizophrenia. *Journal of Nervous and Mental Disease*, **183**, 103–107.

Lysaker, P., Bell, M., Milstein, R., Bryson, G. and Beam-Goulet, J. (1994) Insight and psychosocial treatment compliance in schizophrenia. *Psychiatry*, **57**, 307–315.

Lysaker, P., Bell, M., Bryson, G. and Kaplan, E. (1998) Neurocognitive function and insight in schizophrenia: support for an association with impairments in executive function but not with impairments in global function. *Acta Psyciatrica Scandinavica*, **97**, 297–301.

McEvoy, J.P., Freter, S., Everett, G., Geller, J.L., Appelbaum, P.S., Apperson, L.J. *et al.* (1989) Insight and the clinical outcome of schizophrenics. *Journal of Nervous and Mental Disease*, **177**, 48–51.

McGlashan, T.H. and Carpenter, W.T. (1981) Does attitude toward psychosis relate to outcome? American *Journal of Psychiatry,* **138**, 797–801.

McKee, M., Hull, J.W. and Smith, T.E. (1997) Cognitive and symptom correlates of participation in social skills training groups. *Schizophrenia Research*, **23**, 223–229.

Miller, S., Saccuzzo, D. and Braff, D. (1979) Information processing deficits in remitted schizophrenics. *Journal of Abnormal Psychology*, **88**, 446–449.

Mirsky, A.F., Lockhead, S.J., Jones, B.P., Kugelmass, S., Walsh, D. and Kendler, K.S. (1992) On familial factors in the attentional deficit in schizophrenia: a review and report of two new subject samples. *Journal of Psychiatric Research*, 26, 383–403.

Mueser, K.T., Doonan, R., Penn, D.L., Blanchard, J.J., Bellack, A.S., Nishith, P. and deLeon, J. (1996) Emotion recognition and social competence in chronic schizophrenia. *Journal of Abnormal Psychology*, **105**, 271–275.

Nuechterlein, K.H. (1983) Signal detection in vigilance tasks and behavioral attributes among offspring of schizophrenic mothers and among hyperactive children. *Journal of Abnormal Psychology*, **92**, 4–28.

Nuechterlein, K.H., Dawson, M.E., Gitlin, M., Ventura, J., Goldstein, M.J., Snyder, K.S. *et al.* (1992) Developmental processes in schizophrenic disorders: longitudinal studies of vulnerability and stress. *Schizophrenia Bulletin*, **18**, 387–425.

Penn, D.L., Spaulding, W., Reed, D. and Sullivan, M. (1996) The relationship of social cognition to ward behavior in chronic schizophrenia. *Schizophrenia Research*, **20**, 327–335.

Rutschmann, J., Cornblatt, B. and Erlenmeyer-Kimling, L. (1986) Sustained attention in children at risk for schizophrenia: findings with two visual continuous performance tests in a new sample. *Journal of Abnormal Child Psychology*, **14**, 365–385.

Schneider, F., Gur, R.C., Gur, R.E. and Shtasel, D.L. (1995) Emotional processing in schizophrenia: neurobehavioral probes in relation to psychopathology. *Schizophrenia Research*, **17**, 67–75.

Schwartz, R.C. (1998) The relationship between insight, illness and treatment outcome in schizophrenia. *Psychiatric Quarterly*, **69**, 1–22.

Silverstein, S.M., Schenkel, L.S., Valone, C. and Nuernberger, S.W. (1998) Cognitive deficits and psychiatric rehabilitation outcomes in schizophrenia. *Psychiatric Quarterly*, **69**, 169–191.

Startup, M. (1996) Insight and cognitive deficits in schizophrenia: evidence for a curvilinear relationship. *Psychological Medicine*, **26**, 1277–1281.

Steinhauer, S.R., Zubin, J., Condray, R., Shaw, D.B., Peters, J.L. and Van Kammen, D.P. (1991) Electrophysiological and behavioral signs of attentional disturbance in schizophrenics and their siblings. In: Tamminga, C.A. and Schulz, S.C. (eds), *Advances in Neuropsychiatry and Psychopharmacology, Volume 1: Schizophrenia Research*. Raven Press, New York, pp. 169–178.

Turner, J.L.B. (1964) Schizophrenics as judges of vocal expressions of emotional meaning. In: Davitz, J.R. (ed.), *The Communication of Emotional Meaning*. McGraw-Hill, New York, pp. 129–142.

Voruganti, L.N.P., Heslegrave, R.J. and Awad, A.G. (1997) Neurocognitive correlates of positive and negative syndromes in schizophrenia. *Canadian Journal of Psychiatry*, **42**, 1066–1071.

Walker, E., McGuire, M. and Bettes, B. (1984) Recognition and identification of facial stimuli by schizophrenics and patients with affective disorders. *British Journal of Clinical Psychology*, **23**, 37–44.

Young, D.A., Davila, R. and Scher, H. (1993) Unawareness of illness and neuropsychological performance in chronic schizophrenia. *Schizophrenia Research*, **10**, 117–124.

Young, D.A., Zakzanis, K.K., Bailey, C., Davila, R., Griese, J., Sartory, G. *et al.* (1998) Further parameters of insight and neuropsychological deficit in schizophrenia and other chronic mental disease. *Journal of Nervous and Mental Disease*, **186**, 44–50.

10 Cognitive functioning and negative symptoms in schizophrenia

Jean Addington

Introduction

The 19th century British neurologist Hughlings Jackson was one of the first to use the terms negative and positive symptoms in psychiatry. Jackson speculated that negative symptoms were a result of a disease-induced loss of higher mental functioning (1958). It was not until 1974 that John Strauss and his colleagues (Strauss *et al.*, 1974) suggested that these phenomenologies of positive and negative symptoms represented distinct pathophysiologies within schizophrenia. Crow in the UK, who postulated that there were two syndromes in schizophrenia (1980, 1985), developed this hypothesis more fully. He called these two syndromes type 1 and type 2 schizophrenia. Patients with type 1 had predominantly positive symptoms that were considered to be responsive to neuroleptics, with good premorbid functioning, an acute onset, a better long-term course and outcome, and cognitive deterioration. Type 2 was characterized by mainly negative symptoms that were drug resistant, with poorer premorbid functioning, an insidious onset, a poorer long-term course and outcome, and cognitive deterioration. Crow believed that type 1 reflected reversible hyperdopaminergic activity in a structurally normal brain, and type 2 irreversible neuronal loss in a structurally abnormal brain (1980, 1985).

In the USA, Nancy Andreasen and her colleagues at the University of Iowa were responsible for much of the impetus for empirical work in the area of positive and negative symptoms of schizophrenia (Andreasen, 1982; Andreasen and Olsen, 1982; Andreasen *et al.*, 1986, 1995). Subsequently, over the next decade, a multitude of articles on the positive and negative symptoms of schizophrenia appeared in the literature, particularly after scales for assessing positive and negative symptoms became available. Such studies addressed the phenomenology of positive and negative symptoms and their connections to biology, genetics, family history, treatment responsiveness, long-term course and outcome, and cognitive functioning.

Assessment of negative symptoms

Negative symptoms represent the absence of a behavior or implied function. Consequently, they are one of the more difficult clinical phenomena to measure with acceptable reliability and validity. Several systems, which have been reviewed and compared, have been devised to define positive and negative symptoms (Fenton and McGlashan, 1992). Which symptoms are considered positive or negative varies across these systems. All systems include flat affect and poverty of speech among the negative symptoms, with most systems including anhedonia, apathy and avolition as negative symptoms. Andreasen (1982) defined negative symptoms as impoverished speech and thinking, affective flattening, avolition, anhedonia and impaired attention. Crow's definition included poverty of speech, psychomotor retardation and flat affect (Crow, 1985).

The first scales that were used to assess positive and negative symptoms were general symptom scales such as the Krawiecka Scale (Krawiecka *et al.*, 1977) or the Brief Psychiatric Rating Scale (BPRS) (Overall and Gorham, 1962). In the 1980s, several new scales were developed. The most widely used was the Scale for the Assessment of Negative Symptoms (SANS) (Andreasen, 1982; Andreasen and Olsen, 1982). A later development was the Positive and Negative Syndrome Scale (PANSS) (Kay *et al.*, 1987). This is one of the most widely used scales today.

Negative symptoms formed a more coherent construct than the positive symptoms (Bilder *et al.*, 1984; Liddle, 1987a; Addington and Addington, 1991). Compared with positive symptoms, negative symptoms were seen as more stable, persistent and predictive of long-term outcome (McGlashan and Fenton, 1992). In the acute phases of the illness or in first-episode cases, negative symptoms were less frequent than in the later stages of the illness. Often they co-occurred with other signs of psychosis including positive symptoms (McGlashan and Fenton, 1992).

The association of negative symptoms and cognitive functioning

Cross-sectional studies

In their initial studies, Andreasen and Crow reported that those individuals with schizophrenia who had predominantly negative symptoms evidenced more cognitive impairment than those patients with predominantly positive symptoms. Their work stimulated interest in examining further the associations between cognitive functioning and positive and negative symptoms. As a result, a large number of hypotheses, which were both scientifically interesting and testable, were pursued.

The first group of studies began to examine the possibility that positive and negative symptoms were associated with different patterns of performance deficits on neurocognitive tests and not that negative symptoms were associated uniquely with general cognitive impairment. Many of these studies have been reviewed (Walker and Lewine, 1988; Strauss, 1993). In several of the studies, symptoms were treated as categorical variables, and subjects were divided into subgroups such as positive, negative and mixed. Groups were then compared on their cognitive performance. This design was based on the assumptions that either the symptoms reflected distinct subgroups or that they possibly were etiologically dissimilar.

Several studies, all using the SANS as a measure of negative symptoms, examined a measure of early visual processing, backward masking. In a preliminary study with 14 patients, Green and Walker (1984) demonstrated that negative symptom patients required a significantly longer critical interstimulus interval to identify the stimulus correctly. These results were replicated later in a larger sample (Green and Walker, 1986). Braff (1989) reported that in a sample of 40 hospitalized patients, those classified as negative or mixed performed less well than non-psychiatric control subjects but not less well than positive symptom patients. They did, however, require longer stimulus duration compared with those subjects in the positive symptom group. More recently, using SANS data as categorical variables, Slaghuis and Bakker (1995) compared non-psychiatric controls with positive symptom and negative symptom out-patients on target duration threshold of forward and backward masking of contour by light. Here, the only significant difference reported was between the negative group and the controls. Finally, in a categorical study, Hawkins compared 46 schizophrenia out-patients, 22 bipolar patients and 26 non-psychiatric control subjects on measures of attention, language and IQ (Hawkins *et al.*, 1997). The 21 subjects in the negative group displayed inferior cognitive ability.

Many studies failed to support the hypothesis that positive and negative symptoms defined either a dichotomy or opposite ends of a positive/negative continuum. Therefore, the second group of studies began to consider positive and negative symptoms as continuous variables and used correlational analysis. Such studies do not make the assumption that symptoms reflect subgroups. Furthermore, they make more use of the data. Green and Walker (1985) assessed 44 in-patients on the SANS and on a range of cognitive tests. It was hard to identify any consistent trends from the group comparisons between the negative symptom patients and the positive symptom patients. However, when symptoms were used as continuous variables, the results suggested that negative symptoms were significant predictors of visual memory, motor speed and dexterity tasks. High positive symptoms reportedly were associated with poor scores on certain verbal tasks. The implication was that the various cognitive tests were associated differentially with positive and negative symptoms. Cornblatt and her associates (Cornblatt *et al.*, 1985) examined negative symptoms and attentional processes, and suggested that positive symptoms were associated with distractibility and negative symptoms were related to more complex cognitive deficits.

These initial studies concluded that potentially negative symptoms were associated with poor performance on tests that measure visuomotor and visuospatial skills, and positive symptoms were related to deficits on tests such as verbal memory and distractibility (Green and Walker, 1985; Spring *et al.*, 1991). Patterns of associations between cognitive functioning and negative and positive symptoms appeared to depend on the sensory modality of the cognitive task being used. Of course, these results were not evidence of any underlying processes that may be connecting the symptoms of schizophrenia with cognition. Nevertheless, they were seen as exciting beginnings.

Brain connections

The similarity of negative symptoms to those symptoms seen in the frontal lobe syndromes subsequent to brain injury led to hypotheses that the frontal lobes may play a role in schizophrenia. These potential connections were reinforced by findings by Weinberger (Weinberger, 1987; Berman and Weinberger, 1990) whose data showed that individuals with schizophrenia demonstrated less activation in their frontal lobes during a prefrontal type task. The studies that followed focused on testing hypotheses of potential connections between negative symptoms and specific brain regions, in particular connections between negative symptoms and measures that reflected frontal lobe functioning. However, discrepant results began to emerge.

Breier and his colleagues (Breier *et al.*, 1990) reported a significant relationship between performance on the Wisconsin Card Sorting Test (WCST) and negative symptoms, as well as a significant association between verbal fluency and negative symptoms. Braff *et al.* (1991) found that WCST perseverative errors were significantly correlated with both positive and negative symptoms. Other studies were unable to demonstrate a relationship between either verbal fluency or WCST scores and negative symptoms (Morrison-Stewart *et al.*, 1992). These authors did report an association of verbal memory with negative symptoms. When the PANSS was used in a study with 29 chronic in-patients, negative symptoms were associated with poor performance on the WCST and Trails A, but not with verbal fluency (Berman *et al.*, 1997).

Finally, in a recent study by Addington and Addington (1998a) with first-episode patients, there were some interesting results. A sample of 53 individuals who were experiencing their first episode of schizophrenia or schizophreniform disorder was compared with a sample of 76 multi-episode patients. These first-episode patients had significantly less negative symptoms than the multi-episode patients as assessed by the PANSS. In both groups, negative symptoms were associated with verbal memory and performance on the WCST. Interestingly, in this first-episode sample, as a group, they performed significantly better on the WCST than the more chronic patients. Two-thirds had normal scores on the WCST, with one-third performing as poorly as the more chronic group. It was this third who exhibited significantly more severe negative symptoms.

Three-dimensional models

Crow did not regard type 1 and type 2 schizophrenia as mutually exclusive. Instead, he considered them to be independent dimensions reflecting different underlying pathological processes. Andreasen and Olson (1982) considered positive and negative symptoms as characteristic of two different types of illness. The type 1 and type 2 model has been challenged by Liddle (1987a) because neither a unidimensional nor a two-factor model appeared to account for the correlational patterns previously described. Liddle (1987a) suggested three factors: the psychomotor poverty syndrome, which is essentially negative symptoms; the disorganization syndrome; and the reality distortion syndrome. Other research groups have considered three symptom dimensions and agreed that the symptoms from the SANS and SAPS (Scale for the Assessment of Positive Symptoms) fit well as a three-factor model (Bilder *et al.*, 1985; Liddle, 1987a; Arndt *et al.*, 1991). The SANS components all load on one factor, and the SAPS divides into two independent dimensions. This three-factor model of negative symptoms, delusions/hallucinations and thought disorder appears robust. Addington and Addington (1991) reported similar factors in a sample of clinically stable patients. However, the factors were not as clearly defined when the symptom ratings were obtained 6 months earlier during a period of acute relapse.

Thus, the third group of studies focused on the relationship between symptom dimensions and performance on neurocognitive tests. In one of the first studies looking at symptom dimensions, Bilder identified three clusters of symptoms (Bilder *et al.*, 1985). The first cluster appeared to reflect primarily a disorganization of thought, the second cluster reflected predominantly flat affect and volition, i.e. negative symptoms, and the third cluster represented florid psychotic features. This study, with a sample of 32 in-patients, used the SANS to assess negative symptoms. The neuropsychological assessment consisted of 35 tests covering a wide range of cognition. Cognitive impairment was associated most strongly with the disorganization factor, less with negative symptoms and not with the third factor of florid symptoms. Using similar factors, Liddle (1987b) reported that the psychomotor poverty syndrome, which best reflected negative symptoms, was associated with impaired abstract thinking and long-term memory. In a follow-up study, which specifically examined measures of frontal lobe functioning, Liddle and Morris (1991) reported that measures that reflected frontal lobe functioning, such as verbal fluency, perseverative errors on the WCST, performance on the Stroop and Trails A, were associated with the psychomotor poverty syndrome.

Our data demonstrated that the negative symptom factor was associated with verbal ability, verbal fluency and poor performance on the WCST (Addington *et al.*, 1991). In comparison, a Dutch study with 60 in-patient adolescents (Van Der Does *et al.*, 1993) reported that there was no relationship between negative symptoms assessed by the expanded BPRS and the Dutch version of COGLAB, a computerized battery of cognitive tasks (Spaulding *et al.*, 1989). These studies utilizing symptom dimensions or factors usually revealed significant associations between cognitive functioning and the negative symptom factor. However, it must be noted that there were also strong associations between cognitive impairment and the factor that reflects disorganization. There was no association with the dimension of hallucinations and delusions.

The deficit syndrome

A later definition of negative symptoms was the deficit syndrome. Carpenter and his colleagues (1988) distinguished between two types of negative symptoms, primary and secondary, on the basis of their causative mechanism. Primary negative symptoms are considered to be deficit symptoms. It was proposed that they are a purer form of negative symptoms and are the core enduring feature of the illness. They do require longitudinal observation. Secondary symptoms are considered to be temporary and associated with other factors that are not inherent to schizophrenia, for example depression or side effects from medications. The deficit–non-deficit distinction is stable over time and has long-term predictive validity (Fenton and McGlashan, 1992). There is evidence from several other studies that deficit patients have poorer premorbid adjustment, more neurological signs and more difficulties with eye tracking than non-deficit patients (Buchanan *et al.*, 1990, 1994).

The neuroanatomical substrate of deficit symptoms has been addressed and reviewed in the literature (Buchanan *et al.*, 1990, 1994). There are positron emission tomography studies that support the involvement of the frontal and parietal lobes (Tamminga *et al.*, 1992). There are also functional imaging studies that confirm an association between negative symptoms and decreased glucose utilization or decreased regional cerebral blood flow (rCBF) in the frontal lobes, and between negative symptoms and decreased rCBF in the inferior parietal cortex. It is possible that frontal and parietal cortices have interdependent interconnections and connections with the thalamus and other brain regions implicated in the studies of glucose utilization and, secondly, they are also connected through the involvement in the basal ganglia–thalamocortical circuits. Buchanan *et al.* hypothesized: "the involvement of the dorsolateral prefrontal circuit in the production of deficit symptoms as it is composed of the brain regions, e.g. the dorsolateral prefrontal and inferior parietal cortices and the thalamus, implicated in the pathophysiological features of the deficit syndrome." (Buchanan *et al.*, 1994, p. 806).

Therefore, it was expected that deficit patients would perform more poorly on frontal and parietal cognitive measures than non-deficit patients (Buchanan *et al.*, 1994). In this study, memory tasks, which are considered to be sensitive to temporal lobe regions, were used as control tasks. The two groups were hypothesized not to differ in their performance on these tasks because temporal lobe abnormalities have been implicated in the production of positive symptoms. The sample consisted of 18 deficit out-patients, 21 non-deficit out-patients and 13 control subjects. The pattern of deficit, non-deficit and normal control group differences varied across the tests. Deficit patients performed significantly less well on two of the four frontal measures (Stroop and Trail making test but not WCST or verbal fluency). Deficit patients performed less well on one of the three visuospatial measures of parietal functioning. There were no significant differences between the two schizophrenia subgroups on any of the memory tasks. Deficit patients did have lower WAIS-R general ability scores. Using general ability as a co-variant, the general pattern did not change but magnitudes were reduced to trend instead of significant levels. The non-deficit patients did not differ from non-psychiatric controls on the measures that actually differentiated the deficit and non-deficit patients. Furthermore, since the groups were similar on many clinical and demographic variables, these authors proposed that the observed cognitive differences were due to deficit symptoms.

Recently Buchanan and his colleagues (Buchanan *et al.*, 1997) reported that deficit symptom patients performed less well on the Continuous Performance Test (CPT) and Span of Apprehension task (SPAN) than non-deficit patients and normal controls. Such results support the hypothesis that primary and enduring negative symptoms may represent a core feature of schizophrenia and that it is the patients with enduring negative symptoms that have more difficulty with allocation and activating attention. This supports the idea that although deficits on the CPT and the SPAN are considered to be stable, their association with negative symptoms is with the negative symptoms that remain into a period of remission, i.e. core negative symptoms.

Longitudinal studies

Since negative symptoms are more trait-like than delusions and hallucinations, it would be useful to determine whether the cognitive correlates of negative symptoms are more persistent than those of positive symptoms. Longitudinal studies, however, are rare. In one study, we examined 38 patients during an acute relapse and again 6 months later during a period of relative remission (Addington *et al.*, 1991). Negative symptoms were related to poor performance on verbal reasoning and verbal fluency at both assessment periods. Significant associations of poor cognitive functioning and positive symptoms that were observed in the acute phase were no longer significant during the period of remission after a significant improvement in positive symptoms had occurred. Brekke *et al.* (1995) assessed 40 out-patients using the BPRS as a measure of negative symptoms. At the initial assessment, negative symptoms were associated with poor performance on the Stroop. At the 6 month follow-up assessment, negative symptoms correlated again with the Stroop but also with digit–symbol, a measure of visuomotor processing. These results support the persistence of the connection between negative symptoms and poor cognitive functioning. In a second longitudinal study (Addington *et al.*, 1997), our results were that in a sample of 59 individuals with schizophrenia, neither positive nor negative symptoms were related to a measure of distractibility at either hospitalization for an acute episode or during a period of relative remission 3 months later. This was a measure that previously had been considered to be associated uniquely with positive symptoms.

Vulnerability markers

A further series of longitudinal studies have been published. These studies not only considered the longitudinal relationship between negative symptoms and neurocognitive functioning but also whether certain cognitive deficits that are considered to be vulnerability markers could actually be considered to be negative symptom-linked vulnerability indicators.

From the literature (Nuechterlein and Dawson, 1984), it is evident that certain aspects of information processing are deficient in schizophrenia. One research strategy (Spring *et al.*, 1990) has been to separate deficits that are episode indicators (i.e. impairments that appear with an exacerbation of symptoms and normalize when the symptoms dissipate) from more lasting characteristics that are vulnerability indicators (i.e. impairments that are evident in high risk groups, actively psychotic and remitted schizophrenia patients). Two of the primary measures of visual attention that have been considered to be vulnerability indicators are the CPT (Nuechterlein, 1991; Cornblatt and Kelip, 1994;) and the forced-choice SPAN (Asarnow *et al.*, 1991). These versions of the CPT and the SPAN place a burden on certain aspects of information processing and require a high processing load.

There is a large body of literature that shows that deficits on these two measures have been found in schizophrenia patients who are actively psychotic, who are in remission and in high risk groups (Asarnow *et al.*, 1991; Nuechterlein, 1991). Consistent results have been found more with the CPT than with the SPAN (Harvey *et al.*, 1985). Furthermore, it has been suggested that deficits on the CPT and SPAN may be negative symptom-linked vulnerability indicators. Deficits on the CPT and the SPAN have been reported to be associated with negative but not positive symptoms (Nuechterlein *et al.*, 1986; Asarnow *et al.*, 1991; Strauss *et al.*, 1993). In Strauss' study, however, negative symptoms did not account for variance in SPAN scores after controlling for verbal ability. Ito *et al.* (1997), in a study with 43 in-patients, reported no relationship between negative symptoms and the CPT or the SPAN. This was contrary to previously reported results.

A vulnerability-linked indicator of schizophrenia must also differentiate between schizophrenia patients and other psychiatric patients. Several studies support the relevance of the CPT deficits to schizophrenia as opposed to psychopathology in general (Asarnow and MacCrimmon, 1981; Walker, 1981; Harris *et al.*, 1985; Cornblatt *et al.*, 1989a; Nuechterlein *et al.*, 1992). However, there are inconsistencies in the results (Strauss *et al.*, 1987; Rund *et al.*, 1992).

A further demonstration of vulnerability is that deficits on these measures of attention remain stable regardless of changes in symptoms (Cornblatt and Kelip, 1994). In both multi-episode and first-episode samples, deficits on the CPT and SPAN have been found to remain stable over time despite an improvement in symptoms (Asarnow and MacCrimmon, 1982; Nuechterlein *et al.*, 1986, 1992; Cornblatt *et al.*, 1989b; Winters *et al.*, 1991).

Nuechterlein and his colleagues at UCLA (1986), in a longitudinal study with 40 young patients with a recent onset of schizophrenia, indicated that deficits on the CPT and the SPAN consistently were related to the presence of negative symptoms (BPRS anergia factors). The magnitude of the relationships did not change across assessments of the measures of visual attention. In our study (Addington and Addington, 1997a), schizophrenia subjects, despite a significant improvement in symptoms, showed stable deficits on the CPT and the SPAN from a period of hospitalization for relapse to a period of relative remission 3 months later. There were no associations between the visual attention tasks and positive symptom at either hospitalization or at the 3 month follow-up. At the 3 month follow-up, poor visual attention was significantly associated with high levels of negative symptoms (Addington and Addington, 1997a).

These results supported the conclusion that the deficit in attention was not simply linked to negative symptoms that were present concurrently, which would be expected if attention deficits were secondary to clinical symptomatology (Nuechterlein *et al.*, 1986). One conclusion was that these deficits in visual attention might have trait qualities that are associated with the development of negative symptoms, in particular the negative symptoms that remain into a period of relative remission. These results offer partial support for the hypothesis that deficits in visual attention may be negative symptom-linked vulnerability indicators.

We recently designed a study to test the hypothesis that, if deficits in visual attention are stable and are related to negative symptoms, such attentional deficits would be associated with negative symptoms assessed at a later point during continued remission. Using the same sample as the earlier report (Addington and Addington, 1997a), positive and negative symptoms were re-assessed 12 months after the acute episode. Results of this study confirmed that there were no significant relationships between positive symptoms and visual attention (Addington and Addington, 1998b). Furthermore, in this follow-up study, there were no significant associations between attention which had been assessed at the 3 month mark and negative symptoms assessed at 12 months. Thus the hypothesis that the association between poor performance on the CPT and SPAN and higher levels of negative symptoms would remain constant at later points of assessment during the illness was not supported. An examination of the data revealed that following an acute relapse, improvement in positive symptoms appeared to be achieved by the 3 month period. This was not the case with negative symptoms. The remission of negative symptoms continued until 1 year following the acute relapse.

One possible explanation suggested by Harvey is that cognitive impairment is an autonomous feature of the symptomatology of schizophrenia but it does overlap with negative symptoms (Harvey *et al.*, 1996). These authors published a 1 year follow-up with 174 elderly chronic patients (average age of 75 years) (Harvey *et al.*, 1996). In this study, negative symptoms and cognitive functioning were stable over time. Cognitive impairment was more stable than negative symptoms. There was no evidence of a cross-temporal relationship between cognitive impairment at the initial assessment and negative symptoms at the follow-up. There was a consistent finding, however, of a concurrent correlation between the composite measure of cognitive functioning and negative symptoms. These authors conclude that cognitive functioning and negative symptoms are actually discernible but related constructs.

Another explanation may be that attention is significantly associated with the negative symptoms that remain into a period of remission, as was suggested in our earlier paper. However, it appears that the negative symptoms that remain into remission are those assessed at 12 months and not those assessed at the 3 month follow-up. Buchanan demonstrated that it was the patients with enduring negative symptoms that had more difficulty with allocation and activating attention (Buchanan *et al.*, 1997). This supports the idea that, although deficits on the CPT and the SPAN are considered to be stable, their association with negative symptoms is with the negative symptoms that remain into a period of remission, i.e. core negative symptoms. The implication of our 12 month follow-up study is that cognitive variables under consideration should be measured at the point of remission of negative symptoms. This is more likely to be 12 months rather than 3 months after an acute relapse.

In summary, there are replicated results of associations between negative symptoms and information processing tasks such as backward masking, the CPT and the SPAN. Associations of negative symptoms with verbal ability, verbal and visual memory, visuospatial and motor tasks have also been replicated, as has performance on the WCST and other measures of frontal lobe functioning. There are, however, inconsistent results, with many studies reporting negative findings. Consideration of several methodological issues may contribute to a better understanding of the variation in findings.

Methodological issues

The nature of negative symptoms

One reason for the lack of consistency in results may be the definition of negative symptoms used. A range of measures that assess negative symptoms continues to be used. In many studies, a negative symptom is defined on the basis of one cross-sectional observation. In other studies, consistency across longitudinal observations of varying length, often 1 year, is required. Even if there are comparable definitions, the reliability with which they are applied may vary across studies. Considering symptoms as three factors or dimensions rather than as a positive–negative distinction may be more valid in predicting cognitive impairment. Greater coherence exists among negative symptoms, thus they may be treated usefully as one construct.

Another source of variability in findings derives from the possibility that there may be different types of negative symptoms or that negative symptoms vary depending on the phase of the illness. McGlashan and Fenton (1992) outlined three negative symptom phases that may be separate or that may represent qualitatively different underlying processes at work. The first phase is associated with compromised premorbid functioning and suggests a link between negative symptoms and the vulnerability to schizophrenia. This may be genetic in origin. The second negative symptom process is associated with the acute and/or florid states of schizophrenia. At this time, similarly to positive symptoms, negative symptoms are relatively unstable and may vary with treatments and environmental stress. The third negative symptom process is associated with the longer term more chronic phase of the illness. In this stage, negative symptoms are more prominent, persistent, resistant to intervention and can be functionally disabling.

Clearly, differences in defining the negative syndrome across studies have made cross-study comparisons very difficult. Results may even vary depending on the measure used for negative symptoms. Eighteen years have passed since the publication of Crow's seminal paper, and a consensus has not yet been developed regarding the best means of defining negative symptoms.

Sampling

The power of many of the studies is questionable because sample sizes, particularly in the earlier studies, were often small. However, results reported in small samples have sometimes been replicated in larger samples. Secondly, the research represents a wide range of patients. Samples include acutely ill inpatients, chronically institutionalized in-patients, stable out-patients, geriatric patients and first-episode patients. Nevertheless, there are some consistent results across these different types of patient samples. Thirdly, the majority of the studies are cross-sectional, with few longitudinal studies. Although longitudinal studies have an advantage over cross-sectional designs, studies of schizophrenia symptoms and their correlates may require longitudinal studies that are more than 3 or 6 months, as the Addington study has demonstrated (Addington and Addington, 1998b).

Continuous versus categorical variables

In the early research, more consistent results were reported with continuous variables. However, the issue of continuous versus categorical variables with respect to negative symptoms deserves revisiting. Many patients have both positive and negative symptoms, making it difficult to divide schizophrenia subjects accurately into positive and negative groups. Continuous measures are more appropriate for testing hypotheses concerning the relationship between symptom severity and cognitive impairment. However, if we want to divide schizophrenia subjects into two groups based on the presence or absence of certain criteria (e.g. deficit symptoms) rather than on the severity of negative symptoms and then to compare these two groups on some criteria of interest (e.g. cognitive impairment), then using symptoms as categorical variables is more valid. This avoids the risk of a type II error that might occur in a design using symptoms as continuous variables, because those with high and low symptom levels might exhibit the same cognitive impairment (Buchanan and Carpenter, 1997).

Generalized versus specific cognitive deficit

The search for a characteristic cognitive profile in schizophrenia is a search for a differential deficit. Compared with non-psychiatric controls, schizophrenia patients as a group almost always have poorer performance on neurocognitive tasks. One question that is often asked is whether they perform slightly less well than controls on some cognitive tasks and much less well than controls on other tasks. If two groups appear to differ more on one test than on another, it may reflect a true differential deficit, or it may reflect psychometric differences because one test has more power to discriminate between groups that the other. This issue has been argued in the literature without consensus. Thus, in the research reviewed here, it is possible that observed differences on selected cognitive measures are due to the differential discriminating power of the measures and not due to specific behavioral abnormalities.

Additionally, one hypothesis is that cognitive impairment may reflect some specific deficits against a background of generalized deficits. Therefore, understanding the role of intelligence and general abilities in the cognitive performance of individuals with schizophrenia is important in interpreting cognitive results. A number of investigations have reported significant relationships between intelligence and negative symptoms (Crow, 1985; Addington et al., 1991; Braff et al., 1991). There also appears to be a complex interaction between intelligence and the deficit syndrome. Therefore, it may not be possible to separate the effects of intelligence from more specific impairments on cognitive and information processing tasks using statistical means (Buchanan et al., 1994).

Cognitive deficits and negative symptoms—distinct constructs?

It is possible that cognitive impairment, although related to negative symptoms, is a distinct construct. The observation of cognitive deficits in unaffected family members implies that cognitive impairment reflects more of a vulnerability to the disorder and not just a relationship to the symptoms (Green et al., 1997). The independence of the cognitive symptom construct is supported further by recent work that demonstrated that poor cognitive functioning predicted poor social problem solving (Addington and Addington, 1999). Here it was not possible to assess whether negative symptoms were independent of the relationship between neurocognitive functioning and social functioning. What we were able to demonstrate was that the associations between social problem solving and cognitive functioning were not due entirely to negative symptoms. Moreover, the negative symptoms on the PANSS include items that reflect social contact which may have inflated the relationships between the social functioning measures and negative symptoms. If a narrower measure of negative symptoms had been used, the relationship between symptoms and social outcome may have been reduced.

Another source of evidence that symptom changes are not necessary paralleled by changes in cognitive functioning is studies of pharmacological interventions. Data here are preliminary. In a series of case studies that were part of a randomized control trial for treatment-resistant patients, there were significant changes in cognitive functioning (WCST, CPT, visual recall) for those patients treated with risperidone versus haloperidol. However, there was no change in positive and negative symptoms (Addington and Addington, 1997b). In a trial that demonstrated an advantage for risperidone in improving cognition, improvement in verbal memory remained after controlling for improvement in negative symptoms (Green *et al.*, 1997).

Finally, research examining negative symptoms and cognitive functioning is descriptive and not explanatory. The theoretical basis of the relationship between cognition and negative symptoms is tenuous, with the etiology remaining unclear. Cognitive and negative symptoms of the illness are related on a correlational basis, and positive symptoms appear relatively independent of both. Thus, it is possible that there is a common cause of cognitive deficits and negative symptoms. Harvey (Harvey *et al.*, 1996) gives example of this possibility based on potential etiology. If negative symptoms result from abnormal thalamic activation through connections to the frontal cortex and cognitive deficits result from the same abnormal activation, this time coming through temporoparietal connections, a dysfunction in a single brain region could result in two sets of related but distinct impairments. Another possibility is that negative symptoms and cognitive functioning may result from the same underlying factors, but stressors in the environment have affected both differentially. In this case, associations between negative symptoms and cognitive functioning would be decreased, even if they have similar etiologies.

Conclusions

This chapter has considered the relationship of negative symptoms of schizophrenia to cognitive functioning. Current research has established cognitive deficits as a core feature of schizophrenia. Although no clear pattern linking specific cognitive deficits with different symptoms of schizophrenia has been established consistently, many studies have examined the correlation between performance of individuals with schizophrenia on certain cognitive tasks and their negative symptoms. These cognitive deficits are often associated with negative symptoms, are independent of positive symptoms and are stable across different phases of the illness even when there is a change in symptoms. Our studies as well as others reviewed in this chapter have shown cognitive functioning to be more stable than negative symptoms. However, negative symptoms only seem to account for a small proportion of the variance in cognitive impairment, ~10%. This may account for the overall lack of consistency in the results. Finally, evidence has been presented to suggest that as one of the core features of schizophrenia, cognitive impairment, although related to negative symptoms, is a distinct construct.

References

Addington, J. and Addington, D. (1991) Positive and negative symptoms of schizophrenia: their course and relationship over time. *Schizophrenia Research*, **5**, 51–59.

Addington J. and Addington D. (1997a) Attentional vulnerability indicators in schizophrenia and bipolar disorder. *Schizophrenia Research*, **23**, 197–204.

Addington, J. and Addington, D. (1997b) Neurocognitive functioning in schizophrenia: a trial of risperidone verses haloperidol. A letter to the editor. *Canadian Journal of Psychiatry*, 983.

Addington, J. and Addington, D. (1998a) Neurocognitive functioning in first episode schizophrenia. *Schizophrenia Research*, **29**, 50.

Addington J. and Addington D. (1998b) Visual attention and symptoms in schizophrenia: a one year follow-up. *Schizophrenia Research*.

Addington J. and Addington D. (1999) Neurocognitive and social functioning in schizophrenia. *Schizophrenia Bulletin*, **25**, 173–182.

Addington, J., Addington, D. and Maticka-Tyndale, E. (1991) Cognitive functioning and positive and negative symptoms of schizophrenia. *Schizophrenia Research*, **5**, 123–134.

Addington J., Addington D. and Gasbarre, L. (1997) Distractibility and symptoms in schizophrenia. *Journal of Psychiatry and Neuroscience*, **22**, 180–184.

Andreasen, N.C. (1982) Negative symptoms in schizophrenia: definition and reliability. *Archives of General Psychiatry*, **39**, 784–788.

Andreasen, N.C. and Olsen, S. (1982) Negative versus positive schizophrenia: definition and validation. *Archives of General Psychiatry*, **39**, 789–794.

Andreasen, N.C., Nasrallah, H., Dunn, V., Olsen, S. *et al.* (1986) Structural abnormalities in the frontal system in schizophrenia: a magnetic resonance imaging study. *Archives of General Psychiatry*, **43**, 136–144.

Andreasen, N.C., Arndt, S., Alliger, R.J., Miller, D. and Flaum, M. (1995) Symptoms of schizophrenia: methods, meanings and mechanisms. *Archives of General Psychiatry*, **52**, 341–351.

Arndt, S., Alliger, R.J. and Andreasen, M.C. (1991) The distinction of positive and negative symptoms. *British Journal of Psychiatry*, **158**, 317–322.

Asarnow, R.F. and MacCrimmon, D.J. (1981) Span of Apprehension deficits during post-psychotic stages of schizophrenia. *Archives of General Psychiatry*, **38**, 1006–1011.

Asarnow, R.F. and MacCrimmon, D.J. (1982) Attention/information processing, neuropsychological functioning and thought disorder during the acute and partial recovery phases of schizophrenia: a longitudinal study. *Psychiatry Research*, **7**, 309–319.

Asarnow, R.F., Granholm, E. and Sherman, T. (1991) Span of Apprehension in schizophrenia. In: Steinhauer, S.R., Gruzelier, J.H. and Zubin, J. (eds), *Handbook of Schizophrenia. Neuropsychology, Psychophysiology and Information Processing*. Elsevier, Amsterdam, Vol. 5, pp. 335–370.

Berman, K. and Weinberger, D. (1990) Lateralization of cortical function during cognitive tasks: regional cerebral blood flow studies of normal individuals and patients with schizophrenia. *Journal of Neurology, Neurosurgery and Psychiatry*, **53**, 150–160.

Berman, I., Viegner, B., Merson, A., Allan, E., Pappas, D. and Green, A.I. (1997) Differential relationships between positive and negative symptoms and neuropsychological deficits in schizophrenia. *Schizophrenia Research*, **25**, 1–10.

Bilder, R.M., Mukherjees, Rider, R.O. and Pandurangi, A.K. (1985) Symptomatic and neuropsychological component of defect states. *Schizophrenia Bulletin*, **11**, 409–419.

Braff, D.L. (1989) Sensory input deficits and negative symptoms in schizophrenia patients. *American Journal of Psychiatry*, **146**, 1006–1011.

Braff, D., Heaton, R., Kuck, J., Cullum, M., Moranville, J. Grant, I. and Zisook, S. (1991) The generalized pattern of neuropsychological deficits in outpatients with chronic schizophrenia with heterogeneous Wisconsin Card Sorting Test results. *Archives General Psychiatry*, **48**, 891–898.

Breier, A., Schreiber, G.L., Dyer, J. and Pickar (1990) National Institute of Mental Health longitudinal study of chronic schizophrenia: prognosis and predictors of outcome. *Archives General Psychiatry*, **48**, 239–246.

Brekke, J.S., Raine, A. and Thomson, C. (1995) Cognitive and psychophysiological correlates of positive, negative, and disorganized symptoms in schizophrenia spectrum. *Psychiatry Research*, **57**, 241–250.

Buchanan, R.W. and Carpenter, W.T. (1997) The neuroanatomies of schizophrenia. *Schizophrenia Bulletin*, **23**, 367–372.

Buchanan, R.W., Kirkpatrick, B., Heinrichs, D.W. and Carpenter, W.T. (1990) Clinical correlates of the deficit syndrome of schizophrenia. *American Journal of Psychiatry*, **147**, 290–294.

Buchanan, R.W., Strauss, M.E., Kirkpatrick, R., Holstein, C., Breier, A. and Carpenter, W.T. (1994) Neuropsychological impairments in deficit vs. nondeficit forms of schizophrenia. *Archives of General Psychiatry*, **51**, 804–811.

Buchanan, R.W., Strauss, M.E., Breier, A., Kirkpatrick, B. and Carpenter, W.T. (1997) Attentional impairment in deficit and non-deficit forms of schizophrenia. *American Journal of Psychiatry*, **154**, 363–370.

Carpenter, W.T., Heinrich, D.W. and Wagman, A.M.I. (1988) Deficit and non-deficit forms of schizophrenia: the concept. *American Journal of Psychiatry*, **145**, 578–583.

Cornblatt, B.A. and Kelip, J.G. (1994) Impaired attention, genetics and the pathophysiology of schizophrenia. *Schizophrenia. Bulletin*, **20**, 31–46.

Cornblatt, B.A., Lenzenweger, M.F., Dworkin, R.H. and Erlenmeyer-Kimling, L. (1985) Positive and negative schizophrenic symptoms, attention and information processing. *Schizophrenia Bulletin*, **11**, 397–408.

Cornblatt, B.A., Lenzenweger, M.F. and Erlenmeyer-Kimling, L. (1989a) The CPT, identical pairs version: II contrasting attentional profiles in schizophrenic and depressed patients. *Psychiatry Research*, **29**, 65–85.

Cornblatt, B.A., Winters, L. and Erlenmeyer-Kimling, L. (1989b) Attentional markers of schizophrenia: evidence from the New York high risk study. In: Schulz, S.C. and Tamminga, C.A. (eds), *Schizophrenia: Scientific Progress*. Oxford University Press, New York, pp. 83–92.

Crow, T.J. (1980) Molecular pathology of schizophrenia: more than one disease process. *British Medical Journal*, **280**, 66–68.

Crow, T.J. (1985) The two syndrome concept: origins and current status. *Schizophrenia Bulletin*, **11**, 471–486.

Fenton, W.S. and McGlashan, T.H. (1992) Testing systems for assessment of negative symptoms in schizophrenia . *Archives of General Psychiatry*, **49**, 179–184.

Green, M. and Walker, E. (1984) Susceptibility to backward masking in schizophrenic patients with positive or negative symptoms. *American Journal of Psychiatry*, **141**, 1273–1275.

Green, M. and Walker, E. (1985) Neuropsychological performance and positive and negative symptoms in schizophrenia. *Journal of Abnormal Psychology*, **94**, 460–469.

Green, M. and Walker, E. (1986) Symptoms and correlates of vulnerability to backward masking in schizophrenia. *American Journal of Psychiatry*, **143**, 181–186.

Green, M.F., Neuchterlein, K.H. and Breitmeyer, B. (1997) Backward masking performance in unaffected siblings of schizophrenic patients. *Archives of General Psychiatry*, **54**, 465–472.

Harris, A., Ayers, T. and Leek, M.R. (1985) Auditory Span of Apprehension deficits in schizophrenia. *Journal of Nervous Mental Disorder*, **173**, 650–657.

Harvey, P.D., Weintraub, S. and Neale, J.M. (1985) Span of Apprehension deficits in children vulnerable to psychopathology: a failure to replicate. *Journal of Abnormal Psychology*, **94**, 410–413.

Harvey, P.D., Lombardi, J., Leibman, M., White, L., Parrella, M., Powchiak, P. and Davidson, M. (1996) Cognitive impairment and negative symptoms in geriatric and chronic schizophrenic patients: a follow-up study. *Schizophrenia Research*, **22**, 223–231.

Hawkins, K.A., Hoffman, R.E., Quinlan, D.M., Rakfeldt, J., Docherty, N.M. and Sledge, W.H. (1997) Cognition, negative symptoms, and diagnosis: a comparison of schizophrenic, bipolar, and control samples. *Journal of Neuropsychiatry and Clinical Neurosciences*, **9**, 81–89.

Ito, M., Kanno, M., Mori, Y. and Niwa, S.I. (1997) Attention deficits assessed by continuous performance test and span of apprehension test in Japanese schizophrenic patients. *Schizophrenia Research*, **23**, 205–211.

Jackson, J.H. (1958) Selected writings on John Huglings-Jackson, Vol. 2. *Evolution and Dissolution of the Nervous System*. Various papers, addresses and lectures. Taylor, J. (ed.), Basic Books, New York.

Kay, S.R., Fizbein, A. and Opler, L.A. (1987) The Positive and Negative Syndrome Scale (PANSS) for Schizophrenia. *Schizophrenia Bulletin*, **13**, 261–276.

Krawiecka, M., Goldberg, D. and Vaughan, M. (1977) A standardized psychiatric assessment scale for rating psychiatric patients. *Acta Psychiatrica Scandinavica*, **55**, 299–308.

Liddle, P.F. (1987a) The symptoms of chronic schizophrenia: a re-examination of the positive and negative dichotomy. *British Journal of Psychiatry*, **151**, 145–151.

Liddle, P.F. (1987b) Schizophrenic syndromes, cognitive performance and neurological dysfunction. *Psychological Medicine*, **16**, 49–57.

Liddle, P.F. and Morris, D.L. (1991) Schizophrenia syndromes and frontal lobe performance. *British Journal of Psychiatry*, **158**, 340–345.

McGlashan, T.H. and Fenton, W.S. (1992) The positive–negative distinction in schizophrenia—review of natural history validators. *Archives of General Psychiatry*, **49**, 63–72.

Morrison-Stewart, S.L., Williamson, P.C., Corning, W.C., Ketcher, S.P., Snow, W.G. and Mersky, H. (1992) Frontal and nonfrontal lobe neuropsychological test performance and clinical symptomatology in schizophrenia. *Psychological Medicine*, **22**, 353–359.

Nuechterlein, K.H. (1991) Vigilance in schizophrenia and related disorders. In: Steinhauer, S.R., Gruzelier, J.H. and Zubin, J. (eds), *Handbook of Schizophrenia. Neuropsychology, Psychophysiology and Information Processing*. Elsevier, Amsterdam, Vol. 5, pp. 397–433.

Nuechterlein, K.H. and Dawson, M.E. (1984) Information processing and attentional functioning in the developmental course of schizophrenia. *Schizophrenia Bulletin*, **10**, 160–203.

Nuechterlin, K.H., Edell, W.S., Norris, M. and Dawson, M.E. (1986) Attentional vulnerability indicators, thought disorder and negative symptoms. *Schizophrenia Bulletin*, **12**, 408–426.

Nuechterlein, K.H., Dawson, M.E., Gitlin, M. *et al.* (1992) Developmental processes in schizophrenia disorders: longitudinal studies of vulnerability and stress. *Schizophrenia Bulletin*, **18**, 387–425.

Overall, J.E. and Gorham, D.R. (1962) The brief psychiatric rating scale. *Psychological Reports*, **10**, 799–812.

Rund, B.R., Orbeck, A.L. and Landro, N.I. (1992) Vigilance deficits in schizophrenia and affectively disturbed patients. *Acta Psychiatrica Scandinavica*, **86**, 207–212.

Slaghuis, W.L. and Bakker, V.J. (1995) Forward and backward visual masking of contour by light in positive- and negative-symptom schizophrenia. *Journal of Abnormal Psychology*, **104**, 41–54.

Spaulding, W.D., Storms, L., Goodrich, V. and Sullivan, M. (1986) Applications of experimental psychopathology in psychiatric rehabilitation. *Schizophrenia Bulletin*, **12**, 560–577.

Spring, B., Lemon, M. and Ferguson, P. (1990) Vulnerabilities to schizophrenia: information processing markers. In: Straube, E.R. and Hahlweg, K. (eds), *Schizophrenia: Concepts, Vulnerability and Intervention*. Springer-Verlag, New York, pp. 97–114.

Spring, B., Weinstein, L., Freeman, R. and Thompson, S. (1991) Selective attention in schizophrenia. In: Steinhauer, S.R., Gruzelier, J.H. and Zubin, J. (eds), *Handbook of Schizophrenia. Neuropsychology, Psychophysiology and Information Processing*. Elsevier, Amsterdam, Vol. 5, pp. 371–396.

Strauss, M.E. (1993) Relations of symptoms to cognitive deficits in schizophrenia. *Schizophrenia Bulletin*, **19**, 215–231.

Strauss, J.S., Carpenter, W.T. and Bartko, J.J. (1974) Part III. Speculations on the processes that underlie schizophrenic symptoms and signs. *Schizophrenia Bulletin*, **11**, 61–69.

Strauss, M.E., Prescott, C.A., Gutterman, D.E. and Tune, L.E. (1987) Span of Apprehension deficits in schizophrenia and mania. *Schizophrenia Bulletin*, **4**, 699–704.

Strauss, M.E., Buchanan, R.W. and Hale, J. (1993) Relations between attentional deficits and clinical symptoms in schizophrenic outpatients. *Psychiatry Research*, **47**, 205–213.

Tamminga, C.A., Thaker, G.K., Buchanan, R.W., Kirkpatrick, B., Alphs, L.D., Chase, T.N. and Carpenter, W.T. (1992) Limbic system abnormalities identified in schizophrenia using positron emission tomography with fluorodeoxy glucose and neocortical alterations with a deficit syndrome. *Archives of General Psychiatry*, **49**, 522–530.

Van Der Does, A.W., Dingemans, P.J., Linszen, D.H., Nugter, M.A. and Scholte, W.F. (1993) Symptom dimensions and cognitive and social functioning in recent-onset schizophrenia. *Psychological Medicine*, **23**, 745–753.

Walker, E. (1981) Attention and neuromotor functions of schizophrenics, schizoaffectives and patients with other affective disorders. *Archives of General Psychiatry*, **38**, 1355–1358.

Walker, E. and Lewine, R.J. (1988) Negative symptom distinction in schizophrenia: validity and etiological relevance. *Schizophrenia Research*, **1**, 315–328.

Weinberger, D. (1987) Implications of normal brain development for the pathogenesis of schizophrenia. *Archives of General Psychiatry*, **44**, 660–669.

Winters, L., Cornblatt, B.A. and Erlenmeyer-Kimling, L. (1991) The prediction of psychiatric disorders in late adolescence. In: Walker, E. (ed.), *Schizophrenia: A Life-course Developmental Perspective*. Academic Press, New York, pp. 123–137.

11 Cognitive impairments as causes of positive symptoms in schizophrenia

Mary L. Phillips and Anthony S. David

Introduction

Neuropsychological theories of symptomatology in schizophrenia have linked the abnormal behaviors and cognitive processes demonstrated in patients with the illness with underlying brain dysfunction (David and Cutting, 1994). Several such theories have been developed to explain the deficit syndrome in particular, in which negative symptoms such as reduced motivation, apathy, social withdrawal and alogia occur (Andreasen, 1983).

Neuropsychological impairments associated with negative symptoms or the disorder as a whole have been described in earlier chapters, and theories include the following.

(i) Impairment in working memory, a general-purpose system involved in a wide range of cognitive processes which require the simultaneous storage and processing of information (Baddeley, 1986), and linked with prefrontal lobe function (Goldman-Rakic, 1988).

(ii) A weakening of the influences of stored memories of regularities of previous input on current perception in schizophrenia (Hemsley, 1987), with links proposed between this abnormality in cognitive function and impaired latent inhibition (Lubow *et al.*, 1982; Baruch *et al.*, 1988), an animal model emphasizing the normal inhibition in learning new associations between stimuli in the context of pre-exposure to such stimuli.

(iii) Abnormal lateralization of cognitive function (see Gruzelier, 1996), emphasizing either left (Gur, 1978) or right (Cutting, 1990) hemisphere dysfunction.

Whilst these studies have helped to clarify the nature of the neurocognitive deficit underlying schizophrenia *per se*, it is widely believed that schizophrenia is a heterogeneous condition with different subtypes. There has, therefore, been much interest in the investigation of the neuropsychological basis of the different syndromes and specific symptoms in schizophrenia, with implications for the treatment of individual patients with these specific symptom profiles. Positive symptoms (delusions, hallucinations and thought disorder) are particularly interesting symptoms in schizophrenia in that, unlike negative symptoms, they represent the presence of abnormal experiences rather than the absence or impairment of normal functions. The aim of this chapter is to describe the studies which have investigated the nature of the neuropsychological impairments associated with the presence of positive symptoms in general in schizophrenia, and then those associated with delusions and hallucinations.

Cognitive deficits associated with positive symptom syndromes in schizophrenia

Acute (type I) versus chronic (type II) schizophrenia

A widely accepted classification system for distinguishing different subtypes of schizophrenia emphasizes the presence of either positive or negative symptoms in two syndromes of schizophrenia, type I and type II (Crow, 1980). Type I is associated with positive symptoms, in addition to an acute course and better premorbid function, and type II is associated with negative symptoms, in addition to a more chronic course and poorer premorbid function. Hemsley (1977) has linked positive symptoms with the presence of perceptual abnormalities, e.g. attention to inappropriate stimuli in patients with delusions (see below), and negative symptoms, such as social withdrawal, resulting from attempts by the patient to cope with these unusual experiences. Frith (1987) has argued that the two syndromes are distinguished by the presence of different impairments in the initiation of action. Whereas type II schizophrenia is characterized by a difficulty in forming willed intentions, type I schizophrenia is characterized by abnormal monitoring of the source of willed intention, so that the patient has difficulty in distinguishing self- from non-self-originated intention. As a consequence of this, the patient experiences positive symptoms, including delusions of control and passivity experiences.

Frith (1992) has argued further that the inability to monitor willed intentions can lead to delusions of alien control, auditory hallucinations and thought insertion, as the patients experience their actions, subvocal speech and thoughts, respectively, as originating from an external source not under their control. He also argues that the inability to monitor the beliefs and intentions of others can lead to persecutory delusions, delusions of reference and, on occasions, third person auditory hallucinations (see later). Thus, abnormalities both in generating willed intentions and in monitoring willed intentions and the beliefs and intentions of others may underlie negative and positive symptoms, respectively, in schizophrenia.

Paranoid versus non-paranoid schizophrenia

Another approach has been to classify schizophrenia as either paranoid or non-paranoid on the basis of classification systems such as DSM-IV and ICD-10. Unfortunately, this terminology has also been used to refer to positive and negative symptom syndromes. Thus, although previous researchers have reported that patients with the paranoid subtype of schizophrenia demonstrate less impairment on neurocognitive tasks and greater social adjustment than their non-paranoid counterparts (e.g. Tsuang and Winokur, 1974), the wide range of diagnostic criteria for the paranoid and non-paranoid schizophrenia subtypes has made it extremely difficult to compare the results of different studies investigating neuropsychological function in these two subtypes. In a recent review of the literature from 1975 to 1995 examining the neuropsychological differences between paranoid and non-paranoid subtypes, only limited support was found for the distinction between the two on the basis of cognitive function (Zalewski *et al.*, 1998). The authors reviewed a total of 32 studies in which the two subtypes had been compared in terms of intellectual function, attention, memory, language, visuospatial and motor function, and found no evidence of subtype differences in verbal and visuospatial function, and only limited support for neuropsychological differences in favor of the paranoid subtype in executive function/problem solving, attention, memory and motor skills. In addition to the difficulty with the employment of different diagnostic criteria across studies, Zalewski *et al.* also noted the problem of variability in the level of standardization of the neuropsychological tests employed by the studies, and the additional difficulty associated with the variability across studies of medication effects and severity and chronicity of illness.

The three syndrome approach

Liddle (1987a) examined the relationships between symptoms in 40 patients with chronic schizophrenia, and demonstrated that the symptoms segregated into three syndromes:

(i)   psychomotor poverty (poverty of speech, lack of spontaneous movement and blunting of affect);

(ii) disorganization (inappropriate affect, poverty of content of speech and disturbances in the form of thought); and

(iii) reality distortion (delusions and hallucinations).

This model has been supported by the findings of several other studies examining the relationships between symptoms in schizophrenia (e.g. Bilder *et al.*, 1985; Arndt *et al.*, 1991; Brown and White, 1992).

Examination of the correlations between syndrome severity and performance on a range of neuropsychological tests revealed that each of the syndromes was associated with a specific pattern of neuropsychological impairment (Liddle, 1987b). Whereas the psychomotor poverty syndrome was associated with poor performance in tests of conceptual thinking, object naming and long-term memory, the two syndromes linked with the presence of positive symptoms were associated with a different pattern of cognitive dysfunction. The disorganization syndrome was associated with poor performance in tests of concentration, immediate recall and word learning, and the reality distortion syndrome was associated with poor figure-ground perception.

A similar approach using factor analysis was undertaken by Basso *et al.* (1998) with 62 schizophrenia patients on whom a wide variety of clinical, demographic and neuropsychological measures were available. Negative symptoms were associated with a range of abnormalities such as impaired global IQ, executive function, motor skill, vigilance, attention and memory indices, while disorganization correlated with a subset of these (IQ, attention and motor tasks). Psychotic symptoms did not correlate with the standard tests carried out.

Functional imaging research has linked each syndrome with a different pattern of abnormal cerebral function (Liddle *et al.*, 1992a,b; Ebmeier *et al.*, 1993). The psychomotor poverty syndrome was linked with left-sided prefrontal hypofunction. The disorganization syndrome was associated with decreased perfusion in the right ventral prefrontal cortex and insula, and with increased perfusion in the right anterior cingulate gyrus. The reality distortion syndrome was linked with overactivity in the left medial temporal lobe and underactivity in the left lateral temporal lobe. It was noted that the sites of abnormal cerebral function associated with each syndrome included structures known to be linked to normal performance of the cognitive processes associated with the syndrome.

There has been further support for the distinction amongst these three syndromes in schizophrenia from studies investigating the degree of impairment of theory of mind, the ability to understand the behavior and intentions of others (Premack and Woodruff, 1978), in patients with each of the different syndromes of schizophrenia (Frith, 1992; Corcoran *et al.*, 1995, 1997) (see below). With the employment of novel tasks designed to examine the ability to infer intentions behind indirect speech (Corcoran *et al.*, 1995), and the ability to understand visual jokes (Corcoran *et al.*, 1997), the studies demonstrated that whereas schizophrenic patients with the psychomotor poverty syndrome performed poorly on all tasks, patients with passivity phenomena performed well on inference of intentions from indirect speech, but poorly on understanding of visual jokes. Furthermore, patients with paranoid delusions performed poorly with the visual jokes which required understanding of the mental states of others, but not with visual jokes which could be understood on the basis of physical and semantic analysis. In addition, these patients also performed less well than normal controls on the indirect speech inference task.

Taken together, these findings suggest that whereas patients with predominantly negative symptoms perform poorly on many different tasks relating to social inference, patients with positive symptoms, including paranoid delusions and passivity phenomena, have more selective deficits. These selective deficits may relate to the specific nature of the positive symptoms, with patients with paranoid delusions being impaired in the perception of social information dependent upon inference of the mental states of others, but not in that dependent upon the analysis of physical and semantic information, and patients with passivity phenomena exhibiting a different pattern of impairment.

Cognitive deficits associated with specific positive symptoms

Hallucinations

First of all, there have been no convincing studies to suggest that auditory verbal hallucinations (AVHs) correlate with deficits on standard neuropsychological tests, unlike, for example, negative symptoms (see above and, for a review, see David, 1994a). Cognitive psychologists have therefore taken a more experimental approach. There are two basic theories of hallucinations. The first of these may be described as the 'disinhibition' model, through which cortical activity experienced as hallucinations is 'released' as a consequence of reduced sensory input (Schultz and Melzack, 1991). The second 'cerebral irritation' model implies abnormal cortical excitability in regions associated with 'sensory' memory. This has grown from such dramatic experimental situations as the stimulation of the temporal lobes during neurosurgery (Penfield and Perot, 1963). It is also possible that both disinhibition and irritation processes could operate in a single individual.

Deafness

Does the release explanation have relevance to auditory (as opposed to visual) hallucinations? While hearing impairment detected early in life has been found to be a risk factor for schizophrenia *per se* (O'Neal and Robins, 1958; David *et al.*, 1994), a specific premorbid link with auditory hallucinations has yet to be established. Several cross-sectional studies have supported an association between deafness and paranoia in the elderly, and there have been reports of an association with auditory hallucinations. This is especially clear in the case of unilateral hallucinations (Almeida *et al.*, 1993; Doris *et al.*, 1995; Gordon, 1995). Usually, the hallucination occurs on the deaf side, although exceptions occur, perhaps where they are drug induced (Gilbert, 1993). A consistent association has been found between deafness and musical hallucinations. Reviews by Keshavan *et al.* (1992) and Berrios (1990) show that musical hallucinations in non-psychotic individuals almost invariably implicate hearing loss (Gordon, 1994), sometimes with additional cerebral pathology (Paquier *et al.*, 1992; Fénelon *et al.*, 1993).

Some cases have been described recently which are of interest in this context. A 35-year-old man with otosclerosis was described who first experienced tinnitus, then musical hallucinations and finally AVHs (Marneros *et al.*, 1997), all of which recovered after surgery. Terao and Yukio (1998) report a 63-year-old woman (with a history of ear infection) whose musical hallucinations responded to the anticonvulsant, carbamazepine, and Carroll and Milnes (1998) describe a 27-year-old woman with a left middle-ear infection who experienced left unilateral AVHs and delusions of possession. Finally, positron emission tomography revealed increased right temporal blood flow correlated with intensity of musical hallucinations in a 73-year-old man with moderate bilateral hearing loss (Griffiths *et al.*, 1997).

A reduction in central as opposed to peripheral perceptual sensitivity may be implicated in auditory hallucinations. Mathew *et al.* (1993) measured auditory thresholds in schizophrenic patients rated as hallucinators and found that the usual right ear superiority was lost, suggesting a left temporal lobe dysfunction.

Left or right hemisphere?

The left hemisphere is of course specialized in linguistic production and analysis. However, the 'non-propositional' nature of some AVHs has suggested the right hemisphere as their source. David (1994a) outlined a series of scientific proofs which would support this. For example, an excess of this symptom in left-handed schizophrenics was predicted and has been reported by Tyler *et al.* (1995). A corresponding excess of auditory hallucinations in females in general and female schizophrenic patients was also predicted and reported (Bardenstein and McGlashan, 1990; Tien, 1991; Rector and Seeman, 1992). However, research utilizing the technique of dichotic listening points to *left* hemisphere dysfunction. Dichotic listening entails competition between the right and left hemispheres in the identification of auditory stimuli presented simultaneously, one to each ear. When the stimuli are words or consonant–vowel syllables, input to the left hemisphere predominates, especially in right-handers. This right ear/left hemisphere advantage appears to be attenuated in patients who are hallucination prone (Green *et al.*, 1994; Bruder *et al.*, 1995) and correlates with symptom severity (we have been unable to replicate this in our laboratory; Rossell *et al.*, 1999). The possibility remains, therefore, that relatively intact right hemisphere functioning could support AVHs in schizophrenia. Much neuroimaging work has been devoted to the cerebral localization of activity coincident with hallucinations (for a review, see David, 1999). Recent functional magnetic resonance imaging (fMRI) work has shown that the right hemisphere shows more activity relative to the left in response to external speech (Woodruff *et al.*, 1997), while activity during hallucinations in the single cases studied has a right temporal cortex emphasis (Woodruff *et al.*, 1995; Lennox *et al.*, 1999).

Language and hallucinations

Schizophrenic auditory hallucinations, the characteristic 'voices' talking to or about the subject, have a precise content which is often highly personalized to the voice-hearer (Nayani and David, 1996; Leudar *et al.*, 1997). It has been suggested that consistency of semantic content of AVHs leads the voice-hearer to personify the experience (Hoffman *et al.*, 1994). Often a complex relationship develops between the patient and 'the voices', usually that of the powerless and the powerful, respectively (Chadwick and Birchwood, 1994), although some patients come to value their hallucinations (Miller *et al.*, 1993). Various treatment approaches have arisen out of the fact that hallucinations may arise in predictable contexts and provoke a range of coping strategies, some of which reduce their frequency (Haddock *et al.*, 1993, Slade and Bentall, 1988). As well as being of practical value, this work aids the theoretical understanding of the phenomena (for a review, see Shergill *et al.*, 1998).

Inner speech

The observation that the universal experience of inner speech resembles some AVHs continues to stimulate neurocognitive research. A single case study of a woman with continuous hallucinations in the form of voices addressing and advising her showed that inner speech—as defined as the process by which phonological representations are maintained in short-term memory—could co-exist with AVHs (David and Lucas, 1995). This implies that inner speech may in fact consist of several different processes or that AVHs are not synonymous with inner speech in any simple sense. The same short-term memory tests were used in a group comparison of schizophrenic patients who recently had reported hallucinations versus patients who had not (Haddock *et al.*, 1993). The authors tested a less specific hypothesis than that of David and Lucas, namely that any abnormality of the phonological store could affect monitoring of inner speech adversely, leading to an increased vulnerability to AVHs. The results showed that all patients performed less well than controls on phonological span tasks but there was no significant interaction with the presence or absence of hallucinations, compatible with David and Lucas' conclusions. In contrast, a separate case study suggested that thought echo (a pathological experience akin to hearing voices) does appear to be incompatible with effective short-term or working memory (David, 1994b).

The verbal transformation effect (the sensation that when a word like 'life' is repeated over and over, it turns into 'fly') has been used in this context, and most recent findings suggest that hallucinators are no more prone to the effect than controls. However, Haddock *et al.* (1995) demonstrated that this effect is vulnerable to motivational factors (i.e. suggestion).

Evans *et al.* (2000) carried out an in-depth study of seven patients with no history of AVH and 12 with a strong history of AVH using auditory imagery paradigms which tapped into the functioning of the 'inner ear', the 'inner voice' and the 'inner ear–inner voice' partnership (Smith *et al.*, 1995). These included: parsing meaningful letter strings, pitch judgements of the verbal transformations and a range of tasks requiring phonological judgements. The results showed a wide range of abilities and deficits in both groups, but no clear pattern. Indeed, as a whole, the AVH group were somewhat superior. Analysis of individual cases showed that performance was not impaired consistently on any of the tasks, and, on some, patients achieved maximum scores. These results provide evidence against an abnormality in inner speech and phonological processing in patients vulnerable to AVHs but do not rule out attributional or 'metalinguistic models' (see below) or indeed those more 'physiologically based'—arising out of the functional neuroimaging literature—based on lower level perceptual processes.

Source monitoring

The problem of deciding whether you imagined hearing a voice or heard someone else speaking, and, if the latter, deciding who it was, falls under the rubric of source (or reality) monitoring (Johnson *et al.*, 1988). Hallucinations can therefore be conceived of as failures of source monitoring. The attraction of this approach is that it proposes a kind of 'monitor' which operates with a simple range of algorithms based on such things as the sensory qualities of memories. Let us say that a remembered speech segment fails to attract a 'tag' denoting its source, then an operation is triggered which runs: if the memory is vivid, then I probably said it. A fading memory trace may therefore be mislabeled as 'other'. Some empirical evidence for such a process underlying AVHs has been gathered. The first attempt was by Bentall *et al.* (1991), and the results were somewhat equivocal, with hallucinators being no more prone to monitoring errors than other groups. Morrison and Haddock (1997) introduced an innovation to this paradigm by examining source monitoring for words with emotional content. They found that such words tended to disrupt source monitoring (as suggested by David and Howard, 1994), but only in terms of immediate ratings of subjective ownership—although this is arguably more relevant to hallucinations.

Seal *et al.* (1997) manipulated several task parameters including emotional content, and found trends towards more self-to-other misattributions in hallucinators ($n = 6$) versus non-hallucinators ($n = 11$). Other research using similar methodology has shown that patients with schizophrenia may well be prone to making source monitoring errors (tending to attribute words they have read previously to an external source), but the relationship to hallucinations has not emerged (Vinogradov *et al.*, 1997). Indeed, a confounding effect of low IQ (Vinogradov *et al.*, 1997) and poor verbal memory (Seal *et al.*, 1997) has been problematic, especially in small samples.

Frith's model (1992) proposes that source monitoring is achieved by a corollary discharge-like mechanism. Hence, there should be no confusion as to the source or, more specifically, ownership of a speech act if its occurrence had been signaled at the intention stage. A test of this hypothesis was carried out by Cahill and colleagues (1996) using distorted auditory feedback. The aim was to produce a dissonance between external and 'internal' monitoring. Reliance solely on the external route would lead to the attribution of an alien source to the heard speech. By lowering or raising the pitch of the patients' speech, the authors did indeed induce hallucination-like experiences: patients said the voice they heard was not theirs and was, for example, 'evil', while noting that it coincided with their act of speaking. However, this tendency correlated more strongly with the presence of delusions than hallucinations. Johns and McGuire (1999) repeated the experiment using 10 schizophrenia patients with hallucinations (and delusions) and eight with delusions alone, plus normal volunteers. The results showed that, while uncertainty as to the source of the speech was a feature of both schizophrenia groups, external attribution was more common in the hallucinators, a tendency more evident when derogatory material was heard.

Goldberg *et al.* (1997) used delayed as opposed to distorted auditory feedback on the assumption that the dysfluency this usually causes is due to the mismatch between planned and perceived output. The authors argued that if the planned speech production is not anticipated (due to a disconnection between intentions and the monitored output), then this adverse effect on speech should be *less* in those with hallucinations compared with those without. The results showed the opposite, i.e. speech output was even more affected in the hallucinators.

Indirect psychological evidence for a failure in self-monitoring comes from examining speech repairs, especially when these occur rapidly, often within a word, before external acoustic feedback can have come into play. Leudar *et al.* (1994) found that internal error detection occurred much less commonly in schizophrenic patients compared with normal controls. However, there was no difference between patients with and without AVHs as classified according to Present State Examination ratings (Wing *et al.*, 1974).

Summary

There seems to be a role for sensory defects and 'de-afferentation' in inducing auditory hallucinations, especially those of music. AVHs, the main focus of this section, are constructed within narrow parameters of form and content. So far, a model within language production and reception, and monitoring provides the best explanatory framework. A defect in the self-monitoring or misattribution of the source of inner speech—which itself appears not to be impaired differentially in hallucinators—is an attractive hypothesis which has gained encouraging support from some studies, while others are resolutely negative. This mislabeling requires more precise cognitive dissection to explain its apparently transient nature and interaction with emotive content.

Delusions

Delusions represent a core feature of psychosis, and are especially evident in schizophrenia. There have been several cognitive models proposed to explain delusion formation. One explanation is that they result from the natural interpretations of abnormal experiences (Maher, 1974). For example, a specific deficit in facial recognition has been proposed to account for the presence of delusional misidentification, a delusion in which a familiar (or unfamiliar) person is misidentified consistently by the patient (see below). Furthermore, delusions of alien control have been linked with hyperactivation of the right inferior parietal lobule and cingulate gyrus, brain regions important for visuospatial function (Spence *et al.*, 1997).

Biases or deficits?

Delusions can occur, however, in the absence of abnormal perceptions, and different delusional beliefs can be present in various subjects with similar abnormal perceptions (Chapman and Chapman, 1988). These findings indicate that other cognitive deficits may be responsible for the formation of delusions. Other theories of delusion formation have therefore emphasized abnormalities in attentional bias, such as increased attention to threatening stimuli in patients with persecutory delusions, in which the theme of the delusion is threat against the self (Ullman and Krasner, 1969). Evidence for this includes the significantly longer time that patients with persecutory delusions require to name the print colors of threatening compared with depressive and neutral words in an emotional Stroop test (Bentall and Kaney, 1989), and their demonstrating preferential recall of threat-related propositions in a story recall task (Kaney *et al.*, 1992). It has also been proposed that patients with persecutory delusions have abnormal attributional processes, making external attributions for negative events and internal attributions for positive events (Kaney and Bentall, 1989), and that this acts as a 'self-serving bias' (Kaney and Bentall, 1990).

More recent studies have examined the nature of reasoning biases in patients with delusions about non-persecutory themes. Leafhead *et al.* (1996) employed the emotional Stroop paradigm to investigate the attentional bias in a patient with the Cotard delusion, the belief that one is dead. The patient was found to have increased attention to death-related words. Rossell *et al.* (1998) administered a sentence verification task to patients with delusions. When asked to make real (true)/unlikely/nonsense (untrue) categorization judgements, deluded subjects, whose overall performance matched that of controls, made significantly more incorrect responses to sentences that had an emotional content congruent with their delusional beliefs. These findings suggest that reasoning abnormalities in deluded patients become particularly evident with tasks related to the theme of the delusional belief, and also indicate the presence of disturbed higher order semantic processes in these patients.

Reasoning

Further studies have emphasized abnormalities in hypothesis testing in deluded patients, with patients with persecutory delusions requiring less information before reaching a conclusion than non-deluded controls (Huq *et al.*, 1988; Garety *et al.*, 1991; Dudley *et al.*, 1997) and being more inclined to stick to hypotheses in the presence of negative feedback (Young and Bentall, 1995).

Although recent investigation of logical reasoning ability, including conditional and syllogistic reasoning tasks (Evans *et al.*, 1993), has demonstrated that such reasoning is not impaired in deluded patients, at least no more than in non-deluded patients (Kemp *et al.*,

1997), another study has shown that increasing the emotional content *per se* of such tasks may affect logical reasoning ability in deluded patients to a greater extent than in normal controls (Phillips *et al.*, 1997). It is unclear whether these perceptual and reasoning biases lead to predisposition and formation of persecutory delusions, or maintain delusions once formed. Indeed, the difficulty in distinguishing between the effects of beliefs on current perception and reasoning, and the effects of the latter on belief formation, has been highlighted in the investigation of delusional misidentification, in which it has been argued that abnormal beliefs distort current perceptual experiences in a top-down fashion (Fleminger, 1994).

Finally, David and Howard (1994) employed the reality monitoring methodology described above to study cognitively intact patients with delusional memory. The phenomenal characteristics of the delusional memory were contrasted with a real memorable event and a fantasy. It was found that delusional memories were more vivid and tangible than even real events (although they tended to be 'rehearsed' more mentally), which could lead to reality confusion. However, a detailed case study approach revealed coincident reasoning aberrations as well.

Other approaches to the study of the cognitive deficits associated with positive symptoms in schizophrenia

Studies of face perception

Schizophrenic patients often appear to misinterpret social cues and exhibit poor social skills. One approach to this has been to employ socially salient stimuli to investigate the nature of the cognitive processes underlying positive (and negative) symptoms in schizophrenia. Human faces are ideal stimuli in that they convey a wealth of socially relevant information, such as age, gender, identity and expression (Bruce and Young, 1986).

Several studies have investigated perception of facial expression in schizophrenic patients without distinguishing between different syndromes. Whilst many studies have demonstrated poor judgement of facial emotion in these patients (Novic *et al.*, 1984; Feinberg *et al.*, 1986; Gessler *et al.*, 1989; Gaebel and Woelwer, 1992), a more recent study has found no evidence to support this (Flack *et al.*, 1997). Despite this, another recent study, in which the authors employed an audio-visual affect recognition task designed to test a subject's ability to recognize an affect state from facial expression, voice tone and upper body movement cues has demonstrated that schizophrenic patients are impaired in recognition of affects, in particular negative affects, compared with normal and patient controls (Bell *et al.*, 1997). Other studies have demonstrated that schizophrenic patients perform poorly not only on facial expression perception tasks but on all tasks of facial processing, including facial identity, age and gender perception (Archer *et al.*, 1992; Kerr and Neale, 1993). These studies suggest that there is a generalized performance deficit rather than a specific emotion recognition deficit in schizophrenic patients. It has been suggested further that the generalized performance deficit in facial perception demonstrated in schizophrenic patients may be related to chronicity of illness (Mueser *et al.*, 1997).

The role of the right hemisphere in facial perception has been highlighted by neuropsychological and functional imaging studies (Etcoff, 1984a,b; Sergent, 1988; Sergent *et al.*, 1992; Puce *et al.*, 1995, 1996). Taken together with the findings of impaired facial perception in schizophrenia, this suggests the presence of right hemisphere dysfunction in the illness (Cutting, 1990).

Attempts to differentiate performance in facial expression recognition tasks of different subgroups of schizophrenic patients have provided evidence for the superior ability of paranoid compared with non-paranoid patients in the labeling of negative affects (Kline *et al.*, 1992). One symptom of schizophrenia, delusional misidentification, has been studied extensively by Young and colleagues (e.g. Ellis and Young, 1990). The authors distinguish between the three main types, the Capgras syndrome (familiar person replaced by a physically similar double), the Fregoli syndrome (unfamiliar person replaced by a physically similar familiar person) and the syndrome of intermetamorphosis (another person replaced by someone with physical characteristics and identity familiar to the subject) in terms of specific deficits in facial identity perception.

Visual scan path measurements

Many tests of specific cognitive functions rely upon 'off-line' measures of attention. Monitoring directed attention in subjects in real time—an 'on-line' measurement of attention—has the advantage over off-line measures in that it allows the presence of 'abnormal' information processing strategies in patients, i.e. strategies differing significantly from those employed by normal subjects, to be detected. The measurement of visual scan paths is one method which has potential as a monitor of real-time visual information processing (Phillips and David, 1994).

Whilst measurements of different types of eye movement, including smooth pursuit and saccadic eye movements, have been made in several previous studies of schizophrenic patients, the emphasis in these studies has been in linking eye tracking abnormalities in patients with schizophrenia, in particular those with the deficit syndrome, with underlying dysfunction in specific cortical–subcortical circuits (Henderson *et al.*, 1996; Ross *et al.*, 1997). The visual scan path is, literally, a map which traces the direction and extent of gaze when an individual comprehends a complex scene (Noton and Stark, 1971), i.e. a psycho-physiological 'marker' of sensory input and directional attention on viewing a stimulus. Measurement of visual scan paths in schizophrenic patients is, therefore, not only a measure of the underlying function of the oculomotor apparatus but also an on-line measure of the attentional or cognitive processes involved in the appraisal of visual stimuli in these patients.

A small number of studies have investigated visual scan paths in schizophrenic subjects (see Phillips and David, 1994). A relationship between symptomatology and viewing strategy has been demonstrated in schizophrenic patients, with the presence of positive symptoms associated with increased scanning and negative symptoms with increased staring (Gaebel *et al.*, 1987; Streit *et al.*, 1997). It has also been demonstrated that schizophrenics, on viewing a facial stimulus, initially attend less to facial features compared with normal controls (Gordon *et al.*, 1992). A further study has indicated that schizophrenics have a less efficient viewing strategy compared with normal controls on viewing picture completion figures (Kurachi *et al.*, 1994).

Whilst these studies have demonstrated abnormalities in viewing strategies in schizophrenic patients *per se*, others have aimed to investigate specific abnormalities in the visual scan paths, i.e. specific attentional deficits, in deluded schizophrenic patients compared with non-deluded schizophrenics (Phillips and David, 1994, 1997, 1998). These studies have demonstrated that deluded schizophrenic patients employ abnormal strategies when viewing salient visual stimuli, human faces—viewing non-feature areas to a significantly greater extent than both non-deluded schizophrenics matched for medication, illness duration and negative symptoms, and age-matched normal controls. One interpretation of these findings is that deluded schizophrenic patients rely on less salient visual information when appraising complex stimuli compared with control groups, in support of the theory of abnormal reasoning in this group (Garety *et al.*, 1991).

Conclusions

Linking cognitive abnormalities with positive symptoms has proven to be a challenge. It appears that standard neuropsychological tests lack the specificity and sensitivity to shed light on the cognitive basis of phenomena such as hallucinations and delusions. Negative symptoms, in contrast, seem by their very nature to be eminently reducible to cognitive deficits, although there is a danger of circularity (e.g. reduced verbal fluency correlating with poverty of speech). More successes have been claimed when individual symptoms or symptom complexes have been the focus of investigation. Contrasting individual cases with clear-cut phenomenology and relatively few intellectual impairments is a strategy worth employing. Within-subject designs with and without the symptoms of interest is another potentially powerful approach. Finally, the remit of neuropsychology has benefited from expanding into social psychology and making use of concepts such as attribution and bias. This offers the most promise in unraveling the mysteries of both the form and content of the 'inexplicable' features of psychosis.

References

Almeida, O., Forstl, H., Howard, R. and David, A. (1993) Unilateral auditory hallucinations. *British Journal of Psychiatry*, **162**, 262–264.

Andreasen, N.C. (1983) *The Scale for the Assessment of Negative Symptoms (SANS)*. The University of Iowa, Iowa City.

Archer, J., Hay, D.C. and Young, A.W. (1992) Face processing in psychiatric conditions. *British Journal of Clinical Psychology*, **31**, 45–61.

Arndt, S., Alliger, R.J. and Andreasen, N.C. (1991) The distinction of positive and negative symptoms: the failure of a two dimensional model. *British Journal of Psychiatry*, **158**, 317–322.

Baddeley, A.D. (1986) *Working Memory*. Clarendon Press, Oxford.

Bardenstein, K.K. and McGlashan, T.H. (1990) Gender differences in affective, schizo-affective, and schizophrenic disorders: a review. *Schizophrenia Research*, **3**, 159–172.

Baruch, J., Hemsley, D.R. and Gray, J.A. (1988) Differential performance of acute and chronic schizophrenics in a latent inhibition task. *Journal of Nervous and Mental Disease*, **176**, 598–606.

Basso, M.R., Nasrallah, H.A., Olson, S.C. and Bornstein, R.A. (1998) Neuropsychological correlates of negative, disorganized and psychotic symptoms in schizophrenia. *Schizophrenia Research*, **31**, 99–111.

Bell, M., Bryson, G. and Lysaker, P. (1997) Positive and negative affect recognition in schizophrenia: a comparison with substance abuse and normal control subjects. *Psychiatry Research*, **73**, 73–82.

Bentall, R.P. and Kaney, S. (1989) Content specific information processing and persecutory delusions: an investigation using the emotional Stroop test. *British Journal of Medical Psychology*, **62**, 355–364.

Bentall, R., Baker, G. and Havers, S. (1991) Reality monitoring and psychotic hallucinations. *British Journal of Clinical Psychology*, **30**, 213–222.

Berrios, G. (1990) Musical hallucinations: a historical and clinical study. *British Journal of Psychiatry*, **156**, 188–194.

Bilder, R.M., Mukherjee, S., Rieder, R.O. *et al.* (1985) Symptomatic and neurological components of defect states. *Schizophrenia Bulletin*, **11**, 409–419.

Brown, K.W. and White, T. (1992) Syndromes of chronic schizophrenia and some clinical correlates. *British Journal of Psychiatry*, **161**, 317–322.

Bruce, V. and Young, A.W. (1986) Understanding face recognition. *British Journal of Psychology*, **77**, 305–327.

Bruder, G., Rabinowics, E., Towey, J., Brown, A., Kaufmann, C.A., Amador, X., Malaspina, D. and Gorman, J.M. (1995) Smaller right ear (left hemisphere) advantage for dichotic fused words in patients with schizophrenia. *American Journal of Psychiatry*, **152**, 932–935.

Cahill, C., Silbersweig, D. and Frith, C. (1996) Psychotic experiences induced in deluded patients using distorted auditory feedback. *Cognitive Neuropsychiatry*, **1**, 201–211.

Carroll, A. and Milnes, D. (1998) Unilateral auditory hallucinations in association with ear infection. *Irish Journal of Psychiatric Medicine*, **15**, 31–32.

Chadwick, P. and Birchwood, M. (1994) The omnipotence of voices: a cognitive approach to auditory hallucinations. *British Journal of Psychiatry*, **164**, 190–201.

Chapman, L.J. and Chapman, J.P. (1988) The genesis of delusions. In: Oltmanns, T.F and Maher, B.A. (eds), *Delusional Beliefs*. Wiley, New York, pp. 179–188.

Corcoran, R., Mercer, G. and Frith, C.D. (1995) Schizophrenia, symptomatology and social inference: investigating 'theory of mind' in people with schizophrenia. *Schizophrenia Research*, **17**, 5–13.

Corcoran, R., Cahill, C. and Frith, C.D. (1997) The appreciation of visual jokes in people with schizophrenia: a study of 'mentalizing' ability. *Schizophrenia Research*, **24**, 319–327.

Crow, T.J. (1980) Molecular pathology of schizophrenia: more than one disease process. *British Medical Journal*, **280**, 66–68.

Cutting, J. (1990) *The Right Hemisphere and Psychiatric Disorders*. Oxford University Press, New York.

David, A.S. (1994a) The neuropsychology of auditory–verbal hallucinations. In: David, A.S. and Cutting, J.C. (eds), *The Neuropsychology of Schizophrenia*. Lawrence Erlbaum Associates, Hove, UK, pp. 269–312.

David, A.S. (1994b) Thought echo reflects the activity of the phonological loop. *British Journal of Clinical Psychology*, **33**, 81–83.

David, A.S. (1999) Auditory hallucinations: phenomenology, neuropsychology and neuroimaging up-date. *Acta Psychiatrica Scandinavica*, **395**, 95–104.

David, A.S. and Cutting, J.C. (eds) (1994) *The Neuropsychology of Schizophrenia*. Lawrence Erlbaum Associates, Hove, UK.

David, A.S. and Howard, R. (1994) An experimental phenomenological approach to delusional memory in schizophrenia and late paraphrenia. *Psychological Medicine*, **24**, 515–24.

David, A.S. and Lucas, P. (1993) Auditory–verbal hallucinations and the phonological loop: a cognitive neuropsychological study. *British Journal of Clinical Psychology*, **32**, 431–441.

David, A., Malmberg, A., Lewis, G., Brandt, L. and Allebeck, P. (1994) Are there neurological and sensory risk factors for schizophrenia? *Schizophrenia Research*, **14**, 247–251.

Doris, A., O'Carroll, R.E., Steele, J.D. and Ebmeier, K.P. (1995) Single photon emission computed tomography in a patient with unilateral auditory hallucinations. *Behavioural Neurology*, **8**, 145–148.

Dudley, R.E.J., John, C.H., Young, A.W. and Over, D.E. (1997) Normal and abnormal reasoning in people with delusions. *British Journal of Clinical Psychology*, **36**, 243–258.

Ebmeier, K.P., Blackwood, D.H.R., Murray, C. *et al.* (1993) Single photon emission tomography with 99mTe-exametazime in unmedicated schizophrenc patients. *Biological Psychiatry*, **33**, 487–495.

Ellis, H.D. and Young, A.W. (1990) Accounting for delusional misidentifications. *British Journal of Psychiatry*, **157**, 239–248.

Etcoff, N.L. (1984a) Perceptual and conceptual organisation of facial emotions: hemispheric differences. *Brain and Cognition*, **3**, 385–412.

Etcoff, N.L. (1984b) Selective attention to facial identity and facial emotion. *Neuropsychologia*, **22**, 281–295.

Evans, C., McGuire, P. and David, A.S. (2000) Is auditory imagery defective in patients with auditory hallucinations? *Psychological Medicine*, **30**, 137–148.

Evans, J.St.B.T., Newstead, S.E. and Byrne, R.M.J. (1993) *Human Reasoning*. Lawrence Erlbaum Associates, Hove, UK.

Feinberg, T.E., Rifkin, A., Scaffer, C. and Walker, E. (1986) Facial discrimination and emotional recognition in schizophrenia and affective disorders. *Archives of General Psychiatry*, **43**, 276–279.

Fénelon, G., Marie, S., Ferroir, J.-P. and Guillard, A. (1993) Musical hallucinations: 7 cases. *Revue Neurologique (Paris)*, **149**, 8–9.

Flack, W.F., Cavallaro, L.A., Laird, J.D. and Miller, D.R. (1997) Accurate encoding and decoding of emotional facial expressions in schizophrenia. *Psychiatry*, **60**, 197–210.

Fleminger, S. (1994) Top-down processing and delusional misidentification. In: David, A.S. and Cutting, J.C. (eds), *The Neuropsychology of Schizophrenia*. Lawrence Erlbaum Associates, Hove, UK, pp. 361–379.

Frith, C.D. (1987) The positive and negative symptoms of schizophrenia reflect impairments in the perception and initiation of action. *Psychological Medicine*, **17**, 631–648.

Frith, C. (1992) *Cognitive Neuropsychology of Schizophrenia*. Lawrence Erlbaum Associates, Hove, UK.

Gaebel, W. and Woelwer, W. (1992) Facial expression and emotional face recognition in schizophrenia and depression. *European Archives of Psychiatry and Clinical Neuroscience*, **242**, 46–52.

Gaebel, W., Ulrich, G. and Frick, K. (1987) Visuomotor performance of schizophrenic patients and normal controls in a picture viewing task. *Biological Psychiatry*, **22**, 1227–1237.

Garety, P.A., Hemsley, D.R. and Wessely, S. (1991) Reasoning in deluded schizophrenic and paranoid patients. Biases in performance on a probabilistic inference task. *Journal of Nervous and Mental Disease*, **179**, 194–201.

Gessler, S., Cutting, J., Frith, C.D. and Weinman, J. (1989) Schizophrenic inability to judge facial emotions. A controlled study. *British Journal of Clinical Psychology*, **28**, 19–29.

Gilbert, G. J. (1993) Pentoxifyline-induced musical hallucinations. *Neurology*, **43**, 1621–1622.

Goldberg, T.E., Gold, J.M., Coppola, R. and Weinberger, D.R. (1997) Unnatural practices, unspeakable actions: a study of delayed auditory feedback in schizophrenia. *American Journal of Psychiatry*, **154**, 858–860.

Goldman-Rakic, P.S. (1988) Topography of cognition: parallel distributed networks in primate association cortex. *Annual Review of Neuroscience*, **11**, 136–156.

Gordon, A.G. (1994) Musical hallucinations. *Neurology*, **44**, 986–987.

Gordon, A.G. (1995) Schizophrenia and the ear. *Schizophrenia Research*, **17**, 289–290.

Gordon, E., Coyle, S., Anderson, J. *et al.* (1992) Eye movement response to a facial stimulus in schizophrenia. *Biological Psychiatry*, **31**, 626–629.

Green, M.F., Hugdahl, K. and Mitchell, S. (1994) Dichotic listening during auditory hallucinations in patients with schizophrenia. *American Journal of Psychiatry*, **151**, 357–362.

Griffiths, T.D., Jackson, M.C., Spillane, J.A., Friston, K.J. and Frackowiak, R.S.J. (1997) A neural substrate for musical hallucinosis. *Neurocase*, **3**, 167–172.

Gruzelier, J. (1996) Lateralised dysfunction is necessary but not sufficient to account for neuropsychological deficits in schizophrenia. In: Pantelis, C., Nelson, H.E. and Barnes, T.R.E. (eds), *Schizophrenia. A Neuropsychological Perspective*. Wiley, Chichester, UK, pp. 125–161.

Gur, R.E. (1978) Left hemisphere dysfunction and left hemispheric overactivation in schizophrenia. *Journal of Abnormal Psychiatry*, **87**, 226–238.

Haddock, G., Bentall, R.P. and Slade, P.D. (1993) Psychological treatment of chronic auditory hallucinations: two case studies. *Behavioural and Cognitive Psychotherapy*, **21**, 335–346.

Haddock, G., Slade, P.D. and Bentall, R.P. (1995) Auditory hallucinations and the verbal transformation effect; role of suggestions. *Personality and Individual Differences*, **19**, 301–306.

Hemsley, D.R. (1977) What have cognitive deficits to do with schizophrenic symptoms? *British Journal of Psychiatry*, **130**, 167–173.

Hemsley, D.R. (1987) An experimental psychological model for schizophrenia. In: Hafner, H., Gattaz, W.F. and Janzarik, W. (eds), *Search for the Causes of Schizophrenia*. Springer, Heidelberg, pp. 179–188.

Henderson, L., Crawford, T.J. and Kennard, C. (1996) Neuropsychology of eye movement abnormalities in schizophrenia. In: Pantelis, C., Nelson, H.E. and Barnes, T.R.E. (eds), *Schizophrenia. A Neuropsychological Perspective*. Wiley, Chichester, UK, pp. 259–279.

Hoffman, R.E., Oates, E., Hafner, J., Hustig, H.H. and McGlashan, T.H. (1994) Semantic organization of hallucinated 'voices' in schizophrenia. *American Journal of Psychiatry*, **151**, 1229–1230.

Huq, S.F., Garety, P.A. and Hemsley, D.R. (1988) Probabilistic judgements in deluded and non-deluded subjects. *Quarterly Journal of Experimental Psychology*, **40A**, 801–812.

Johns, L.C. and McGuire, P.K. (1999) Verbal self-monitoring and auditory hallucinations in schizophrenia. *Lancet*, **353**, 469–470.

Johnson, M.K., Foley, M.A. and Leach, K. (1988) The consequence for memory of imagining in another person's voice. *Memory and Cognition*, **16**, 337–342.

Kaney, S. and Bentall, R.P. (1989) Persecutory delusions and attributional style. *British Journal of Medical Psychology*, **62**, 191–198.

Kaney, S. and Bentall, R.P. (1990) Persecutory delusions and the self-serving bias. Evidence from a contingency judgement task. *Journal of Nervous and Mental Disease*, **180**, 773–780.

Kaney, S., Wolfenden, M., Dewey, M.E. and Bentall, R.P. (1992) Persecutory delusions and the recall of threatening and non-threatening propositions. *British Journal of Clinical Psychology*, **31**, 85–87.

Kemp, R., Chua, S., McKenna, P. and David, A.S. (1997) Reasoning and delusions. *British Journal of Psychiatry*, **170**, 398–405.

Kerr, S.L. and Neale, J.M. (1993) Emotion perception in schizophrenia: specific deficit or further evidence of generalised poor performance? *Journal of Abnormal Psychology*, **102**, 312–318.

Keshavan, M.S., David, A.S., Steingard, S. and Lishman, W.A. (1992) Musical hallucinations: a review and synthesis. *Neuropsychiatry, Neuropsychology and Behavioural Neurology*, **3**, 211–223.

Kline, J.S., Smith, J.E. and Ellis, H.C. (1992) Paranoid and nonparanoid schizophrenic processing of facially displayed affect. *Journal of Psychiatric Research*, **26**, 169–182.

Kurachi, M., Matsui, M., Kiyoko, K., Suzuki, M., Tsunoda, M. and Yamaguchi, N. (1994) Limited visual search on the WAIS picture completion test in patients with schizophrenia. *Schizophrenia Research*, **12**, 75–80.

Leafhead, K.M., Young, A.W. and Szulecka, T.K. (1996) Delusions demand attention. *Cognitive Neuropsychiatry*, **1**, 5–16.

Lennox, B.R., Bert, S., Park, B.G., Jones, P.B. and Morris, P.G. (1999) Spatial and temporal mapping of neural activity associated with auditory hallucinations. *Lancet*, **353**, 644.

Leudar, I., Thomas, P. and Johnston, M. (1994) Self-monitoring in speech production: effects of verbal hallucinations and negative symptoms. *Psychological Medicine*, **24**, 749–761.

Leudar, I.; Thomas, P.; McNally, D. and Glinski, A. (1997) What voices can do with words: pragmatics of verbal hallucinations. *Psychological Medicine*, **27**, 885–898.

Liddle, P.F. (1987a) The symptoms of chronic schizophrenia: a re-examination of the positive–negative dichotomy. *British Journal of Psychiatry*, **151**, 145–151.

Liddle, P.F. (1987b) Schizophrenic syndromes, cognitive performance and neurological dysfunction. *Psychological Medicine*, **17**, 49–57.

Liddle, P.F., Friston, K.J., Frith, C.D. *et al.* (1992a) Patterns of cerebral blood flow in schizophrenia. *British Journal of Psychiatry*, **160**, 179–186.

Liddle, P.F., Friston, K.J., Frith, C.D. *et al.* (1992b) Cerebral blood flow and mental processes in schizophrenia. *Journal of the Royal Society of Medicine*, **85**, 224–227.

Lubow, R.E., Weiner, I. and Feldon, J. (1982) An animal model of attention. In: Spiegelstein, M.Y. and Levy, A. (eds), *Behavioural Models and the Analysis of Drug Action*. Elsevier, Amsterdam, pp. 89–107.

Maher, B.A. (1974) Delusional thinking and perceptual disorder. *Journal of Individual Psychology*, **30**, 85–95.

Marneros, A., Beyenburg, S. and Berghaus, A. (1997) Unilateral hallucinations and other psychotic symptoms due to otosclerosis. *Psychopathology*, **30**, 89–92.

Mathew, V.M., Gruzelier, J.H. and Liddle, P.F. (1993) Lateral asymmetries in auditory acuity distinguish hallucinating from nonhallucinating schizophrenic patients. *Psychiatry Research*, **46**, 127–138.

Miller, L.J., O'Connor, E. and DiPasquale, T. (1993) Patients' attitudes toward hallucinations. *American Journal of Psychiatry*, **150**, 584–588.

Morrison, A.P. and Haddock, G. (1997) Cognitive factors in source monitoring and auditory hallucinations. *Psychological Medicine*, **27**, 669–679.

Mueser, K.T., Penn. D.L., Blanchard, J.J. and Bellack, A.S. (1997) Affect recognition in schizophrenia: a synthesis of findings across three studies. *Psychiatry*, **60**, 301–308.

Nayani, T. H. and David, A. S. (1996) The auditory hallucination: a phenomenological survey. *Psychological Medicine*, **26**, 177–189.

Noton, D. and Stark, L. (1971) Eye movements and visual perception. *Scientific American*, **224**, 35–43.

Novic, J., Luchins, D.J. and Perline, R. (1984) Facial affect recognition in schizophrenia: is there a differential deficit? *British Journal of Psychiatry*, **144**, 533–537.

O'Neal, P. and Robins, L.N. (1958) Childhood patterns predictive of adult schizophrenia: a 30-year follow-up study. *American Journal of Psychiatry*, **115**, 385–391.

Paquier, P., van Vugt, P., Bal, P., Cras, P., Parizel, P.M., van Haesendonck, J., Creten, W. and Martin, J.J. (1992) Transient musical hallucinosis of central origin: a review and clinical study. *Journal of Neurology, Neurosurgery, and Psychiatry*, **55**, 1069–1073.

Penfield, W. and Perot, P. (1963) The brain's record of auditory and visual experience: a final summary and conclusion. *Brain*, **86**, 568–693.

Phillips, M.L. and David, A.S. (1994) Understanding the symptoms of schizophrenia using visual scan paths. *British Journal of Psychiatry*, **165**, 673–675.

Phillips, M.L. and David, A.S. (1997) Visual scan paths are abnormal in deluded schizophrenics. *Neuropsychologia*, **35**, 1, 99–105.

Phillips, M.L. and David, A.S. (1998) Abnormal visual scan paths: a psychophysiological marker of delusions in schizophrenia. *Schizophrenia Research*, **29**, 235–245.

Phillips, M.L., Howard, R. and David, A.S. (1997) A cognitive neuropsychological approach to the study of delusions in late-onset schizophrenia. *International Journal of Geriatric Psychiatry*, **12**, 892–901.

Premack, D. and Woodruff, G. (1978) Does the chimpanzee have a theory of mind? *Behavioural and Brain Sciences*, **4**, 515–526.

Puce, A., Truett, A., Gore, J.C. and McCarthy, G. (1995) Face-sensitive regions in human extrastriate cortex studied by functional MRI. *Journal of Neurophysiology*, **74**, 1192–1199.

Puce, A., Truett, A., Asgari, M., Gore, J.C. and McCarthy, G. (1996) Differential sensitivity of human visual cortex to faces, letterstrings, and textures: a functional magnetic resonance imaging study. *Journal of Neuroscience*, **16**, 5205–5215.

Rector, N.A. and Seeman, M.V. (1992) Auditory hallucinations in women and men. *Schizophrenia Research*, **7**, 233–236.

Ross, D.E., Thaker, G.K., Buchanan, R.W., Kirkpatrick, B., Lahti, A.C., Medoff, D., Bartko, J.J., Goodman, J. and Tien, A. (1997) Eye tracking disorder in schizophrenia is characterised by specific ocular motor defects and is associated with the deficit syndrome. *Biological Psychiatry*, **42**, 781–796.

Rossell, S.L, Shapleske, J. and David, A.S. (1998) Sentence verification and delusions: a content-specific deficit. *Psychological Medicine*, **28**, 1189–1198.

Rossell, S.L., Shapleske, J., Woodruff, P.W.R. and David, A.S. (1999) The functional asymmetry of auditory–verbal hallucinations. Abstracts of the VIIth International Congress on Schizophrenia Research, Santa Fe, New Mexico, USA. *Schizophrenia Research*, **36**, 181.

Schultz, G. and Melzack, R. (1991) The Charles Bonnet syndrome: 'phantom visual images'. *Perception*, **20**, 809–825.

Seal, M.L., Crowe, S.F. and Cheung, P. (1997) Deficits in source monitoring in subjects with auditory hallucinations may be due to differences in verbal intelligence and verbal memory. *Cognitive Neuropsychiatry*, **2**, 273–290.

Sergent, J. (1988) Face perception and the right hemisphere. In: *Thought Without Language*. L. Weiskrantz (ed.) Oxford University Press, pp. 108–131.

Sergent, J., Ohta, S. and MacDonald, B. (1992) Functional neuroanatomy of face and object processing. A positron emission tomography study. *Brain*, **115**, 15–36.

Shergill, S.S. Murray, R.M. and McGuire, P.K. (1998) Auditory hallucinations: a review of psychological treatment. *Schizophrenia Research*, **32**, 137–150.

Slade, P. and Bentall, R. (1988) *Sensory Deception: A Scientific Analysis of Hallucination*. Croom Helm, London.

Smith, J.D., Wilson, M. and Reisberg, D. (1995) The role of subvocalisation in auditory imagery. *Neuropsychologia*, **33**, 1433–1454.

Spence, S.A., Brooks, D.J., Hirsch, S.R. et al. (1997) A PET study of voluntary movement in schizophrenic patients experiencing passivity phenomena (delusions of alien control). *Brain*, **120**, 1997–2011.

Streit, M., Woelwer, W. and Gaebel, W. (1997) Facial-affect recognition and visual scanning behaviour in the course of schizophrenia. *Schizophrenia Research*, **24**, 311–317.

Terao, T. and Yukio, T. (1998) Carbamazepine treatment in a case of musical hallucinations with temporal lobe abnormalities. *Australian and New Zealand Journal of Psychiatry*, **32**, 454–456.

Tien, A.Y. (1991) Distributions of hallucinations in the population. *Social Psychiatry and Psychiatric Epidemiology*, **26**, 287–292.

Tsuang, M.T. and Winokur, G. (1974) Criteria for subtyping schizophrenia: clinical differentiation of hebephrenic and paranoid schizophrenia. *Archives of General Psychiatry*, **81**, 43–47.

Tyler, M., Diamond, J. and Lewis, S. (1995) Correlates of left-handedness in a large sample of schizophrenic patients. *Schizophrenia Research* **18**, 37–41.

Ullman, L.P. and Krasner, L. (1969) *A Psychological Approach to Abnormal Behaviour*. Prentice-Hall, Englewood Cliffs, NJ.

Vinogradov, S., Willis-Shore, J., Poole, J.H., Marten, E., Ober, B.A. and Shenaut, G.K. (1997) Clinical and neurocognitive aspects of source monitoring errors in schizophrenia. *American Journal of Psychiatry*, **154**, 1530–1537.

Wing, J.K. Cooper, J.E. and Sartorius, N. (1974) *Measurement and Classification of Psychiatric Symptoms*. Cambridge University Press.

Woodruff, P., Brammer, M., Mellers, J., Wright, I., Bullmore, E. and Williams, S. (1995) Auditory hallucinations and perception of external speech. *Lancet*, **346**, 1035.

Woodruff, P.W.R., Wright, I.C., Bullmore, E.T., Brammer, M.J., Howard, R.J., Williams, S.C.R., Shaplerke, J., Rossell, S., David, A.S., McGuire, P.K. and Murray, R.M. (1997) Auditory hallucinations and the temporal cortical response to speech in schizophrenia: a functional magnetic resonance imaging study. *American Journal of Psychiatry*, **154**, 1676–1682.

Young, H.F. and Bentall, R.P. (1995) Hypothesis testing in patients with persecutory delusions: comparison with depressed and normal subjects. *British Journal of Clinical Psychology*, **34**, 353–369.

Zalewski, C., Johnson-Selfridge, M.T., Ohriner, S., Zarella, K. and Seltzer, J.C. (1998) A review of neuropsychological differences between paranoid and nonparanoid schizophrenia patients. *Schizophrenia Bulletin*, **24**, 127–145.

12 Cognitive functioning in schizophrenic patients with comorbid substance use disorders

Mark R. Serper and James C.-Y. Chou

Introduction

Substance abuse is a major health concern in schizophrenia because of the remarkably high comorbidity of the two disorders (Regier *et al.*, 1990). Alcohol, cannabis and/or cocaine use disorders have been found to be present in almost half of all schizophrenic patients presenting for psychiatric treatment (Barbee *et al.*, 1989; Galanter *et al.*, 1992) and these are among the most frequently and heavily abused substances by schizophrenic patients (Regier *et al.*, 1990; Herman *et al.*, 1991; Cuffel *et al.*, 1993). Moreover, schizophrenic patients with any substance use disorder are also two to three times more likely to be nicotine dependent (Ziedonis *et al.*, 1997). Although the use patterns and the effects of smoking cigarettes are strikingly different from those of alcohol, cannabis or cocaine abuse, all these psychoactive substances have a significant impact on patients' symptomatic and cognitive functioning. In this chapter, we review the available research examining the effects that these substance use disorders have on schizophrenic patients' neurocognitive functioning and review methodological considerations needed for future research.

Neurocognitive consequences of abuse

Substance abuse may significantly complicate schizophrenic illness in a myriad of domains, including schizophrenic onset, symptom severity and expression, adaptive and social functioning, as well as treatment response and long-term outcome (e.g. Drake *et al.*, 1990; Osher *et al.*, 1994; Shaner *et al.*, 1995; Serper *et al.*, 1995, 1999; Wilkens, 1997). However, despite the high rates of comorbidity, and the large volume of research examining the prevalence rates and clinical effects of substance abuse on schizophrenic patients, surprisingly little research has been conducted examining the effects of substance abuse on schizophrenic patients' neurocognitive functioning. Consequently, the extent to which comorbid substance abuse compounds existing cognitive deficits in schizophrenic patients and/or results in additional deficits above their baseline impairment is not well understood. It has been commonly assumed, nevertheless, that substance abuse by schizophrenic patients results in profound cerebral injury that can adversely effect patients' symptomatic, cognitive and adaptive functioning (Tracy *et al.*, 1995) and subsequently lead to increased violent behavior (e.g. Cuffel *et al.*, 1994).

Cognitive effects of abuse in the general population

In non-schizophrenic patients, the deleterious consequences of substance abuse on addicts' cognitive functioning has been well documented, particularly the effects of chronic alcoholism. Studies examining chronic alcohol dependence in non-schizophrenic individuals find multiple neurological deficits associated with heavy, chronic abuse (see Hales and Yudofsky, 1987). The resulting cognitive deficits can be profound, with the most notable impairments occurring in learning and memory functions (Lishman 1981; Loberg, 1986; Sullivan *et al.*, 1997). However, other domains of cognitive dysfunction, including perceptual impairment and deficits in complex motor tasks, often accompany memory impairment (Loberg, 1986). Very extreme chronic abuse can result in general amnestic syndromes.

Past studies examining the deleterious consequences of cocaine abuse on cognitive functions, while not nearly as extensive as the alcoholism literature, suggest that deficits occur primarily in the addicts' learning and memory ability. Many past reports have found, for example, that cocaine abusers demonstrate significant memory impairment (Ardila *et al.*, 1991; O'Malley *et al.*, 1992; Berry *et al.*, 1993; Mittenberg and Motta, 1993; Beatty *et al.*, 1995), but many of these same studies find relatively mild or intact attentional (e.g. Ardila *et al.*, 1991; Mittenberg and Motta, 1993; Beatty *et al.*, 1995), executive (O'Malley *et al.*, 1992), visuospatial/constructional (Manscherck *et al.*, 1990; Ardila *et al.*, 1991) and global intellectual functioning (Mittenberg and Motta, 1993). Other reports, in contrast, have yielded mixed results. Beatty *et al*, (1995), for example, found that recently cocaine-abstinent patients suffer impaired memory and intact attention, but had difficulty on tasks involving executive functioning and psychomotor speed. One commonality across these studies appears to be that cocaine abuse results in mild to moderate chronic impairment of recent and delayed memory ability.

While still significantly less research exists examining the effects of cannabis abuse on addicts' cognitive functioning compared with either alcohol or cocaine abuse, deleterious consequences have been reported. Cannabis dependence, for example, has been associated with subacute encephalopathy in heavy and chronic users (Castle and Ames, 1996). In terms of neuropsychological effects, acute cannabis abuse has been associated with impairments in attention, psychomotor speed and short-term memory (Millsaps *et al.*, 1993; Lundquist, 1995; Castle and Ames, 1996). The residual effects of long-term cannabis abuse remain, to date, inconclusive.

Nicotine, unlike the other psychoactive substances, may actually enhance cognitive functioning. Nicotine appears to play an important role in modulating dopamine and glutamate transmission in the prefrontal cortex and associated medial–frontal striatal structures, resulting in enhanced synaptic transmission in these areas (Vidal, 1994; Arendash *et al.*, 1995). Sustained nicotine administration has been associated with improved learning and memory performance in rats (Arendash *et al.*, 1995; Socci *et al.*, 1995) and humans with and without Alzheimer's disease (Whitehouse and Kalaria, 1995; Wilson *et al.*, 1995). However, the chronic effects of heavy smoking on cognitive performance have not been well elucidated.

Impact of substance abuse on cognitive functioning of schizophrenic patients

Since drug addiction alters cognitive functioning in the general population, it appears highly likely that abuse would interact with the already compromised cognitive abilities of schizophrenic patients. Only a small handful of studies, surprisingly, have been conducted that have examined directly the impact of substance use disorders on schizophrenic patients' neurocognitive functioning. These studies, moreover, differ sharply in methodology, assessment strategies and the class or classes of abused drug(s) under examination. As a result, studies examining the effects of substance abuse on schizophrenic paitents' cognition have yielded inconsistent, and sometimes contradictory, findings.

In terms of nicotine dependence, schizophrenic patients who smoke cigarettes appear to demonstrate enhanced cognitive performance relative to their non-smoking counterparts. Sandyk (1993) found that schizophrenic patients who smoke performed significantly better on the Mini-Mental State Examination compared with non-smoking schizophrenic patients. In a more comprehensive study, Levin *et al.* (1996) examined haloperidol-treated schizophrenic patients who smoked over four different assessment intervals after overnight cigarette deprivation. On each testing occasion, conducted on consecutive mornings, patients received nicotine skin patches of varied dosages and were tested 3 h after administration. Nicotine dose-related improvements in memory, complex reaction time on a spatial rotation task and attentional functioning using the Continuous Performance Test (CPT) were reported. In another report, smoking had been found to normalize deficits in auditory sensory gating in schizophrenia (Adler *et al.*, 1993). Schizophrenic smokers had a marked but brief improvement in P50 auditory gating immediately after smoking. In terms of the mechanism of action, nicotine may enhance cognitive functioning in schizophrenic patients in much the same way as some novel antipsychotic medications have been found to improve cognition (e.g. Green *et al.*, 1997; Sax *et al.*, 1998). Recent models attribute schizophrenic patients' cognitive impairment to hypodopamingeric functioning in the prefrontal cortex and its associated meso-cortical dopaminergic projections (e.g. Bilder *et al.*, 1992; Cohen and Servan-Scheiver, 1992). Nicotine, specifically, may enhance glutamate transmission in the prefrontal cortex, which may amplify glutamatergic and dopaminergic activity in the basal ganglia and the corpus striatum (Clarke and Pert, 1985; Vidal, 1994).

In contrast to the effects of nicotine, cocaine-abusing schizophrenic patients appear to manifest attentional and cognitive impairment relative to their non-abusing counterparts. Sevy *et al.* (1990) reported that significant cognitive deficits were associated with cocaine-abusing individuals with schizophrenia. Deficits in schizophrenic patients who abused cocaine were detected on tests of verbal memory, conceptual encoding and recall, but not on tests of attention to sequences or spontaneous psychomotor speed compared with schizophrenic patients without a history of cocaine use. Additionally, Sevy and colleagues (1990) point out that the cocaine-abusing patients were by and large polysubstance abusers. Recomputation of the analyses for each other substance of abuse did not account for the differences on the cognitive tests, suggesting that the deficits in encoding, memory and recall were specific to cocaine abuse.

Similarly, Serper *et al.* (2000) have found that schizophrenic individuals with comorbid cocaine abuse manifest specific deficits on measures of learning and memory, but, like the findings of Sevy *et al.* (1990), not on attentional tasks or on executive function tasks, when compared with non-abusing schizophrenic patients. In this study, schizophrenic individuals with comorbid cocaine abuse/dependence demonstrated difficulty in their initial encoding of word list information, in their rate of acquisition over successive learning trials, in their total learning and in their ability to retain the information that they did acquire compared with their non-abusing counterparts. While past studies repeatedly have found that non-abusing schizophrenic patients display significant learning and memory impairment relative to normals (e.g. Gold *et al.*, 1992; Paulsen *et al.*, 1995), information that is acquired has been found to be fairly well retained over time (e.g. Paulson *et al.*, 1995). Schizophrenic patients who recently have abused cocaine, in marked contrast, appear not to retain previously acquired information and suffer much higher rates of memory loss compared with their non-abusing counterparts.

In marked contrast, Cleghorn *et al.* (1991) reported that schizophrenic patients abusing one or more substances did not differ from non-abusing schizophrenic individuals on a wide variety of neuropsychological measures, including memory, attention, verbal fluency, learning and problem solving. Similarly, a study by Addington and Addington (1997) also failed to find differences between schizophrenic patients who abuse substances and their non-abusing counterparts across a wide range of cognitive functions including verbal ability, attention, executive functioning, and verbal and visual memory. Both the Cleghorn *et al.* (1991) and the Addington and Addington (1997) groups utilized extensive and thorough neuropsychological test batteries. The Cleghorn *et al.* report, for example, utilized <60 well known and standardized neuropsychological measures. The Addington and Addington study also utilized commonly used and standardized tests including the Wisconsin Card Sorting Test, the CPT, the forced-choice Span of Apprehension task, parts of the Wechsler Adult Intelligence Scale (revised) and the Wechsler Memory Scale (revised). Sevy *et al.* (1990), in contrast to the studies of Addington and Addington and Cleghorn *et al.*, did not include tasks commonly used in neuropsychological or schizophrenia research (e.g. the Verbal Ability Test), limiting its generalizability, and the Serper *et al.* study (2000), while including tasks commonly used in schizophrenia research (e.g. WCST, California Verbal Learning Test, CPT and digit span task), utilized only four neurocognitive tests.

Class of abused drug

Perhaps of greater importance when accounting for differences in studies is the issue of specification and examination of the class of abused drugs. Both the Cleghorn *et al.* study and the Addington and Addington report included schizophrenic patients who had a history of abusing a wide variety of different substances or multiple substances. In the Cleghorn *et al.* (1991) report, substance abuse was categorized as either present or absent based on patient self-report. No reference was made to previous history of street drug or alcohol abuse, urine drug toxicology or family verification in either the abusing or non-abusing samples, all of which would enhance reliability of substance abuse and dependence diagnosis. Addington and Addington (1997) provide a detailed account and document patients' abuse status, including medical chart documentation and past referral for dual diagnosis treatment. It was reported that the abuser group's drug history included a mix of alcohol dependence (13 subjects), cannabis dependence (five subjects), alcohol and cannabis dependence (12 subjects) and different combinations of drugs including alcohol and crack dependence, codeine dependence, benylin dependence and alcohol and barbiturate dependence (four subjects).

Both the Sevy *et al.* (1990) and Serper *et al.* (2000) studies, in contrast, found specific memory deficits in cocaine-abusing schizophrenic patients relative to their non-abusing counterparts, but relatively well preserved functioning in other cognitive domains. Consequently, specification and examination of the class(es) of abused drug(s) are needed in order to sort out the unique neurobiological effects which different substances have on schizophrenic patients' neurocognitive functioning and to determine their impact on the cognitive functioning of these patients.

Distinguishing acute from residual effects of substance use

Distinguishing between the potentially transitory effects of acute intoxication and drug withdrawal from the long-term or residual consequences of chronic abuse remains a crucial but unresolved issue in the literature. It has been found, for example, in non-schizophrenic alcoholics, that certain cognitive and memory deficits secondary to recent alcohol abuse reverse themselves during periods of abstinence (e.g. O'Leary *et al.*, 1977; Hester *et al.*, 1980; Kish *et al.*, 1980). Similar findings were also found to be correlated with increased regional cerebral blood flow associated with alcohol abstinence (Berglund *et al.*, 1982). Since certain alcohol-related spatial and executive neuropsychological impairments may be transient, the possibility exists that longitudinal assessment of performance may distinguish the progressive cognitive deficits associated with schizophrenia over the lifespan (e.g. Harvey *et al.*, 1995) from the potentially more reversible alcohol-related impairments. It is unknown if alcoholic schizophrenic patients, like non-schizophrenic alcoholics, manifest a resilience to recover from cortical injury associated with recent alcohol abuse. The need exists for a longitudinal investigation to examine whether alcohol abuse by schizophrenic patients induces residual cognitive impairment during long-term alcohol abstinence and symptom remission.

Similarly, in a comprehensive review of the status of research on the long-term cognitive effects of cannabis abuse, Pope *et al.* (1995) point out the need to distinguish acute effects of intoxication from residual neuropsychological effects of heavy cannabis abuse. Pope *et al.* argue that although the acute neurotoxic effects (12–24 h after immediate use) on attention, psychomotor speed and memory are fairly well documented, long-term effects of cannabis on neuropsychological functioning and the central nervous system have not been validated adequately.

In terms of cocaine abuse, there is some evidence from experimental and naturalistic studies that the acute effects of psychostimulants may actually improve schizophrenic patients' neurocognitive functioning by enhancing dopamine activation in medial–frontal neural pathways (e.g. Goldberg *et al.*, 1991; Bilder *et al.*, 1992). There is also evidence in normal subjects that cognitive enhancement endures hours after the euphoric effects of cocaine intoxication have subsided (Stillman *et al.*, 1993). Yet psychostimulant-induced symptomatic or cognitive enhancement appears to be highly transitory. Cocaine abstinence following binge use is associated with dopaminergic (DA) and serotoninergic (5-HT) depletion (e.g. Dackis and Gold, 1985; McDougle *et al.*, 1992; Parsons, *et al.*, 1995; Volkow *et al.*, 1997) within hours after use. In terms of the neuropsychological effects of cocaine abstinence-induced DA and 5-HT depletion, animal studies reveal that impaired learning and memory consolidation occur after destruction of the DA or the 5-HT neurotransmitter systems (Dubrovina and Ilyutchenok, 1996; Meneses and Hong, 1997). Reduced DA tone has also been associated with memory and other cognitive impairment in humans (e.g. Volkow *et al.*, 1998). Both the Serper *et al.* (2000) and the Sevy *et al.* (1990) studies (in addition to almost every study cited above examining cognitive functioning in non-schizophrenic cocaine addicts) were conducted during acute phases of cocaine abstinence and therefore presumably during periods of DA and 5-HT depletion. This raises the possibility that cocaine-abusing schizophrenic patients' learning and memory deficits would reverse themselves with abstinence. However, since little longitudinal research has been conducted, it remains unclear if learning and memory deficits would persist after more prolonged cocaine abstinence and normalization of neurotransmitter levels.

Conclusions and future directions

It is apparent that the substance-induced effects on schizophrenic patients' cognitive functioning is not only mediated by the type of abused drug(s) but also by the duration, frequency and quantity of previous use. Future researchers need to assess these variables when examining the impact which various substances have on patients' cognitive functioning. Another issue concerns the complex neurobiological interaction of various substance with schizophrenic illness. It is relatively unknown whether cognitive deficits resulting from chronic substance abuse combine in additive or synergistic ways with the neurocognitive impairments inherent in schizophrenic illness.

To further our understanding of the effects which various substance abuse disorders have on schizophrenic patients' cognitive functioning, future researchers may wish to: (i) subdivide patients according to the class of abused drug or drugs; (ii) collect information on drug use patterns such as the duration and frequency of abuse; (iii) assess patients' cognitive functioning at various time points over schizophrenic illness (e.g. during acute psychosis and remission); and (iv) collect this same information at various stages of substance dependency (e.g. intoxication, withdrawal, acute and prolonged abstinence). In general, the majority of studies conducted to date indicate that substance use disorders play a significant role in the course of illness, symptom presentation, treatment response and neurocognitive functioning of schizophrenic patients.

Acknowledgements

This chapter was supported, in part, by a NARSAD Young Investigator Award and USPHS grant MH 57793 from the National Institute of Mental Health to Dr Serper.

References

Addington, J. and Addington, D. (1997) Substance abuse and cognitive functioning in schizophrenia. *Journal of Psychiatry and Neuroscience*, **22**, 99–104.

Adler, LE., Hoffer, L., Wiser, A. and Freedman, R. (1993) Normalization of auditory physiology by cigarette smoking schizophrenic patients. *American Journal of Psychiatry*, **150**, 1856–1861.

Ardila, A,, Rossselli, M. and Strumwasser, S. (1991) Neuropsychological deficits in chronic cocaine abusers. *International Journal of Neuroscience*, **57**, 73–79.

Arendash, G.W., Sengstock, G.J., Sanberg, P.R. and Kem, W.R. (1995) Improved learning and memory in aged rats with chronic administration of the nicotinic receptor angonist GTS-21. *Brain Research*, **674**, 252–259.

Barbee, J.G., Clark, P.D., Crapanzano, M.S., Heintz, G.C. and Kehoe, C.E. (1989) Alcohol and substance abuse among schizophrenic patients presenting to an emergency psychiatric service. *Journal of Nervous and Mental Disease*, **177**, 400–407.

Beatty, W.W., Katzung, V.M., Moreland, V.J. and Nixon, S.J. (1995) Neuropsychological performance of recently abstinent alcoholics and cocaine abusers. *Drug and Alcohol Dependence*, **37**, 247–253.

Berglund, M., Risberg, J. and Bliding, A. (1982) Evidence of right hemisphere dysfunction in alcoholism. Presented at the *First Nordic Neuropsychological Symposium*. Helsinki, Finland.

Berry, J, Van-Gorp, W., Herzberg, D.S. and Hinkin, C. (1993) Neuropsychological deficits in abstinent cocaine abusers. *Drug and Alcohol Dependence*, **32**, 231–237.

Bilder, R.M., Lieberman, J.A., Kim, Y., Alvir, J.M. and Reiter, G. (1992) Methylphenidate and neuroleptic effects on oral word production in schizophrenia. *Neuropsychiatry, Neuropsychology and Behavioral Neurology*, **5**, 262–271.

Castle, D.J. and Ames, F.R. (1996) Cannabis and the brain. *Australian and New Zealand Journal of Psychiatry*, **30**, 179–183.

Clarke, P.B. and Pert, A. (1985) Autoradiographic evidence of nicotine receptors on nigrostriatal and mesolimbic dopaminergic neurons. *Brain Research*, **348**, 355–358.

Cleghorn, J.M., Kaplan, R.D., Szechtman, B., Szechtman, H, Brown, G.M. and Franco, S. (1991) Substance abuse and schizophrenia: effect on symptoms but not on neurocognitive function. *Journal of Clinical Psychiatry*, **52**, 26–30.

Cohen, J.D. and Servan-Schreiber, D. (1992) Context, cortex and dopamine: a connectionist approach to behavior and biology in schizophrenia. *Psychological Review*, **99**, 45–77.

Cuffel, B.J., Shumway, M., Chouljian, T.L. and Macdonald, T. (1994) A longitudinal study of substance use and community violence in schizophrenia. *Journal of Nervous and Mental Disease*, **182**, 704–708.

Dackis, C.A. and Gold, M.S. (1985) New concepts in cocaine addiction: the dopamine depletion hypothesis. *Neuroscience and Biobehavioral Review*, **9**, 447–469.

Drake, R.E., Osher, F.C., Noordsy, D.L. *et al.* (1990) Diagnosis of alcohol use disorders in schizophernia. *Schizophrenia Bulletin*, **16**, 57–68.

Dubrovina, N.I. and Ilyutchenok, R.Y. (1996) Dopamine and opioid regulation of the memory retrieval recovery in mice. *Behavioural Brain Research*, **79**, 23–29.

Galanter, M., Egelko, S., de-Leon, G. and Rohrs, C. (1992) Crack/cocaine abusers n the general hospital: assessment and initiation of care. *American Journal of Psychiatry*, **149**, 810–815.

Gold, J.M., Randolph, C., Carpenter, C.J., Goldberg, T.E. and Weinberger, D.R. (1992) Forms of memory failure in schizophrenia. *Journal of Abnormal Psychology*, **101**, 487–494.

Goldberg, T.E., Bigelow, L.B., Weinberger, D.R., Daniel, D.G. and Kleinman, J.E. (1991) Cognitive and behavioral effects on coadministration of dextroamphetamine and haloperidol in schizophrenia. *American Journal of Psychiatry*, **148**, 78–84.

Green, M.F., Marshall, B.D., Wirshing, W.C., Ames, D., Mader, S.R., McGurk, S., Kern, R.S. and Mintiz, J. (1997) Does risperidone improve verbal working memory in treatment resistant schizophrenics? *American Journal of Psychiatry*, **154**, 799–804.

Hales, R.E. and Yudofsky, S.C. (1987) *Textbook of Neuropsychiatry.* American Psychiatric Press, Washington, DC.

Harvey, P.D., Lombardi, J., Kincaid, M., White, L., Parrella, M., Powchik, P. and Davidson, M (1995) Cognitive functioning in chronically hospitalized schizophrenic patients: age-related changes and age disorientation as a predictor of impairments. *Schizophrenia Research*, **17**, 15–24.

Herman, M., Galanter, M. and Lifshutz, H. (1991) Combined substance abuse and psychiatric disorders in homeless and domiciled patients. *American Journal of Drug and Alcohol Abuse*, **17**, 415–422.

Hester, R.K., Smith J.W. and Jackson, T.R. (1980) Recovery of cognitive skills in alcoholics. *Journal of Studies on Alcoholism*, **41**, 363–367.

Kish, G.B., Hagen, J.M., Woody, M.W. and Harvey, H.L. (1980) Alcoholic's recovery from cerebral impairment as a function of duration of abstinence. *Journal of Clinical Psychology*, **36**, 584–589.

Levin, E.D., Wilson, W., Rose, J.E. and McEvoy, J. (1996) Nicotine–haloperidol interactions and cognitive performance in schizophrenics. *Neuropsychopharmacology*, **15**, 429–436.

Lishman, W.A. (1981) Cerebral disorders in alcoholism: syndromes of impairment. *Brain*, **104**, 1–21.

Loberg, T. (1986) Neuropsychological findings in early and middle phases of alcoholism. In: Grant, I. and Adams, K. (eds), *Neuropsychological Assessment of Neuropsychiatric Disorders.* Oxford University Press, New York, pp. 415–440.

Lundquist, T. (1995) Specific though patterns in chronic cannabis smokers observed during treatment. *Life Sciences*, **56**, 2141–2144.

Manscherck, T.C., Magert, L., Schneyer, C., Weinstein, C., Laughery, J., Rosenthal., J. Celada, T. and Berner, J. (1990) Freebase cocaine and memory. *Comprehensive Psychiatry*, **31**, 369–375.

McDougle, C.J, Price, L.H., Palumbo, J.M., Koston, T.R., Heninger, G.R. and Kleber, H.D. (1992) Dopaminergic responsivity during cocaine abstinence: a pilot study. *Psychiatry Research*, **43**, 77–85.

Meneses, A. and Hong, E. (1997) A pharmacological analysis of serotonergic receptors: effects of their activation of blockade in learning. *Progress in Neuropsychopharmacology and Biological Psychiatry*, **21**, 273–296.

Millsaps, C.L., Azrin, R.L. and Mittenberg, W. (1995) Neuropsychological effects of chronic cannabis use on the memory and intelligence of adolescents. *Journal of Child and Adolescent Substance Abuse*, **3**, 47–55.

Mittenberg, W. and Motta, S. (1993) Effects of chronic cocaine abuse on memory and learning. *Archives of Clinical Neuropsychology*, **8**, 477–483.

O'Leary, M.R., Radford, L.M., Chaney, E.F. and Schau, E.J. (1977) Assessment of cognitive recovery in alcoholics by use of the Trail Making Test. *Journal of Clinical Psychology*, **33**, 579–582.

O'Malley, S., Adamse, M., Heaton, R.K. and Gawin, F.H. (1992) Neuropsychological impairment in chronic cocaine abusers. *American Journal of Drug and Alcohol Abuse*, **18**, 131–144.

Osher, F.C., Drake, R.E., Noordsy, D.L. and Teague, G.B. (1994) Correlates and outcomes of alcohol use disorder among rural outpatients with schizophrenia. *Journal of Clinical Psychiatry*, **55**, 109–113.

Parsons, L.H., Koob, G.F. and Weiss, F. (1995) Serotonin dysfunction in the nucleus accumbens of rats during withdrawal after unlimited access to intravenous cocaine. *Journal of Pharmacology and Experimental Therapy*, **274**, 1182–1191.

Paulsen, J.S., Heaton, R.K., Sadek, J.R., Perry, W., Delis, D.C., Braff, D., Kuck, J., Zisook, S. and Jeste, D.V. (1995) The nature of learning and memory impairments in schizophrenia. *Journal of the International Neuropsychological Society*, **1**, 88–99.

Pope, H.G., Gruber, A.J. and Yurgelun-Todd, D. (1995) The residual neuropsychological effects of cannabis: the current status of research. *Drug and Alcohol Dependence*, **38**, 25–34.

Regier, D.A., Farmer, M.E., Rae, D.S., Locke, B.Z., Keith, S.J., Judd, L.L. and Goodwin, F.K. (1990) Comorbidity of mental disorders with alcohol and other drug abuses. *Journal of the American Medical Association*, **264**, 2511–2518.

Sandyk, R. (1993). Cigarette smoking: Effects on cognitive functions and drug-induced parkinsonism in chronic schizophrenia. *International Journal of Neuroscience*, **70**, 193–197.

Sax, K.W., Strakowski, S.M. and Keck, P.E. (1998) Attentional improvement following quetiapine furmate treatment in schizophrenia. *Schizophrenia Bulletin*, **33**, 151–155.

Serper, M.R., Alpert, M., Richardson, N.A., Dickson, S., Allen, M. and Werner, A. (1995) Clinical effects of recent cocaine use in acute schizophrenia. *American Journal of Psychiatry*, **152**, 1464–1469.

Serper, M.R., Chou, J.C-Y, Allen, M.H., Czobor, P. and Cancro, R. (1999) Symptomatic overlap of cocaine intoxication and acute schizophrenia at emergency presentation. *Schizophrenia Bulletin*, **25**, 387–394.

Serper, M.R., Bergman, A., Copersino, M.L., Chou, J.-C.Y., Richarme, D. and Canero, R. (2000). Learning and memory impairment in cocaine dependant and comorbid schizophrenic patients. *Psychiatry Research*, **93**, 387–394.

Sevy, S., Kay, S.R., Opler, L.A. and van Praag, H.M. (1990) Significance of cocaine history in schizophrenia. *Journal of Nervous and Mental Disease*, **178**, 642–647.

Shaner, A., Mintz, J., Eckman, T.A., Roberts, L.J., Wilkens, J.N., Tucker, D.E. and Tsuang, J. (1995) Disability income, cocaine use and repeated hospitalizations among schizophrenic cocaine abusers: a government-sponsored revolving door? *New England Journal of Medicine*, **333**, 777–783.

Socci, D.J., Sanberg, P.R. and Arendash, G.W. (1995) Nicotine enhances Morris water maze performance of young and aged rats. *Neurobiology of Aging*, **16**, 857–861.

Stillman, R., Jones, R.T., Moore, D., Walker, J. and Welm, S. (1993) Improved performance four hours after cocaine. *Psychopharmacology*, **110**, 415–420.

Sullivan, E.V., Shear, P.K., Zipursky, R.B., Sager, H.J. *et al.* (1997) Patterns of content, contextual, and working memory impairments in schizophrenics and nonamnesic alcoholism. *Neuropsychology*, **11**, 195–206.

Tracy, J.I., Josiassen, R. and Bellack, A.S. (1995) Neuropsychology of dual diagnosis: understanding the combined effects of schizophrenia and substance use disorders. *Clinical Psychology Review*, **15**, 67–97.

Vidal, C. (1994) Nicotine potentiation of glutamatergic synapses in the prefrontal cortex: new insights into the analysis of the role of nicotinic receptors in cognitive functions. *Drug Development Research*, **31**, 120–126.

Volkow, N.D., Wang, G.J., Fowler, J.S. *et al.* (1997) Decreased striatal dopaminergic responsiveness in detoxified cocaine-dependent subjects. *Nature*, **386**, 830–833.

Volkow, N.D., Gur, R., Wang, G.J. *et al.* (1998) Association between decline in brain dopamine activity with age and cognitive and motor impairment in healthy individuals. *American Journal Psychiatry*, **155**, 344–349.

Whitehouse, P.J. and Kalaria, R.N (1995) Nicotinic receptors and neurodegenerative dementing diseases: basic research and clinical implications. *Alzheimer Disease and Associated Disorders*, **9** (Suppl. 2), 3–5.

Wilkens, J.N. (1997) Pharmacotherapy of schizophrenic patients with comorbid substance abuse. *Schizophrenia Bulletin*, **23**, 215–228.

Wilson, A.L., Langley, L.K., Monley, J., Bauer, T. *et al.* (1995) Nicotine patches in Alzheimer's disease: pilot study on learning, memory and safety. *Pharmacology, Biochemistry and Behavior*, **51**, 509–514.

Ziedonis, D.M. and George, T.P. (1997) Schizophrenia and nicotine use: report of a pilot smoking cessation program and review of neurobiological and clinical issues. *Schizophrenia Bulletin*, **23**, 247–254.

Section 3:
Treatment for cognitive impairments

13 Cognitive effects of typical antipsychotic treatment: another look

Crystal R. Blyler and James M. Gold

Introduction

The introduction of several new 'atypical' or new generation antipsychotic compounds in the last decade represents a major advance in schizophrenia therapeutics. Evidence suggests that some of these compounds, particularly clozapine, may be differentially effective for a significant percentage of treatment-resistant patients, and the presence of fewer undesirable side effects relative to traditional antipsychotics may enhance treatment compliance (Kane *et al.*, 1988; Buchanan *et al.*, 1998). These drugs, therefore, may be superior antipsychotics, both because of true differential efficacy and because increased compliance with treatment reduces the relapse risk associated with medication discontinuation. Far less clear, however, is whether these newer compounds are more than better antipsychotics, i.e. the data are much less compelling regarding whether these compounds are truly differentially effective in the treatment of the cognitive impairments that are characteristic of schizophrenia (Buchanan *et al.*, 1994). In light of evidence that cognitive deficits are critically important mediators of functional disability (Green, 1996), the establishment of whether these newer compounds truly act as cognitive enhancers rather than being simply better antipsychotics is necessary. In formulating the issue in this way, we do not mean to in any way diminish the importance of antipsychotic effects. Clearly, such effects are crucial in the clinical management of the illness. If the goal of treatment is to have a major impact on long-term functional outcome, however, the problem of cognitive impairment remains a major hurdle in the evaluation of the broad scope of drug efficacy.

Earlier reviews: conclusions and limitations

Because of ethical issues involved in withholding medical treatments from those who need them, the cognitive effects of the new antipsychotics are most often reported as relative effects compared with those of traditional neuroleptics. In order to evaluate the cognitive impact of the newer agents, therefore, the accumulated literature on typical agents must be considered. The large literature on traditional antipsychotics, dating from the earliest clinical trials of chlorpromazine in the 1950s through to the late 1980s, has been subjected to several extensive narrative reviews. The reviews of Heaton and Crowley (1981), Medalia *et al.* (1988), Spohn and Strauss (1989), Cassens *et al.* (1990), King (1990) and Bilder *et al.* (1992) have come to remarkably similar conclusions. Based on these reviews, chronic treatment with conventional agents appears to have limited cognitive benefits and costs. Specifically, positive effects have been noted on aspects of selective/sustained attention, and mild negative effects have been observed on aspects of motor function, consistent with evidence that these agents cause extrapyramidal symptoms, and, possibly, on memory, which appears to be attributable primarily to the use of adjunctive anticholinergic agents (Tune *et al.*, 1982). Practically speaking, the greatest importance of the finding of limited cognitive benefits and costs of traditional agents was to support the hypothesis that neurocognitive deficits in schizophrenia result from the disease process rather than from iatrogenic treatment effects. Theoretically, past reviews have also supported the idea that the positive symptoms and cognitive abnormalities associated with the illness are at least partially, if not largely, dissociable. There is little dispute that conventional agents are effective in the treatment of positive psychotic symptoms, and the absence, or near absence, of cognitive improvement despite marked symptomatic change strongly suggests that these two dimensions of the illness represent distinct domains of pathology.

Despite the consistency of their conclusions, the reviews of the early literature should be re-examined critically for several reasons. First, all reviewers, including one of the present authors (J.M.G.), noted the remarkably poor methodological quality of the literature, raising the possibility that the results of these studies might not provide an adequate foundation for the theoretical interpretations that have been based on them. Many of the studies used very small samples, and conclusions typically were based on null hypothesis testing with inadequate power to detect even fairly large effects. Second, several aspects of the findings themselves remain puzzling and provocative. If neuroleptic treatment improves aspects of sustained attention (Orzack *et al.*, 1967; Spohn *et al.*, 1977), for example, one would expect other cognitive benefits to accrue simply by an improvement in the ability to stay on task and respond selectively to targets and distractors. In addition, studies of medication effects on cognition almost inevitably confound direct cognitive effects, if such exist, with symptomatic effects. Numerous studies have documented significant correlations between higher symptom levels and poorer cognition (for a review, see Strauss, 1993). Although typically modest in size, the fact that such correlations have been reported frequently might lead one to expect that a diminution of symptom severity with medication would be accompanied by some cognitive benefit. The failure to document such positive effects in the older literature is puzzling, perhaps explained by limited power to detect small changes, or limited variance as the most severely symptomatic subjects may not have been able to complete the cognitive testing. If such confounds do not explain the paradoxical lack of cognitive benefit of symptomatic change, a more complicated possibility arises: typical agents might have cognitive costs that are hidden and balanced by symptomatic effects. This possibility would be consistent with subjective complaints of patients receiving neuroleptic medications, such as feelings of cognitive slowing.

Despite historical findings that neuroleptics have little effect on cognition in schizophrenic patients, several other lines of evidence suggest that dopaminergic blockade does have cognitive consequences. Studies in both normal and schizophrenic subjects have documented cognitive benefits associated with dopamine agonists (Goldberg *et al.*, 1991; Luciana *et al.*, 1992; Dolan *et al.*, 1995; Muller *et al.*, 1998). Conversely, disorders which involve dopamine depletion, such as Parkinson's disease and phenylketonuria (PKU), present with cognitive deficits often attributed to a disruption of frontal lobe function (Lees and Smith, 1983; Taylor *et al.*, 1986; Welsh *et al.*, 1990; Diamond *et al.*, 1994). Recent animal and computational modeling research has established an important role for dopamine in the processing of reward and error information, fundamental processes involved in new learning (Cohen and Servan-Schreiber, 1992; Schultz *et al.*, 1993; Montague *et al.*, 1996). Krimer *et al.* (1998) recently reported evidence that dopamine neurotransmission may be involved in the regulation of local cerebral cortical blood flow. In a study comparing the cerebral metabolism of patients studied both when taking haloperidol and when medication free for 30 days, Holcomb *et al.* (1996) noted large regional changes in brain metabolism as a function of drug state, including medication-related increases in the thalamus and putamen and decreases in the anterior cingulate and frontal cortex. It is hard to imagine that such a dramatic rearrangement of the cortical metabolic landscape would not have some cognitive consequences, either positive or negative.

These data form the empirical and conceptual background that is critical to consider in evaluating new data on both the typical and new generation antipsychotic agents. In our view, the essential question is, are the new agents cognitive enhancers, or were the typical neuroleptics actually worse for many cognitive functions than previously was appreciated? If the latter is the case, the apparent advantage of the newer agents might be best interpreted as reflecting a lack of deleterious effect rather than as a direct cognitive enhancement.

Studies published since 1990

Here, we review the studies published since 1990 (i.e. those published since the previously cited series of reviews) that examined the relationship between traditional neuroleptic medication and cognitive functioning in schizophrenia. Earlier reviews identified a number of important methodological limitations of the older literature, including lack of operational diagnostic criteria, non-random assignment to treatment, failure to control for adjunctive medication status and failure to consider the role of practice effects on performance. We reviewed the most recent literature to determine (i) whether the methodology of studies has improved so that the findings may be more trustworthy; and (ii) whether the findings of newer studies are consistent with those of the older literature.

Twenty eight studies were included altogether, and they consisted of four different types of research design (Tables 13.1 and 13.2). The largest group of studies (13) employed a within-subjects design in which comparisons of cognitive functioning were made between time periods when research subjects were on neuroleptic medication and times when they were on greatly reduced doses or no medication. Ten studies employed a between-subjects design in which the cognition of patients who were taking medication was compared with that of different patients who were taking considerably less or no medication. Three studies examined the relationship between medication dosage or blood levels and tests of cognition. The remaining three studies were mixed designs that incorporated aspects of more than one of

Table 13.1 Research designs that allow for the clearest and easiest interpretation of findings

Citation	N	Medications	Tests	Medication effects
Within-subjects designs				
With counterbalanced crossover design to control for practice effects				
Pigache (1993)	20	Chlorpromazine 500 mg (300–900)	Auditory CPT	Improved
Salo et al. (1997)	7	Antipsychotics, some investigational	Stroop negative priming, RT, errors, and within-trial interference and facilitation	Mixed: mostly no effect; normalized negative priming
Mixed designs				
Randomized to medication status				
Gilbertson and van Kammen (1997)	12 medication maintenance, 9 neuroleptic-withdrawn	Haloperidol 11 ± 4 mg (4–20)	WMS-R verbal and visual memory, attention; Boston Remote Memory, verbal and visual; Trails A and B; non-degraded CPT	Mixed: mostly no effect; improved WMS-R memory; worsened verbal remote recall
Levine et al. (1997)	10 chlorpromazine, 10 perphenazine, 10 placebo	Perphenazine: 8 mg, Chlorpromazine: 100 mg	Word Association Test	Mixed: improved RTs; no effect on uncommon word associations
Between-groups designs				
Randomized to medication status				
Earle-Boyer et al. (1991)	17 unmedicated, 17 medicated, 19 normal controls	Haloperidol 20 mg	Auditory and visual CPT (3-letter words or nonsense syllables; 2-stimulus target sequence); penny-placing; peg displacement	Mixed: mostly no effect; improved non-lexical errors
Levin et al. (1996)	6 low dosage, 6 medium dosage, 3 high dosage	Haloperidol low 1.59 ± 1 mg, medium 4.67 ± 2.42 mg, high 10 ± 3.46 mg	Simple and spatial rotation RT, delayed matching to sample, modified Sternberg memory test, Conners' CPT	Mixed: no effect on simple RT, Sternberg, or CPT; worsened spatial rotation RT and delayed matching to sample
Serper et al. (1990)	4 medicated, 4 unmedicated	Haloperidol 10 mg b.i.d.	Non-degraded CPT, word-list shadowing	Mixed: no effect on first trial errors; improved learning over trials

these research techniques. (Salo *et al.*, 1997 separately analyzed data on the same subjects using first a between-subjects design and then a within-subjects design; this study, therefore, was included in both categories.)

Adequacy of methodology

Within-subjects and mixed designs

Within-subject designs most closely approximate everyday clinical practice in which patients are assessed first under one drug condition and then another, with the goal of determining whether the drug is associated with better performance or clinical response. In order to attribute the observed change confidently to the treatment condition, the confounding effect of repeated assessment, i.e. practice effects, on test performance must be ruled out. Practice effects must be accounted for even when no change between assessments is observed because an absence of practice effects in patient groups may indicate that the medication conditions significantly disrupt the ability to learn.

As noted by Lezak (1995), practice effects typically are most evident on tasks that involve speeded responding, learning or an 'unfamiliar response mode,' or on problem-solving tasks that have a 'single solution' (p. 129). Many of the tasks that are used with the greatest frequency in studying the impact of medication on schizophrenia have the characteristics that are associated most with susceptibility to practice effects, and practice effects can be quite large. In reliability studies of the third versions of the Wechsler Adult Intelligence Scale (WAIS-III) and Wechsler Memory Scales (WMS-III; Psychological Corporation, 1997), healthy young adults typically gained an average of 5 points in full-scale IQ (FSIQ) and 13 points on the General Memory Index on repeated testing. Practice effects in special populations can vary somewhat unpredictably. They may be reduced, for example, in elderly normal subjects and in some neurologically compromised groups (Lezak, 1995). Contrary to expectations, however, robust practice effects have been demonstrated in patients with temporal lobe epilepsy, a patient population with prominent memory and learning deficits that one might hypothesize would attenuate practice effects (Sawrie *et al.*, 1996).

Of the 13 within-subjects studies included in this review, seven neither controlled for nor made reference to possible practice effects (Table 13.2). Neither Gold and Hurt (1990) nor Finkelstein *et al.* (1997) controlled for practice effects within their studies, but both referenced data from previous studies that addressed practice effects of the tests employed in normal healthy subjects. Both Verdoux *et al.* (1995) and Censits *et al.* (1997) compared medication-related change in patient performance with the change in performance of normal controls over the same period of time. Although comparison with normal controls over time allows analysis of differences in practice effects between medicated patients and controls, this strategy is inadequate for distinguishing between the effects of medication and possible disease effects of schizophrenia on the ability to learn from practice. In order to control ideally for practice effects in within-subjects analyses of medication effects on cognition, mixed designs should be used in which unmedicated patients are compared with medicated patients over the same time interval. All three of the mixed design studies included in this review employed such a technique, but Serper *et al.* (1990) did not assign patients randomly to groups so that pre-

Table 13.2 Studies for which alternative interpretations of presumed medication effects are possible due to inadequate research designs

Citation	N	Medications	Tests	Medication effects
Within-subjects designs				
With normal controls for practice effects				
Censits et al. (1997)	30 first episode 30 previously treated	Typicals previously treated: 601 ± 47 mg CPZEQ first episode: 260 ± 47 mg CPZEQ 3 on clozapine: 320 ± 25 mg CPZEQ	WCST; Stroop; Trails; WAIS-R digit span, digit–symbol, bock design; CPT; logical memory; CVLT; WMS design reproduction; verbal fluency; Animal and Boston Naming; WRAT-R reading; Token Test; line orientation; Rosen Drawing Test; Reitan–Klove Sensory–Perceptual Exam; finger–thumb opposition; finger tapping	No effect
Verdoux et al. (1995)	18	Typicals 641 ± 678mg CPZEQ	WCST, verbal fluency, Stroop, Rey figure, WAIS-R digit–symbol	No effect
With reference to practice effects in healthy subjects				
Finkelstein et al. (1997)	24 neuroleptic-naive 20 neuroleptic withdrawn 44 normal controls	Typicals 310 ± 255 mg CPZEQ	Gordon distractibility CPT	No effect
Gold and Hurt (1990)	19	2 dosage groups of haloperidol	WAIS	Improved, but probably due to practice effects
With no controls for practice effects				
Allen et al. (1997)	22	Haloperidol 10.2 ± 4.05 mg (4–20)	Trails, Letter Cancellation, WMS-R forward and backward digit span, degraded CPT, WCST	No effect
Bilder et al. (1992)	13	Neuroleptics (6 oral, 7 injectible) 351 ± 269 mg CPZEQ (50–1000)	Verbal fluency	Improved, but probably due to practice effects

Study	Sample	Medication	Tests	Effect
Cannon et al. (1994)	7 first episode neuroleptic-naïve 8 previously treated (all must have eligible siblings)	Not reported; 'clinically determined' doses	Gordon CPT vigilance and distractibility; WCST categories and perseverations; WAIS-R vocabulary, block design, digit–symbol; verbal fluency; naming; Comprehension of Complex Ideational Material; sentence repetition; reading recognition; WMS logical memory, paired associates, design reproduction; CVLT; facial recognition; Trails A and B; Stroop word, color, color–word; finger–thumb opposition; finger tapping; digit span; Rosen Drawing Test; Token Test; Reitan–Klove Sensory–Perceptual Exam	No effect
Lee et al. (1994)	23 non-treatment-resistant	Typicals	WAIS-R digit–symbol, Consonant Trigram (attention), verbal fluency, Verbal List Learning recall, WCST, WISC-R Maze	Mixed: mostly no effect; improved verbal list learning recall
Seidman et al. (1993)	11	Typicals 521 ± 529 mg CPZEQ before reduction 78 ± 32 mg CPZEQ after reduction	WAIS-R vocabulary, block design, picture arrangement; WRAT-R spelling; finger tapping; Rey figure; Graphic Sequencing Test; auditory CPT; WMS; verbal fluency; WCST; Porteus Mazes; Visual–Verbal Test; dichotic digits	Mixed: mostly no effect; worsened left ear accuracy on dichotic digits
Strauss and Kliese (1990)	8	Haloperidol 16 ± 8 mg	Short Test for General Intelligence, Short Syndrome Test (concentration/memory)	Worsened
Zahn et al. (1994)	14	Mostly fluphenazine; 1–2 thioridazine 23 ± 15 mg	Simple (fixed foreperiod) warned RT; two modality RT regular, choice, and sensory dominance	No effect
Serper et al. (1994)	12 medicated stable out-patients 13 unmedicated acute in-patients	Haloperidol 20 mg	Digit span, distraction and non-distraction conditions	Improved

Table 13.2 – *Continued*

Citation	N	Medications	Tests	Medication effects
Between-groups designs *Not randomized to medication status*				
Barch et al. (1996)	75 medicated 25 unmedicated	52 haloperidol; 2 'medication'; 21 'antipsychotics'; 589 ± 461 mg CPZEQ	Semantic priming (unrelated RT minus related RT) at various stimulus onset asynchronies (SOAs)	Mixed: worsened RT overall; med status no effect on priming; higher dose improved priming for 4/5 SOAs
SOAs				
Bedard et al. (1996)	12 medicated 11 drug-naïve	Haloperidol mean 11.2 mg	Mirror drawing	Worsened
Cleghorn et al. (1990)	37 medicated 27 unmedicated	Typicals 'low to moderate' doses	WAIS; Continuous Reaction Time (CRT); + 60 measures from Halstead-Reitan and other commonly used tests, including verbal fluency, Rey figure, Trails, WCST, Pegboard, Tapping, Spatial Block span, Porteus Mazes Rey figure, Pegboard,	Mixed: mostly no effect; improved immediate logical memory recall and RTs on slowest 20 trials of CRT; worsened delayed recall of Porteus Mazes
David (1995)	50 on neuroleptics (40 schizophrenia, 10 major affective disorders) 18 off neuroleptics (6 schizophrenia, 12 major affective disorders)	Neuroleptics; 20 mg flupenthixol decanoate intramuscular per month to 800 mg CPZEQ/day	Stroop positive and negative priming	Mixed: no effect on positive priming; improved negative priming
Nestor et al. (1991)	13 medicated 12 unmedicated	Neuroleptics mean 789 mg CPZEQ	CPT, regular and degraded	Mixed: no effect on undegraded CPT; improved degraded over course of 3 trials
Salo et al. (1997)	10 medicated 14 unmedicated	Antipsychotics; 12 in investigational drug study seeking fewer side effects	Stroop negative priming, RTs, errors, and within-trial interference and facilitation	Mixed: mostly no effect; normalized negative priming
Servan-Schreiber et al. (1996)	21 medicated 17 unmedicated (11 first-episode) 11 non-psychotic major depressive in-patients	Neuroleptics 'standard' doses	Non-degraded A-X CPT with long and short interstimulus intervals (ISIs)	Mixed: no effect on d' for long ISI; worsened d' for short ISI

Correlational studies (Not randomized to medication dosage)

Study	N	Treatment	Tests	Outcome
Cutmore and Beninger (1990)	26	Typicals (2 unmedicated) 11.95 ± 2.25 mg/kg CPZEQ/day prolactin levels 30.65 ± 8.22 µg/l	Paired associates; money loss avoidance task; rotary pursuit; button pressing; simple reaction time	Mixed: worsened all but paired associates
Sweeney et al. (1991a)	39 (15 first episode)	High potency neuroleptics	Finger tapping, Trails, digit–symbol, digit span, block design, line orientation, verbal fluency, Rey AVLT, WMS-R visual memory, WCST	Worsened
Sweeney et al. (1991b)	44	36 fluphenazine, 8 other neuroleptics 760.2 ± 646.3 mg CPZEQ (100–3500)	Finger tapping, Trails A and B, digit–symbol, digit span, block design, line orientation, verbal fluency, Rey auditory verbal learning, WCST, auditory digit span (distracter)	Worsened

existing differences between the groups might account for the medication effects that they found. An alternative to the mixed design that also controls for practice effects in a within-subjects analysis is the counterbalanced crossover design in which half of the patients are tested first on medication and half are tested first off medication. Two of the studies that we reviewed, those of Pigache (1993) and Salo *et al.* (1997), employed this method.

Between group designs

A total of 10 studies in Tables 13.1 and 13.2 employed between-groups designs. Only three of these studies randomly assigned patients to groups that received or did not receive medication (Table 13.1). The remaining seven between-group studies are difficult to interpret because the cognitive differences between the groups could be due to any number of factors, other than medication, that might differentiate the groups. Unmedicated patients in David's (1995) study, for example, were 8 years older, had IQs 4–5 points higher and were more likely to be female and affective disordered rather than schizophrenic than were his medicated patients. In non-randomized studies, the reasons that patients are not receiving standard medication therapy might differentiate them systematically from medicated patients. Sources of unmedicated patients, for example, typically include those who enter the hospital for acute psychotic exacerbations due to presumed neuroleptic non-compliance, those on 'drug holiday' (Cleghorn *et al.*, 1990) or those who are withdrawn from typical neuroleptics in order to begin atypical medication trials (Salo *et al.*, 1997). These patients may differ from other patients in the extent to which they experience debilitating side effects or in their cognitive organization and memory, which might lead them to forget to take oral medications. In many of the studies, a significant number of the unmedicated patients were first-episode or neuroleptic-naive patients who may have experienced fewer episodes, been hospitalized less and been ill for a shorter length of time than medicated comparisons (Cleghorn *et al.*, 1990; Barch *et al.*, 1996; Bedard *et al.*, 1996; Servan-Schreiber *et al.*, 1996). In addition, first-episode samples probably include a greater proportion of good prognosis cases than do the chronically ill patient samples drawn from tertiary care centers with whom they are often compared. The overall severity of illness of neuroleptic-naive samples that include patients with a substantial illness duration probably differs from that observed in chronically treated samples. Nestor *et al.* (1991) did not describe how their patients came to be neuroleptic withdrawn.

Correlational analyses of medication dosage effects

We have included in Table 13.2 several studies which report correlation of drug dose with cognitive performance. Such correlations are very difficult to interpret because drug dose was not assigned randomly, and subjects treated with higher doses may have more difficult to treat forms of the illness. The cognition–dose correlations, therefore, may actually represent the correlation of cognition with illness severity and/or treatment responsiveness.

Our approach to the literature

We have divided the recent literature into two groups of studies. Table 13.1 shows those studies with research designs that allow for the clearest and easiest interpretation of findings.

These include within-subjects designs that have taken account of possible practice effects, between-groups designs in which patients were randomized to medication status, and mixed designs that fit both criteria. Despite the limitations of the remaining designs (Table 13.2), we have included them in our review because such studies are usually cited in the literature when drug effects are discussed. In our view, the evidence from such studies is at best suggestive and, at worst, misleading.

Prior reviews have tended to classify cognitive tests according to which concepts or areas of brain functioning the tests are presumed to measure. Most of the tests, however, involve multiple cognitive skills. As a result, different authors have, at times, classified the same tests under different headings, and findings from different tests falling under the same presumed skill area are often contradictory. We have opted to organize our review around specific tests wherever possible in order to enhance clarity of reporting. Within each test, we will emphasize the findings of those studies with the most interpretable research designs, i.e. those in Table 13.1, wherever possible.

Two of the studies, those of Cannon *et al.* (1994) and Censits *et al.* (1997), were not conducive to the type of categorization used in this review because they did not report individual findings for each test. They administered a large battery of neuropsychological tests, many of which were also used in the studies reviewed below, which they grouped into seven or eight functional domains. They reported their results in terms of profile analyses based on composite z-scores for each of the domains. Both studies employed within-subjects designs with initial testing conducted off medication, and both reported that the overall level and shape of the profile of the patients when medicated did not differ significantly from the profile's level and shape when unmedicated, despite significant clinical improvement with medication. In addition, Censits *et al.* found no practice effects on the neuropsychological tests for a normal control group retested after an interval similar to that of the patients. This lack of practice effects may be explained by the unusually long time period between tests (mean 19 months; range 6–32 months). Censits *et al.* also found no significant correlations between medication dose and any of the eight functions at either test period.

Wechsler Adult Intelligence Scale (WAIS)

Nine studies, none of which are included among the best designed studies of Table 13.1, have examined subtests of the WAIS. Using a within-subjects design, Gold and Hurt (1990) found that FSIQ, verbal IQ (VIQ) and performance IQ (PIQ), as well as scores on most of the subtests, were higher when patients were tested on medication than when tested 26 days earlier during drug washout. These improvements, however, were in the expected range of practice effects previously documented for the WAIS. Verdoux *et al.* (1995) similarly found that digit–symbol performance of patients significantly improved after 1–3 months on medication but that the improvement did not differ significantly from that of normal subjects retested after the same interval. None of the other studies that employed within-subjects designs controlled for practice effects, but all failed to find significant medication effects on WAIS subtest performances, including vocabulary, block design, digit span and digit–symbol (Seidman *et al.*, 1993; Lee *et al.*, 1994; Allen *et al.*, 1997). In a non-randomized between-subjects design, Cleghorn *et al.* (1990) also found no medication effects on VIQ, PIQ and FSIQ.

Only Serper *et al.* (1994), also using a non-randomized design, found a positive effect of traditional neuroleptics on WAIS subtest performance. They found that haloperidol improved performance on a distractor version of digit span after 1 week of treatment compared with an unmedicated baseline, whereas performance of medication-maintained patients did not change over the same time period. The change in distractibility for the medicated group could not be accounted for by changes in symptoms. This result is consistent with prior reports of medication-related performance enhancement in distraction conditions (Harvey and Pedley, 1989).

Negative effects were found by Sweeney *et al.* (1991a), who found that higher doses of neuroleptics were correlated with poorer performance on digit–symbol, block design and digit span. All three subtests, however, were also related negatively to benztropine dosage. Sweeney *et al.* (1991b) found that all of these correlations, as well as a negative correlation between antipsychotic dose and the distractor version of digit span, were non-significant when the effects of symptoms and anticholinergic medications were controlled.

Overall, the best designed and the majority of these studies found that typical neuroleptics have no effect on WAIS performance.

Wechsler Memory Scale (WMS) and similar memory tests

Gilbertson and van Kammen (1997) reported results from the only memory study that employed random assignment to medication condition and accounted for practice effects. At first testing, all patients had been taking haloperidol for 6 weeks. Second testing occurred after half of the patients had been administered placebo for 3 weeks and half had been maintained on haloperidol in a double-blind fashion. None of the patients were given any additional medications during the study. Both groups performed better on the revised WMS verbal and visual memory scales at retesting, with less improvement observed in the drug-withdrawn group. These findings suggest that typical neuroleptics had a beneficial effect on recent memory tests relative to medication withdrawal. No significant group or group ? session interaction effects were found for WMS attention.

Seven other studies with less adequate research designs also examined the effects of traditional neuroleptics on the types of memory measured by the WMS. Three of these employed within-subjects designs that did not account for practice effects. Seidman *et al.* (1993) found no significant effects of 80% dose reductions on either visual or verbal memory or visual copy. Verdoux *et al.* (1995) also found no significant effect of medication on Rey figure recall or copy compared with normal controls retested after the same length of time. In contrast, Lee *et al.* (1994) found improved verbal list learning recall among patients retested on medication three times in a 12 month period. In a between-subjects non-randomized design, Cleghorn *et al.* (1990) found no medication effects on a general memory quotient or on the copy phase of the Rey figure, poorer delayed recall of the Rey figure among medicated than among unmedicated patients, and improvement among medicated patients relative to unmedicated patients on immediate recall of passages. None of the three correlational studies that examined memory tasks resembling those on the WMS found any significant relationships of memory to medication dosage or blood prolactin levels (Cutmore and Beninger, 1990; Sweeney *et al.*, 1991a,b).

The findings of Gilbertson and van Kammen (1997) suggest that in the absence of concomitant anticholinergic medication, traditional neuroleptics may have some overall positive effect on the types of verbal and visual memory assessed via the WMS. The nature of the direct effect of neuroleptics on memory, however, is unclear because the studies generally have not controlled adequately for indirect effects of symptom reduction following neuroleptic use.

Continuous Performance Test (CPT)

One of the few replicated positive findings in the older literature was that medication improved performance on the CPT (Spohn and Strauss, 1989). The more recent literature, including a total of 10 studies, presents a more complicated and conflicting picture. Half of these studies used randomized designs and/or controlled for practice effects. In the simplest version of the task, subjects are presented with a series of numbers flashed one at a time on a computer screen, and they are asked to press a button when they see a particular letter. Using this version of the task in the most rigorous experimental design, Gilbertson and van Kammen (1997) found no difference between neuroleptic-maintained and neuroleptic-withdrawn patients in their improvement in A', a measure of sensitivity derived from the CPT, over a 3 week interval. In a double-blind within-subjects crossover design using an auditory version of the CPT, Pigache (1993) found that medication decreased errors of omission, but had no effect on errors of commission or latency to respond.

Three studies used randomized between-groups designs to assess the effect of typical neuroleptics on the CPT. Levin *et al.* (1996) used Connors' CPT in which subjects were to respond to each letter as it flashed on the screen except for X, for which they were to withhold responding. They found no significant effects of three different dose levels of haloperidol on any index of performance accuracy or reaction time. Using a version of the CPT in which subjects were asked to respond whenever they detected a particular two-number sequence, Serper *et al.* (1990) found that medicated and unmedicated patients did not differ in number of errors at initial testing, but that medicated patients had improved their error rate to the level of that of normal controls by the fourth week of testing, whereas unmedicated patients had not. Medicated patients, therefore, were better able to learn from experience. Earle-Boyer *et al.* (1991) used a version of the CPT in which stimuli were either three-letter words or three-letter nonsense syllables presented in either the visual or auditory modality; subjects were asked to detect a particular sequence of two stimuli. They found no differences between medicated and unmedicated patients in errors for word stimuli presented in either sensory modality, but medicated patients made significantly fewer errors for nonsense stimuli in both modalities.

Overall, therefore, the results of the best designed studies suggest that medication may have some positive effects on CPT performance. Because every study used a different version of the task, it is difficult to specify the parameters that differentiate findings of improvement from findings of no change. Results of the studies with less adequate research designs (Nestor *et al.*, 1991; Seidman *et al.*, 1993; Servan-Schreiber *et al.*, 1996; Allen *et al.*, 1997; Finkelstein *et al.*, 1997) generally tend to support the conclusion that medication either leads to performance enhancement or has no effect. Three of the four studies that reported correlations between CPT performance and symptoms found that better performance was related to lower symptom levels (Pigache, 1993, Servan-Schreiber *et al.*, 1996 and Finkelstein *et al.*, 1997 found this relationship; Gilbertson and van Kammen, 1997 found no significant relationship). The possible positive effects of medication on CPT performance, therefore, may be mediated through symptomatic improvements.

Wisconsin Card Sorting Test (WCST)

Six studies have examined the effect of traditional neuroleptics on performance on the WCST. None of these studies controlled adequately for practice effects or randomized medication status. Neither the three within-subjects designs (Lee *et al.*, 1994; Verdoux *et al.*, 1995; Allen *et al.*, 1997) nor Cleghorn *et al.*'s (1990) between-subjects design detected any effects of typical neuroleptics on WCST performance. Sweeney *et al.* (1991a), however, found that dosage of neuroleptics was significantly correlated with completing fewer categories ($r = -0.38$ or -0.56) and making more perseverative errors ($r = 0.28, 0.46$) on the WCST. Sweeney *et al.* (1991b) found a similar significant effect on perseverative errors ($r = 0.43$) when level of symptoms and the effects of concomitant medications were statistically controlled. The limitations of the study designs employed here prohibit us from drawing firm conclusions regarding the effect of traditional neuroleptics on WCST performance. The strongest statement we can make is that the pattern of results tentatively suggests that traditional antipsychotics either have no effect on or possibly worsen WCST performance in a dose-related fashion.

Verbal fluency

Seven studies have examined the effects of traditional neuroleptics on verbal fluency, but none of them controlled adequately for practice effects or randomized medication status; thus, the conclusions drawn from these studies should be taken as only tentative. Four of the studies employed within-subjects designs. Verdoux *et al.* (1995) found that although the verbal fluency of schizophrenic patients slightly but significantly improved after 1–3 months on medication, the improvement was not significantly greater than that of normal subjects who were retested after the same length of time. Bilder *et al.* (1992) tested patients on medication first and found that they produced more words ~3–6 weeks later when tested off medication. As in Verdoux *et al.*, this result most probably represents strong practice effects because the patients were retested on verbal fluency 12 times. Seidman *et al.* (1993) found no significant effects of a 80–90% dose reduction 14–70 weeks later when practice effects would have less impact. Lee *et al.* (1994) found no significant changes relative to baseline in number of words produced after 6 weeks, 6 months or 12 months of treatment with neuroleptics. Using a between-subjects design, Cleghorn *et al.* (1990) also found no significant effect of neuroleptics on verbal fluency. In two correlational studies, Sweeney *et al.* (1991a,b) found that a small association between higher doses of neuroleptics and poorer performance on verbal fluency was not significant when symptoms and anticholinergic dose were statistically controlled.

The results of these studies converge on the conclusion that traditional neuroleptics have no discernible effect on verbal fluency. This lack of effect is particularly striking because verbal fluency is one of the measures for which there is consistent evidence that new generation agents may enhance performance relative to conventional agents (Buchanan *et al.*, 1994; Lee *et al.*, 1994; Hoff *et al.*, 1996). Several of the studies cited here have demonstrated clear practice effects on verbal fluency that may be responsible for findings of 'cognitive enhancement' in studies of the atypical neuroleptics. True effects of both typical and atypical medications on verbal fluency are particularly important to determine in the future through the use of better research designs that randomize treatment groups and/or account for practice effects.

Stroop test

Three studies have examined the relationship of traditional neuroleptics to performance on the Stroop test. Verdoux *et al.* (1995) found no significant effect of medication on word reading or color naming speed on the Stroop. Similarly, using the color naming condition only in a non-randomized between-group design, Salo *et al.* (1997) demonstrated no significant effects of medication on overall speed nor a significant interaction of medication status with the degree of congruence between the word and the color of ink. Salo *et al.* also examined priming effects by subtracting reaction times for the second trial of related pairs from reaction times for the second trial of unrelated pairs of stimuli. Related pairs were those in which the color name for the first trial corresponded to the color of ink on the second trial (e.g. RED printed in blue ink followed by GREEN printed in red ink); in unrelated pairs, there was no overlap of color of either word or ink. Medicated schizophrenic patients reacted more slowly to related pairs of words than to unrelated words, producing a negative priming effect that was similar in magnitude to that of healthy control subjects. Unmedicated patients, on the other hand, reacted more quickly to related than to unrelated words pairs, producing a positive priming effect. In seven of the same patients who were tested both off and on medication, Salo *et al.* found similar medication effects. Although the medicated patients performed more like normal control subjects, it is not conceptually clear whether the failure of unmedicated patients to show negative priming means that they performed less well or better than medicated patients and controls.

David (1995) defined negative priming trials in the way that Salo *et al.* (1997) defined related pairs. Rather than comparing related trials with unrelated trials, however, David compared negative priming trials with what he called positive priming trials in which either the color or the word were the same in both trials. In a non-randomized between-subjects design that included groups of both schizophrenic and affective disordered patients either on or off neuroleptic medication, David found that, for the negative priming/related pairs trials, the reaction times of medicated patients were faster, i.e. more similar to those of normal controls, than were those of unmedicated patients. The reaction times of medicated and unmedicated groups did not appear to differ for the positive priming trials.

Overall, these three studies suggest that traditional neuroleptics have no effect on Stroop word reading or color naming speed. The conflicting methodologies and definitions employed by David (1995) and Salo *et al.* (1997) do not allow us to draw conclusions regarding the effect of antipsychotics on negative priming in the Stroop at this time.

Trails

Five studies have examined the effects of traditional neuroleptics on Trails A and B. In the best designed of these, Gilbertson and van Kammen (1997) found no significant differences between medicated and unmedicated patients in either Trails A or B. The less adequate research designs of Cleghorn *et al.* (1990) and Allen *et al.* (1997) also found no effect of medication on Trails performance. In two correlational studies, Sweeney *et al.* (1991a,b) found that higher doses of neuroleptics were significantly associated with slower completion of Trails A and B, even when symptoms and anticholinergic effects were statistically controlled. Taken together, these findings suggest that traditional neuroleptics either have no effect on or possibly worsen performance on Trails.

Mazes

Three studies have examined the relationship of traditional neuroleptics to maze performance. Two within-subjects studies that did not control for practice effects found no difference in maze performance between medication states (Seidman *et al.*, 1993; Lee *et al.*, 1994). Cleghorn *et al.* (1990) found that non-randomized medicated patients entered significantly more blind alleys on the Porteus Mazes than did unmedicated patients. The results of these studies tentatively suggest that typical neuroleptics have little effect on maze performance. The older literature contained some evidence of a negative medication effect (Medalia *et al.*, 1988). Further controlled study of this issue, therefore, appears warranted.

Simple reaction time

Three studies have examined the effects of traditional neuroleptics on simple reaction time. In a repeated measures between-subjects design in which patients were randomized to one of three different dose levels of haloperidol, Levin *et al.* (1996) found no significant effects of dose on time to press a button upon seeing a descending snowflake on a computer screen. Zahn *et al.* (1994) also found no effect on a simple warned reaction time test when patients were tested first on fluphenazine, then on placebo 2–3 weeks later. In a correlational study that statistically controlled for symptom level, Cutmore and Beninger (1990) found that higher neuroleptic dose in chlorpromazine equivalents was significantly associated with increased time to release a button in response to a light stimulus. Together, these three studies suggest that traditional neuroleptics either have no effect on or, possibly, may slow simple reaction time.

Manual motor tests

Prior reviews have suggested that typical neuroleptics might be associated with decrements in fine motor performance. Six new studies have examined the effects of traditional neuroleptics on some form of manual motor performance. In the best designed of these, Earle-Boyer *et al.* (1991) found no significant differences between patients who were randomized to medicated or unmedicated conditions in either number of pegs displaced in 15 s or time to place 12 pairs of pennies into two boxes simultaneously with each hand. All medicated patients were also receiving 2 mg/day benztropine.

Using a non-randomized between-subjects design, Cleghorn *et al.* (1990) found that number of finger taps produced did not differ between medicated and unmedicated patients for either hand, but that medicated patients performed significantly more slowly on a Pegboard task than did unmedicated patients when using both hands. Fewer than half of the medicated patients were receiving anticholinergics. Seidman *et al.* (1993) found no effects of neuroleptic dose reduction on finger tapping over 14–70 weeks. None of the patients were receiving anticholinergics at either testing.

In a correlational study, Sweeney *et al.* (1991a) found that higher doses of neuroleptics were significantly associated with fewer finger taps produced at 1 year follow-up, but not at initial hospital discharge. In a similar study by Sweeney *et al.* (1991b), finger tapping was significantly related to benztropine dose but not to antipsychotic dose. In a correlational study that statistically controlled for symptom level, Cutmore and Beninger (1990) found that higher neuroleptic dose in chlorpromazine equivalents was associated with less time on target and less improvement in performance with practice on rotary pursuit. They also found that higher blood prolactin levels were associated with fewer responses in a 30 s speeded button press task. One third of their patients were also taking anticholinergic medication.

Overall, the results of these studies suggest that the traditional neuroleptics either have no effect on or possibly worsen manual motor performance. Poorer motor performance may result from motor side effects of the neuroleptics that traditionally are treated by adjunctive anticholinergic medications.

Miscellaneous other tests

Since 1990, 22 other cognitive tasks have been included in only a single study or used by a single laboratory that has examined the relationship of traditional neuroleptics to cognition. No relationship to medication was found for 10 of these measures, including spatial block span (Cleghorn *et al.*, 1990); judgement of line orientation (Sweeney *et al.*, 1991a,b); Visual–Verbal Test misses, Graphic Sequencing Test errors and WRAT-R spelling (Seidman *et al.*, 1993); Consonant Trigram, a measure of attention (Lee *et al.*, 1994); three different conditions of Two Modality reaction time (Zahn *et al.*, 1994); a modified Sternberg memory test (Levin *et al.*, 1996); letter cancellation (Allen *et al.*, 1997); and visual remote recall of famous faces (Gilbertson and van Kammen, 1997). Negative effects were found for eight of the additional measures, including a money loss avoidance task (Cutmore and Beninger, 1990); the Short Test for General Intelligence and the Short Syndrome Test, a test of concentration (Strauss *et al.*, 1990); left ear, but not right ear, accuracy in detecting dichoticly presented digits (Seidman *et al.*, 1993); mirror drawing (Bedard *et al.*, 1996); spatial rotation reaction time and delayed matching to sample (Levin *et al.*, 1996); and verbal remote recall of famous events (Gilbertson and van Kammen, 1997). Three additional measures have been found to be improved by traditional neuroleptics, including the slowest 20 trials of the Continuous Reaction Time test, in which subjects moved a pen left or right in response to a moving square (Cleghorn *et al.*, 1990); automatization of word list shadowing over repeated testing (Serper *et al.*, 1990); and reaction time in a word association task (Levine *et al.*, 1997). Barch *et al.* (1996) found mixed results on a semantic priming test in which medicated and unmedicated patients did not differ. Within the medicated group, however, medication dose in chlorpromazine equivalents was significantly positively associated with priming for the four smallest stimulus onset asynchronies (SOAs) but negatively associated with priming for the longest SOA.

In summary, the large majority of studies found that traditional neuroleptics either had no effect on or worsened cognitive functioning as assessed by these additional unique measures. Given the inherent flaws in every study, however, definitive conclusions should not be drawn regarding tasks that have not been examined by multiple research groups.

Conclusions

The more recent literature on conventional antipsychotic effects on cognition closely resembles the older literature in several important respects: (i) there is still little compelling evidence that conventional antipsychotics provide cognitive benefits; (ii) there is limited direct evidence that such treatments exact a cognitive cost; and (iii) there are a number of clear demonstrations of a lack of cognitive change concomitant with symptomatic improvement (Cannon *et al.*, 1994; Verdoux *et al.*, 1995; Censits *et al.*, 1997; Finkelstein *et al.*, 1997). More recent studies have provided less consistent evidence of a medication-related enhancement of the attentional functions assessed by versions of the CPT, and less evidence of fine motor decrements.

The interpretation of these findings remains largely a matter of opinion. There are few rigorous, well-controlled studies in the entire literature, and conflicting findings abound. As noted above, the nature of conventional antipsychotic effects on cognition has become an important issue for the interpretation of studies examining the new generation of compounds. In our view, the possibility remains that conventional agents may not be as benign as the 'no effect' findings might suggest. Many studies demonstrate a lack of practice-related improvement or any benefit from dramatic improvements in clinical state on tasks that have been shown in some studies to be sensitive to state-related change. Thus 'no effect' may represent the lack of an expected positive effect, although this inference cannot be made with great confidence.

Measurement approaches

One possible explanation for the apparent dissociation of clinical benefit and lack of cognitive change is that we have simply been measuring the wrong things. As noted by Bilder *et al.* (1992), the measures used in most studies reflect a 'round up the usual suspects approach'. Although clinical neuropsychological measures have been useful in documenting impairment among patients, such measures may not be sensitive to the detection of change. There are several reasons to suspect this might be the case. First, multiple lines of evidence indicate that most cognitive measures are assessing stable traits, both in patients and in normal subjects. If such is the case, then we may be trying to document subtle state-related changes with stable trait measures. Indeed, one may suggest paradoxically that the use of instruments with high test–retest reliabilities is problematic because such instruments are not sensitive to subtle state changes, the type which are the object of study. Second, the majority of variance observed among schizophrenic patients on most traditional ability measures reflects individual differences unrelated to the presence or severity of their illness. This is seen most clearly in the NIMH study of monozygotic twins discordant for schizophrenia. Although each sick twin scored systematically less well than their own well twin, many of the sick twins had superior scores when compared with the well twin from another family (Goldberg *et al.*, 1990). The results of this twin study suggest that, of the total score variance observed, only a small portion may be attributable directly to illness features. Any treatment-related changes would have to occur in this 'illness-associated' variance, but, unfortunately, this portion of the variance is relatively small. Very large sample sizes would be necessary, therefore, to detect even moderate sized effects. Such sample sizes are difficult to achieve with the schizophrenic population.

The solution to the problem of test sensitivity is not the complete abandonment of traditional clinical neuropsychological measures. Such measures have a rich history and, in some instances, documented relationships to functional outcome. Including some of these measures in an assessment battery, therefore, is reasonable. New measures, however, that are designed to be sensitive directly to the presumed action of the compounds under investigation should also be developed.

The problem of practice effects

As noted previously, the literature is predominated by test–retest designs which do not control adequately for practice effects. Several of the published studies and several of the currently ongoing multisite clinical trials involve three or four testing occasions, each of which is compared with a baseline level of performance. No published data that we are aware of are available to serve as a guide as to normative practice effects on the batteries that have been selected using this number of testing occasions. Given the magnitude of practice effects in normal subjects tested with the WMS-III twice, approaching a full standard deviation (Psychological Corporation, 1997), studies clearly must control explicitly for practice effects. Such effects are not simply error variance. Performance enhancements as a function of previous exposure are clear learning effects, and any evidence of differential learning from experience as a function of drug treatment condition is of great interest.

Confounding of symptomatic change, treatment effects and cognitive change

The recent literature contains examples of significant relationships between cognitive performance and clinical state (e.g. Sweeney *et al.*, 1991a; Pigache, 1993; Servan-Schreiber *et al.*, 1996). As we noted earlier, this observation raises the possibility that cognitive improvement due to reduction of symptoms balances out and hides a direct negative effect of conventional agents on cognition. Although most of the studies included in this review reported some measure of symptoms, most did not use these data adequately to control for the effect of symptoms in the mediation of the relationship between medication and cognition. Demonstrations of a lack of cognitive change concomitant with symptomatic improvement (Cannon *et al.*, 1994; Verdoux *et al.*, 1995; Censits *et al.*, 1997; Finkelstein *et al.*, 1997) may suggest, at first glance, a dissociation between cognitive and symptom effects. The studies of Cannon *et al.* and Censits *et al.*, however, show how misleading this interpretation can be.

Both of these studies found no significant changes with medication on a large battery of cognitive tests, despite significant symptomatic improvement. Nevertheless, Censits *et al.* noted significant correlations between cognitive and symptomatic improvement in their sample of 60 patients. Correlations of similar magnitude were found by Cannon *et al.*, but were not statistically significant in their sample of 15 patients. The seemingly contradictory findings of no zero-order relationship between medication and cognition in the presence of symptom changes that are related to cognition could be explained by our hypothesis that the indirect positive effect of medication on cognition via improved symptoms is balanced out by a direct negative effect of medication on cognition.

Some authors have attempted to show a dissociation between medication effects on cognition and symptoms by demonstrating that the zero-order relationships between symptoms and cognition or between symptoms and medication are statistically non-significant (Earle-Boyer *et al.*, 1991; David, 1995; Bedard *et al.*, 1996; Allen *et al.*, 1997). This strategy presumably is based on the reasoning that if either of these relationships is truly zero, then one would not need to control statistically for symptoms in order to find the direct relationship between medication and cognition. Studies in which such non-significant relationships are found, however, often do not have large enough sample sizes or sufficient power to prevent type II errors. Non-significance, therefore, usually does not justify accepting that a relationship is truly zero so that, in most cases, symptoms should be statistically partialled out of the relationship between medication and cognition regardless of the significance of the zero-order correlations. Only three of the studies included in this review statistically controlled for symptom level, with mixed results (Cutmore and Beninger, 1990; Sweeney *et al.*, 1991b; Barch *et al.*, 1996).

An alternative approach to controlling for symptom effects is to ensure that symptom levels are truly equivalent between medicated and unmedicated states. Four of the studies reviewed here used this technique (Serper *et al.*, 1990; Nestor *et al.*, 1991; Seidman *et al.*, 1993; Gilbertson and van Kammen, 1997). Ensuring the equivalence of symptoms, however, can pose difficulties for the generalizability or interpretation of a study. Seidman *et al.* (1993), for example, ensured symptom comparability by including data from only the 22% of patients who did not relapse after 80% neuroleptic reduction. Likewise, Gilbertson and van Kammen (1997) excluded three subjects because of symptom exacerbation during their study. This method of subject selection clearly results in studying an unusual group of patients who are either treatment resistant or are able to remain stable without medication. In some cases, equivalent symptoms may suggest that the medication dose or duration of treatment employed in the study was clinically inadequate. As such, it may also be inadequate for effecting cognitive change. Studies that artificially ensure the equivalence of symptoms between untreated and treated groups may provide useful information about subgroups of patients when within-subjects designs are employed and adequate dosage and duration are ensured. They do not substitute adequately, however, for examining the direct effects of medication on cognition in more representative samples.

Several of the recent studies have attempted to control for symptom effects by correlating change in symptoms with change in cognitive functioning across change in medication status in within-subjects designs (e.g. Serper *et al.*, 1994; Finkelstein *et al.*, 1997). Most often, this strategy is used to imply that if no significant relationship exists between cognitive change and symptomatic change, then symptoms cannot be responsible for the relationship between medication and cognition. This type of analysis is problematic for several reasons. First, the conclusions are based on arguing the null hypothesis, which, as discussed above, is generally precluded due to small samples sizes and limited power. Second, the distributions of change scores typically are not normal, and the relationships between change scores usually are not linear. When these assumptions of the statistical test are violated, the correlations are invalid. Third, to perform a correlational analysis, the scores for each subject should be free to take on any possible value of the variables being studied. Change scores, however, are dependent on baseline scores. Due to floor and ceiling effects, patients with more extreme baseline scores will have a restricted range of possible change scores. Fourth, the correlation between change scores does not represent adequately the relationship of interest. In our view, the relationship between medication and cognition represents the sum of a direct effect of medication on cognition and an indirect effect mediated by symptom level. We wish to determine the strength and direction of the direct effect, a number that may be derived from more complex multivariate analyses but which is not produced by correlations of change.

New study designs

Treatment with antipsychotic agents has become the standard of care for nearly all patients with schizophrenia. Further large-scale, double-blind placebo-controlled studies of conventional agents, the type of study design that would be needed to provide more definitive data, are unlikely to be forthcoming. Further investigation of conventional agents will, therefore, need to be conducted using less than optimal study designs. In our view, two designs have been underutilized: (i) studies that manipulate dose, through random assignment of dose either across subjects or within subject; and (ii) studies that compare the magnitude of practice effects across medication conditions. Dose manipulation designs would be informative for everyday clinical practice if such designs were to produce clear evidence that higher doses exact cognitive costs. Ideally, documentation of a dose effect on a biological measure of interest, such as drug plasma levels, would be available to control for the large individual differences in drug metabolism. Few data are available currently to address this question.

The study of practice effects is also relevant to guide clinical practice. The challenge facing rehabilitation programs is to teach patients, typically in an incremental fashion, a new series of skills. Few studies in the literature have examined repeated performance over time as a function of drug condition. The study by Serper *et al.* (1990) demonstrating the role of neuroleptics in the enhanced acquisition of divided attention performance is an example of such a study. Such studies may be more informative for clinical practice than the more frequent design of comparing different drug conditions with a standardized baseline.

Conclusions

In examining the more recent literature on conventional neuroleptic effects on cognition, we are reminded of one of the famous quotes attributed to Yogi Berra, "It's like déjà vu all over again". The recent literature resembles the older literature fairly closely, in terms of both reported results and the limited methodological quality of the bulk of studies. Along with an increased appreciation for the role of cognitive impairment in mediating functional outcome in schizophrenia, interest has increased in evaluating the cognitive impact of the new generation of antipsychotics. The design of these studies should be enhanced by a reading of the literature on typical antipsychotics. Despite close to 40 years of study, definitive answers regarding the cognitive impact of traditional neuroleptics remain elusive. Hopefully, a new generation of studies on atypical antipsychotics will allow for the field to answer the basic question of whether treatment enhances the cognitive performance of patients.

References

Allen, D.N., Gilbertson, M.W., van Kammen, D.P., Kelley, M.E., Gurklis, J.A. and Barry, E.J. (1997) Chronic haloperidol treatment does not affect structure of attention in schizophrenia. *Schizophrenia Research*, **25**, 53–61.

Barch, D.M., Cohen, J.D., Servan-Schreiber, D., Steingard, S., Steinhauer, S.S. and van Kammen, D.P. (1996) Semantic priming in schizophrenia: an examination of spreading activation using word pronunciation and multiple SOAs. *Journal of Abnormal Psychology*, **105**, 592–601.

Bedard, M.-A., Scherer, H., Delorimier, J., Stip, E. and Lalonde, P. (1996) Differential effects of D_2- and D_4-blocking neuroleptics on the procedural learning of schizophrenic patients. *CanadianJournal of Psychiatry*, **4**, 21S–24S.

Bilder, R.M., Turkel, E., Lipschultz-Broch, L. and Lieberman, J.A. (1992) Antipsychotic medication effects on neuropsychological functions. *Psychopharmacology Bulletin*, **28**, 353–366.

Buchanan, R.W., Holstein, C. and Breier, A. (1994) The comparative efficacy and long-term effect of clozapine treatment on neuropsychological test performance. *Biological Psychiatry*, **36**, 717–725.

Buchanan, R.W., Breier, A., Kirkpatrick, B., Ball, P. and Carpenter, W.T., Jr (1998) Positive and negative symptom response to clozapine in schizophrenic patients with and without the deficit syndrome. *American Journal of Psychiatry*, **155**, 751–760.

Cannon, T.D., Zorrilla, L.E., Shtasel, D., Gur, R.E., Gur, R.C., Marco, E.J., Moberg, P. and Price, R.A. (1994) Neuropsychological functioning in siblings discordant for schizophrenia and healthy volunteers. *Archives of General Psychiatry*, **51**, 651–661.

Cassens, G., Inglis, A.K., Appelbaum, P.S. and Gutheil, T.G. (1990) Neuroleptics: effects on neuropsychological function in chronic schizophrenic patients. *Schizophrenia Bulletin*, **16**, 477–499.

Censits, D.M., Ragland, J.D., Gur, R.C. and Gur, R.E. (1997) Neuropsychological evidence supporting a neurodevelopmental model of schizophrenia: a longitudinal study. *Schizophrenia Research*, **24**, 289–298.

Cleghorn, J.M., Kaplan, R.D., Szechtman, B., Szechtman, H. and Brown, G.M. (1990)

Neuroleptic drug effects on cognitive function in schizophrenia. *Schizophrenia Research*, **3**, 211–219.

Cohen, J.D. and Servan-Schreiber, D. (1992) Context, cortex, and dopamine: connectionist approach to behavior and biology in schizophrenia. *Psychology Review*, **99**, 45–77.

Cutmore, T.R.H. and Beninger, R J. (1990) Do neuroleptics impair learning in schizophrenic patients? *Schizophrenia Research*, **3**, 173–186.

David, A.S. (1995) Negative priming (cognitive inhibition) in psychiatric patients: effect of neuroleptics. *Journal of Nervous and Mental Disease*, **183**, 337–339.

Diamond, A., Ciaramitaro, V., Donner, E., Djali, S. and Robinson, M.B. (1994) An animal model of early-treated PKU. *Journal of Neuroscience*, **14**, 3072–3082.

Dolan, R.J., Fletcher, P., Frith, C.D., Friston, K.J., Frackowiak, R.S. and Grasby, P.M. (1995) Dopaminergic modulation of impaired cognitive activation in the anterior cingulate cortex in schizophrenia. *Nature*, **378**, 180–182.

Earle-Boyer, E.A., Serper, M.R., Davidson, M. and Harvey, P.D. (1991) Continuous performance tests in schizophrenic patients: stimulus and medication effects on performance. *Psychiatry Research*, **37**, 47–56.

Finkelstein, J.R.J., Cannon, T.D., Gur, R.E., Gur, R.C. and Moberg, P. (1997) Attentional dysfunctions in neuroleptic-naive and neuroleptic-withdrawn schizophrenic patients and their siblings. *Journal of Abnormal Psychology*, **106**, 203–212.

Gilbertson, M.W. and van Kammen, D.P. (1997) Recent and remote memory dissociation: medication effects and hippocampal function in schizophrenia. *Biological Psychiatry*, **42**, 585–595.

Gold, J.M. and Hurt, S.W. (1990) The effects of haloperidol on thought disorder and IQ in schizophrenia. *Journal of Personality Assessment*, **54**, 390–400.

Goldberg, T.E., Ragland, D., Torrey, E.F., Gold, J.M., Bigelow, L.B. and Weinberger, D.R. (1990) Neuropsychological assessment of monozygotic twins discordant for schizophrenia. *Archives of General Psychiatry*, **47**, 1066–1072.

Goldberg, T.E., Bigelow, L.B., Weinberger, D.R., Daniel, D.G. and Kleinman, J.E. (1991) Cognitive and behavioral effects of the coadministration of dextroamphetamine and haloperidol in schizophrenia. *American Journal of Psychiatry*, **148**, 78–84.

Green, M.F. (1996) What are the functional consequences of neurocognitive deficits in schizophrenia? *American Journal of Psychiatry*, **153**, 321–330.

Harvey, P.D. and Pedley, M. (1989) Auditory and visual distractibility in schizophrenia: clinical and medication status correlations. *Schizophrenia Research*, **2**, 295–300.

Heaton, R.K. and Crowley, T.J. (1981) Effects of psychiatric disorders and their somatic treatment on neuropsychological test results. In: Filskov, S.B. and Boll, T.J. (eds), *Handbook of Clinical Neuropsychology*. Wiley Press, New York, pp. 481–525.

Hoff, A.L., Faustman, W.O., Wieneke, M., Espinoza, S., Costa, M., Wolkowitz, O. and Csernansky, J.G. (1996) The effects of clozapine on symptom reduction, neurocognitive function, and clinical management in treatment-refractory state hospital schizophrenic inpatients. *Neuropsychopharmacology*, **15**, 361–369.

Holcomb, H.H., Cascella, N.G., Thaker, G.K., Medoff, D.R., Dannals, R.F. and Tamminga, C.A. (1996) Functional sites of neuroleptic drug action in the human brain: PET/FDG studies with and without haloperidol. *American Journal of Psychiatry*, **153**, 41–49.

Kane, J., Honigfeld, G., Singer, J., Meltzer, H. and The Clozaril Collaborative Study Group (1988) Clozapine for the treatment-resistant schizophrenic: a double-blind comparison with chloromazine. *Archives of General Psychiatry*, **45**, 789–796.

King, D.J. (1990) The effect of neuroleptics on cognitive and psychomotor function. *British Journal of Psychiatry*, **157**, 799–811.

Krimer, L.S., Muly, E.C., Williams, G.V. and Goldman-Rakic, P.S. (1998) Dopaminergic regulation of cerebral cortical microcirculation. *Nature Neurosciences*, **1**, 286–289.

Lee, M.A., Thompson, P.A. and Meltzer, H.Y. (1994) Effects of clozapine on cognitive function in schizophrenia. *Journal of Clinical Psychiatry*, **55** (9, Suppl. B), 82–87.

Lees, A.J. and Smith, E. (1983) Cognitive deficits in the early stages of Parkinson's disease. *Brain*, **106**, 257–270.

Levin, E.D., Wilson, W., Rose, J.E. and McEvoy, J. (1996) Nicotine–haloperidol interactions and cognitive performance in schizophrenics. *Neuropsychopharmacology*, **15**, 429–436.

Levine, J., Caspi, N. and Laufer, N. (1997) Immediate effects of chlorpromazine and perphenazine following neuroleptic washout on word association of schizophrenic patients. *Schizophrenia Research*, **26**, 55–63.

Lezak, M.D. (1995) *Neuropsychological Assessment*. 3rd edn. Oxford University Press, New York.

Luciana, M., Depue, R.A., Arbisi, P. and Leon, A. (1992) Facilitation of working memory in humans by a D2 receptor agonist. *Journal of Cognitive Neuroscience*, **4**, 58–68.

Medalia, A., Gold, J.M. and Merriam, A. (1988) The effects of neuroleptics on neuropsychological test results of schizophrenics. *Archives of Clinical Neuropsychology*, **3**, 249–271.

Montague, P.R., Dayan, P. and Sejnowski, T.J. (1996) A framework for mesencephalic dopamine systems based on predictive Hebbian Learning. *Journal of Neuroscience*, **6**, 1936–1947.

Muller, U., von Cramon, Y. and Pollmann, S. (1998) D1- versus D2-receptor modulation of visuospatial working memory in humans. *Journal of Neuroscience*, **18**, 2720–2728.

Nestor, P.G., Faux, S.F., McCarley, R.W., Sands, S.F., Horvath, T.B. and Peterson, A. (1991) Neuroleptics improve sustained attention in schizophrenia: a study using signal detection theory. *Neuropsychopharmacology*, **4**, 145–149.

Orzack, M.H., Kornetsky, C. and Freeman, H. (1967) The effects of daily administration of carphenazine on attention in the schizophrenic patient. *Psychopharmacologia*, **11**, 31–38.

Pigache, R.M. (1993) The clinical relevance of an auditory attention task (PAT) in a longitudinal study of chronic schizophrenia, with placebo substitution for chlorpromazine. *Schizophrenia Research*, **10**, 39–50.

The Psychological Corporation (1997) *WAIS-III (Wechsler Adult Intelligence Scale-Third Edition), WMS-III (Wechsler Memory Scale-Third Edition)*. Harcourt Brace & Company, San Antonio.

Salo, R., Robertson, L.C., Nordahl, T.E. and Kraft, L.W. (1997) The effects of antipsychotic medication on sequential inhibitory processes. *Journal of Abnormal Psychology*, **106**, 639–643.

Sawrie, S.M., Chelune, G.J., Naugle, R.I. and Luders, H.O. (1996) Empirical methods for assessing meaningful neuropsychological change following epilepsy surgery. *Journal of The International Neuropsychological Society*, **2**, 556–564.

Schultz, W., Apicella, P. and Ljungberg, T. (1993) Responses of monkey dopamine neurons to reward and conditioned stimuli during successive steps of learning a delayed response task. *Journal of Neuroscience*, **13**, 900–913.

Seidman, L.J., Pepple, J.R., Faraone, S.V., Kremen, W.S., Green, A.I., Brown, W.A. and Tsuang, M.T. (1993) Neuropsychological performance in chronic schizophrenia in response to neuroleptic dose reduction. *Biological Psychiatry*, **33**, 575–584.

Serper, M.R., Bergman, R.L. and Harvey, P.D. (1990) Medication may be required for the development of automatic information processing in schizophrenia. *Psychiatry Research*, **32**, 281–288.

Serper, M.R., Davidson, M. and Harvey, P.D. (1994) Attentional predictors of clinical change during neuroleptic treatment in schizophrenia. *Schizophrenia Research*, **13**, 65–71.

Servan-Schreiber, D., Cohen, J.D. and Steingard, S. (1996) Schizophrenic deficits in the processing of context: a test of a theoretical model. *Archives of General Psychiatry*, **53**, 1105–1112.

Spohn, H.E. and Strauss, M.E. (1989) Relation of neuroleptic and anticholinergic medication to cognitive functions in schizophrenics. *Journal of Abnormal Psychology*, **98**, 367–380.

Spohn, H.E., Lacoursiere, R.B., Thompson, K. and Coyne, L. (1977) Phenothiazine effects on psychological and psychophysiological dysfunction in chronic schizophrenics. *Archives of General Psychiatry*, **34**, 633–644.

Strauss, M.E. (1993) Relations of symptoms to cognitive deficits in schizophrenia. *Schizophrenia Bulletin*, **19**, 215–231.

Strauss, W.H. and Klieser, E. (1990) Cognitive disturbances in neuroleptic therapy. *Acta Psychiatrica Scandinavica*, **82**, 56–57.

Sweeney, J.A., Haas, G. L., Keilp, J.G. and Long, M. (1991a) Evaluation of the stability of neuropsychological functioning after acute episodes of schizophrenia: one-year follow up study. *Psychiatry Research*, **38**, 63–76.

Sweeney, J.A., Keilp, J.G., Haas, G.L., Hill, J. and Seiden, P.J. (1991b) Relationships between medication treatments and neuropsychological test performance in schizophrenia. *Psychiatry Research*, **37**, 297–308.

Taylor, A.E., Saint-Cyr, J.A. and Lang, A.E. (1986) Frontal lobe dysfunction in Parkinson's disease. *Brain*, **109**, 845–883.

Tune, L.E., Strauss, M.E., Lew, M.F., Breitlinger, E. and Coyle, J.T. (1982) Serum levels of anticholinergic drugs and impaired recent memory in chronic schizophrenic patients. *American Journal of Psychiatry*, **139**, 1460–1462.

Verdoux, H., Magnin, E. and Bourgeois, M. (1995) Neuroleptic effects on neuropsychological test performance in schizophrenia. *Schizophrenia Research*, **14**, 133–139.

Welsh, M.C., Pennington, B.F., Ozonoff, S., Rouse, B. and McCabe, E.R.B. (1990) Neuropsychology of early-treated phenylkentonuria: specific executive function deficits. *Child Development*, **61**, 1697–1713.

Zahn, T.P., Pickar, D. and Haier, R.J. (1994) Effects of clozapine, fluphenazine, and placebo on reaction time measures of attention and sensory dominance in schizophrenia. *Schizophrenia Research*, **13**, 133–144.

14 The central cholinergic system and cognitive dysfunction in schizophrenia

Susan R. McGurk and Peter Powchik

Introduction

Cognitive impairment of varying degrees of severity is seen in virtually all patients with chronic schizophrenia (Gold and Harvey, 1993). In some cases, the impairment is quite mild, detectable only by neuropsychological examination, and perhaps only in comparison with an identical twin. In other cases, the impairment is obvious and severe enough to warrant an additional diagnosis of dementia (Davidson *et al.*, 1995). Unlike psychotic symptoms, cognitive deficits in schizophrenia do not remit spontaneously nor are they ameliorated by treatment with typical antipsychotic drugs (for a review, see Cassens *et al.*, 1990).

Few areas of cognitive functioning are spared in schizophrenia. However, the most severe deficits are seen in executive functioning, attention and memory. Of these, memory, in its various constructs, is the most directly linked to cholinergic function. Although muscarinic receptor function has been linked most closely to memory processes, nicotinic receptors may also play a role, especially in schizophrenia. This chapter will focus on cholinergic contributions to cognitive dysfunction in schizophrenia. It will not address the body of evidence implicating acetylcholine (ACh) in either positive or negative symptoms.

The central cholinergic system

The central ACh system is exceedingly complex. The vast majority of cholinergic synapses in the human brain arise from projections from deep brain structures. Only in the striatum are cholinergic connections provided by interneurons. One current nomenclature identifies eight distinct groups of cholinergic cells that project to virtually all areas of the brain (Mesulam, 1995). A thorough discussion of the structure and function of the ACh system is beyond the scope of this chapter, but the following points should be noted.

In the nomenclature introduced by Mesalum (1995), the major projections of the cholinergic system can be identified as Ch1–Ch8 (see Table 14.1). As indicated in Table 14.1, the primary source of ACh in the cerebral cortex and amygdala are the projections from Ch4, which include, but are not synonymous with, the nucleus basalis of Meynert (nbM). The

Table 14.1 Projections of the cholinergic system

Cholinergic group	Origin	Major projections	Minor projections
Ch1	Medial septal nucleus	Hippocampus	Thalamus; striatum
Ch2	Vertical nucleus of the diagonal band	Hippocampus	Thalamus; striatum
Ch3	Horizontal limb of the diagonal band nucleus	Olfactory bulb	Thalamus; striatum
Ch4	Region of the nucleus basalis of Meynert	Cerebral cortex; amygdala	Thalamus; striatum
Ch5	Pediculopontine nucleus of the rostral brainstem	Thalamus	Cerebral cortex; striatum
Ch6	Laterodorsal tegmental of the rostral brainstem	Thalamus	Cerebral cortex; striatum
Ch7	Medial habenula nucleus	Interpenduncular	
Ch8	Parabigeminal nucleus	Superior colliculus	Thalamus

hippocampus receives cholinergic projections from Ch1 and Ch2. The cholinergic innervation of the striatum arises almost exclusively from interneurons, but these striatal structures also receive input from Ch1–Ch4 and, in primates, from Ch5 and Ch6 (Smith and Parent, 1986).

Mesopontine projections (i.e. those arising from Ch5 and Ch6) to thalamic, cortical and striatal structures are of interest in schizophrenia because of their potential involvement in several neurophysiological processes that are disrupted in persons with schizophrenia. Among these are disruptions in the sleep–wake cycle, eye tracking and sensory gating abnormalities, and motor dysfunction (Garcia-Rill *et al.*, 1995).

Generally speaking, the direct effect of cholinergic transmission is excitatory, primarily by increasing the susceptibility of neuronal firing at the postsynaptic site. However, the net effect of cholinergic stimulation may be inhibitory because firing of the postsynaptic neuron may cause an inhibition at its target. Such variability in the net effect of cholinergic stimulation can make it difficult to predict the effect of either enhancement or antagonism of cholinergic neurotransmission. This difficulty in prediction has implications for understanding the effects on cognition of treatment for psychosis and therapies aimed at ameliorating cognitive dysfunction.

Cognitive dysfunction in schizophrenia

Significance of cognitive dysfunction

The presence and severity of positive symptoms generally have been believed to be significant determinants of outcome in schizophrenia. This may have become an especially closely held notion after the advent of effective treatments for positive symptoms (e.g. drugs such as chlorpromazine and haloperidol) with the resultant release from hospital of many patients who otherwise could not be discharged. However, there is increasing evidence that cognitive functioning, and not positive symptoms, is the major determinant of outcome in schizophrenia. The evidence which supports this conclusion was summarized in a recent review of the literature indicating that certain domains of cognitive functioning account for significant variance in functional outcomes (Green, 1996). Specifically, performance on measures of vigilance, secondary verbal memory and executive functioning were found to be strong determinants of community functioning, including independent living skills and occupational status, social skills and ability to benefit from psychiatric rehabilitation.

Although most areas of cognition are impaired in schizophrenia, learning and memory is the cognitive domain most highly influenced by cholinergic neurotransmission. This is true not only for persons with schizophrenia but also for normal populations. For example, the deficits produced in learning and memory by anticholinergic agents in unmedicated persons with schizophrenia are quite similar to deficits in learning and memory demonstrated in normal populations (Spohn and Strauss, 1989).

Cholinergic transmission has additional relevance in schizophrenia because the most common treatment of extrapyramidal side effects in this patient group is the co-administration (along with antipsychotic drugs) of drugs with strong anticholinergic (specifically, anti-muscarinic) properties. The doses of these agents given, most notably of benztropine mesylate, are sufficient to impair learning and memory deficits further in patients with schizophrenia, with higher doses causing more severe memory impairments (Tune *et al.*, 1982; Strauss *et al.*, 1990). For example, in a comparison of normal subjects and schizophrenia patients treated with either neuroleptics alone or neuroleptics with anticholinergics, normal subjects and schizophrenic patients treated with neuroleptics alone showed no disparity between verbal recall and recognition (Calev, 1983). However, schizophrenia patients treated with anticholinergic agents performed significantly less well than the other two groups on the recall task than on the recognition task. A study comparing the same schizophrenia patients when at higher and lower anticholinergic levels demonstrated significantly less verbal recall on the occasion of higher serum anticholinergic levels (Strauss *et al.*, 1990).

Post-mortem studies of cognitive dysfunction in schizophrenia

Although recognized as a brain disorder, post-mortem studies of schizophrenia have generally found little in the way of gross neuropathology (e.g. Arnold *et al.*, 1994). Indeed, the lack of findings in the early part of the 20th century prompted one investigator to deem schizophrenia to be the 'graveyard of neuropathologists'. A major review of the recent findings in neuropathological investigations in schizophrenia was presented recently by Bogerts (1993). Cognitive impairment was recognized as inherent to schizophrenia at the time when it was differentiated from bipolar disorder <100 years ago, prompting the 'dementia' in *dementia praecox*. Neuropathological correlates of clinical dementia had been described since around the same time. Curiously, though, few neuropathological studies have focused on determining the correlates of cognitive impairment in schizophrenia. Nonetheless, given the prevalence of severe cognitive impairment in elderly persons with schizophrenia, it is reasonable to search for a biological basis for this impairment.

Perhaps the most widely identified neuropathological abnormalities associated with cognitive deficits are those seen in Alzheimer's disease (AD), namely senile plaques and neurofibrillary tangles. There have been some reports of increased incidence of AD-like neuropathology in elderly persons with schizophrenia (Prohovnik *et al.*, 1993), but most post-mortem studies fail to show such neuropathology (e.g. Purohit *et al.*, 1993; Arnold *et al.*, 1994). Even potentially early markers of AD-like pathology such as Alz-50 antigen are not present in tissue from cognitively impaired persons with schizophrenia (Powchik *et al.*, 1993). Consistent with this is the lack of increased apolipoprotein E4 allele frequency in similar patients (Powchik *et al.*, 1997).

Another consistently identified deficit in AD is a reduction in the activity of the presynaptic enzyme choline acetyltransferase (ChAT) which is required for the production of ACh. In brain tissue derived from persons with AD, cortical ChAT activity is correlated with nbM cell loss (Etienne *et al.*, 1986). Reduction in ChAT is correlated with length of illness in AD and with severity of cognitive impairment (Bowen *et al.*, 1976, 1982; Davies *et al.*, 1976; Perry *et al.*, 1977; Reisine *et al.*, 1978; Richter *et al.*, 1980). Given the importance of cholinergic activity in cognitive processes, a reduction in ChAT activity, which might be seen in the absence of overt AD-like neuropathology, is a reasonable candidate for examination in cognitive impairment in schizophrenia. One post-mortem series compared 95 elderly persons with schizophrenia, with cognitive impairment ranging from questionably demented to profoundly demented, with 135 cases of confirmed AD and 20 normal controls (Purohit *et al.*, 1993; Haroutunian *et al.*, 1999). Despite severe to profound dementia in many of the patients with schizophrenia, and in marked contrast to the cases of confirmed AD, there was no overall reduction in ChAT activity in the schizophrenia patients. Nonetheless, there was a modest, but statistically significant correlation between ChAT activity and cognitive impairment as measured by the Clinical Dementia Rating Scale (CDR). The CDR is a composite scale that takes into account several different aspects of cognitive and functional capacity. This would seem to suggest that although there is no overt reduction in ChAT activity, the level of cholinergic activity nonetheless is related to cognitive function and, in turn, activities of daily living.

Cognitive correlates of cholinergic function

Considerable evidence exists suggesting an important role for ACh in various aspects of learning and memory. Interference with cholinergic neurotransmission either by lesioning ACh-containing neurons or blocking ACh receptors impairs learning and memory processes in humans and laboratory animals. Interruption of cholinergic transmission has been accomplished by pharmacological manipulation using selective cholinergic antagonists such as scopolamine, or by lesions of the cholinergic projections from the nucleus basalis magnocellularis to the neocortex and from the medial septal nucleus to the hippocampus. Data from by these types of studies provide validity for the causal link between breakdown of cholinergic transmission and disturbances in performance on tasks requiring the acquisition and retention of new information. Additionally, experimental damage of cholinergic cortical projections provides a mechanism to explore possible treatments for diseases of the cholinergic system, such as AD. Although the neuropathology of schizophrenia does not indicate that it is a disease of the cholinergic system, cognitive deficits associated with this disorder are severe, and in some cases warrant the diagnosis of dementia (Davidson *et al.*, 1995).

This section will describe the cognitive effects in animals of lesions of the cholinergic basal forebrain and medial septum, and of cholinergic antagonists. Specifically, short-term memory has been shown to be impacted adversely by interruption of the cholinergic system.

Short-term memory

Short-term memory in animals has been assessed using a variety of paradigms that involve spatial, object or visual recognition tasks, such as active and passive avoidance procedures and spatial memory paradigms (e.g. T-maze and multi-armed radial mazes) in rats, and delayed match-to-sample paradigms in monkeys. Short-term memory has also been referred to as working memory, which is defined as the ability to hold information 'on-line' across a relatively brief delay (Goldman-Rakic, 1994). Working memory most commonly is assessed in non-human primates using delayed response tasks, and in rats using the radial arm maze. These paradigms require the cross-temporal maintenance of information, usually a spatial location. Short-term and working memory are largely analogous terms in that they reflect the ability to remember recently acquired information.

Centrally acting muscarinic antagonists, such as atropine and scopolamine, and nicotinic antagonists, such as mecamylamine, reliably produce deficits in animals on tasks requiring memory for recent events. For example, in non-human primates, scopolamine and atropine impaired performance on position discrimination (Ridley *et al.*, 1984), delayed match-to-sample tasks (Penetar and McDonough, 1983), delayed spatial alternation (Levin and Simon, 1998) and delayed response tasks (Bartus and Johnson, 1976; Liu and Su, 1993). In several of these studies, an interaction of dose and delay was demonstrated, with the greatest memory deficits demonstrated under conditions requiring longer retention intervals and larger doses of the anticholinergic agents. Because central nervous system stimulants such as amphetamine or methylphenidate were not shown to reduce the memory impairment caused by scopolamine, it is unlikely that the performance deficits can be attributed to arousal or attention impairments (for a review, see Bartus *et al.*, 1987). Additionally, impairments in short-term memory in monkeys produced by cholinergic antagonists have been partially, but reliably, reversed by acetylcholinesterase inhibitors such as physostigmine (Penetar and McDonough, 1983; Murray and Fibiger, 1985; Fibiger, 1986) and donepezil (Rupniak *et al.*, 1997).

Similarly, cholinergic antagonists have been demonstrated to impair performance on a variety of measures of short-term memory in rats and mice. Impairments have been demonstrated in delayed spatial alternation (Heise *et al.*, 1975), spatial working memory (Eckerman *et al.*, 1979; Stevens, 1981; Levy *et al.*, 1983; McGurk *et al.*, 1988; Levin, 1990) and T-maze reversal learning (Alpern and Marriott, 1973). As with primates, cholinergic agonists, such as physostigmine, were shown to reverse these impairments (e.g. Alpern and Marriott, 1973).

Initial evidence of the importance of extrinsic sources of ACh to the hippocampus in working memory was provided by lesions of the fimbria-fornix. These lesions result in loss of ACh to the hippocampus and produce profound impairment in working memory tasks (Olton and Papas, 1979). Additionally, lesions of the nbM, which destroy rising cholinergic pathways to the cortex, impaired spatial memory in rats (Murray and Fibigier, 1985) and object discrimination learning in marmosets (Ridley *et al.*, 1994). These impairments were reversed by administration of arecoline (Ridley *et al.*, 1986), physostigmine (Murray and Figiber, 1985) and AF102b, a muscarnic M1 receptor agonist (Dawson and Iverson, 1993). Fetal marmoset grafts containing ACh-rich tissue in the basal forebrain also reversed impairments caused by lesions of the nbM (Ridley *et al.*, 1994)

Working versus reference memory

The radial arm maze presents an opportunity to examine two types of spatial memory: working versus reference memory. Spatial working memory is reflected in the acquisition of the win–shift rule wherein successful performance is measured by the avoidance of arms where food has already been retrieved during a session. When a subset of arms are never baited across trials, avoidance of these arms reflects reference memory. Thus, working memory reflects the variable task aspects that occur within trials, and reference memory reflects the constant aspects of the task across trials. It appears that spatial working memory is composed of flexible stimulus–response associations that change from trial to trial and are highly susceptible to interference. Cholinergic antagonists degrade working, but not reference, memory as measured by the radial arm maze and other spatial memory tasks (Brito *et al.*, 1983; Levy *et al.*, 1983; Beatty and Beirley, 1985; Lydon and Nakajima, 1992). Overall, working memory, and not reference memory, is impaired following the administration of scopolamine or atropine, although the specificity of this effect may depend on the level of training of subjects and dose of drug. For example, rats trained to a higher criterion of learning showed impairment on reference and working memory aspects of a task following scopolamine administration (Lydon and Nakajima, 1992) whereas, at a lower criterion of learning, scopolamine produced only working memory errors.

Lesion studies have demonstrated differential involvement of the nbM and the medial septal nucleus in these two types of spatial memory in rats. Damage to the septal–hippocampal system resulted in profound working memory impairments (Olton and Papas, 1979), whereas damage to the nbM produced a relatively selective impairment in reference memory (Murray and Fibiger, 1985; Kesner *et al.*, 1987). Lesions of the nbM projection to the neocortex produced a transient impairment in working memory and more durable impairment in reference memory (Kesner *et al.*, 1987; McGurk and Butcher, 1987; McGurk *et al.*, 1991). Arecoline was found to reverse the working memory deficits produced by these lesions (McGurk *et al.*, 1991). These data may indicate that the septal–hippocampal cholinergic system is involved in the acquisition and maintenance of recent memories, and therefore possibly the locus of the effects of scopolamine, whereas the cholinergic neocortex is the locus of the encoded spatial memory or spatial rules. Additionally, the similarity of scopolamine-induced working memory impairments to those produced by lesions of the cholinergic projections to the hippocampus have been noted (Eckerman *et al.*, 1979).

Human studies of cholinergic functioning and cognition

Normals

Pharmacological blockade of central cholinergic neurons leads to memory impairments in normal subjects. Scopolamine produces a transient amnestic effect which has long been noted from its applications in surgery as a premedicant. Overall, scopolamine appears to disrupt memory consolidation rather than primary memory, as measured by the digit span subtest of the WAIS-R. This may reflect a relative sparing of attentional processes subsequent to scopolamine administration. For example, scopolamine was found to impair working memory and secondary memory, but not attention nor retrieval from semantic memory (Vitiello *et al.*, 1997). However, scopolamine has been shown to impair performance on certain types of attention, such as vigilance, which is reflected in the capacity to sustain attention to a series of target stimuli over several minutes.

Tasks of secondary memory are particularly vulnerable to the effects of scopolamine. Delayed recall is grossly impaired, which is evident on tasks such as list learning or paired associates which gauge the efficiency of new learning.

Scopolamine impaired immediate selective recall as measured by the Buschke Selective Reminder paradigm. This deficit was reversed by physostigmine but not neostigmine (Prohovnik *et al.*, 1997). Scopolamine was found to increase non-list intrusions as well as reducing the number of correctly recalled items (Broks *et al.*, 1988). In this study, scopolamine did not impair immediate or secondary spatial memory. However, other investigators have found impairment for scopolamine on visual memory at higher doses (Liljequist and Mattila, 1979).

Schizophrenia

Memory

It has long been noted that persons with schizophrenia have difficulty with the acquisition and retention of new information. This is true for information of both a verbal and visual nature. A generalized deficit in neurocognitive functioning in schizophrenia has been postulated. However, even in studies that have demonstrated a generalized neuropsychological deficit in schizophrenic patients, memory scores have been significantly worse than all other cognitive areas measured (e.g. Saykin *et al.*, 1991).

Converging lines of evidence substantiate selective memory impairments in schizophrenia. For example, when identical twins discordant for schizophrenia have been studied, the twin with schizophrenia scored on average 23 points lower on the Wechsler Memory Scale (WMS-R) than the non-ill twin (Goldberg *et al.*, 1993a). Additionally, poor memory performance may not be directly attributable to a generalized intellectual deficit. For example, Gold and colleagues demonstrated that 70% of schizophrenia patients in their sample obtained a relatively lower score on the WMS-R than on the WAIS-R, suggesting a differential memory impairment in the majority of patients (Missar *et al.*, 1994). Lastly, deficits in measures of memory have been dissociated from deficits in attention. Because performance on measures of memory invariably is worse than impairment on attentional measures, this argues against attentional dysfunction as an explanation for poor performance on memory tests

In addition to deficits in secondary memory, schizophrenia subjects also have deficits in working memory. Recent studies have demonstrated impairments in both verbal and spatial working memory. Park and Holzman (1992) demonstrated that schizophrenic subjects performed significantly less well on a computerized measure of spatial working memory compared with subjects with bipolar disorder and age- and education-matched controls. Computerized spatial working memory tests are similar to delayed response tasks used in non-human primates in that they require subjects to retain the location of a target across a brief delay. Similarly, verbal working memory tests require subjects to hold in mind verbal information over a brief delay. Green *et al.* (1997) demonstrated that treatment-resistant schizophrenia patients performed significantly less well than age- and education-matched controls on the Digit Span Distractibility Test. This test measures the ability to recall a string of numbers after a brief delay. Interestingly, patients receiving benztropine performed similarly to those patients who did not. However, spatial working memory performance was significantly more impaired in subjects receiving benztropine compared with those who did not receive it (McGurk *et al.*, 1996), whereas spatial reference memory was not. This finding is consistent with animal literature indicating that spatial working memory is more sensitive to interruption in cholinergic transmission than is spatial reference memory.

Sensory gating

Sensory gating abnormalities, i.e. deficits in the ability to filter sensory stimuli, were described as a pathophysiological feature of schizophrenia nearly four decades ago (McGhie and Chapman, 1961). These deficits have been investigated as a clue to mechanisms of psychopathology and cognitive dysfunction by several groups (Braff *et al.*, 1992; Griffith *et al.*, 1998). A commonly used paradigm in schizophrenia is the P50 auditory event-related potential (AEP). Compared with normal subjects, persons with schizophrenia tend to demonstrate a higher test/conditioning amplitude response ratio—a phenomenon that is seen in up to 50% of non-schizophrenic first-degree relatives of persons with schizophrenia (Adler *et al.*, 1982, Clementz *et al.*, 1997).

There is evidence that the P50 AEP can be influenced by nicotine. Administration of nicotine (via nicotine gum) to schizophrenia patients and their non-smoking relatives tended to normalize the test/conditioning/amplitude response ratio (Adler *et al.*, 1992). There are a variety of nicotinic receptors (for an overview, see Dalack *et al.*, 1998), but converging evidence implicates a central role of the α-bungarotoxin-sensitive α-7 nicotinic receptor in the P50 gating response (Griffith *et al.*, 1998).

In addition to sensory gating, nicotinic receptors may play a role in other cognitive deficits in schizophrenia. Evidence for this is provided by Levin *et al.* (1996) who administered nicotine to haloperidol-treated patients with schizophrenia. Improvements were noted in several areas of cognition, including attention, reaction time and memory.

Pharmacological treatment of schizophrenia and the impact on cognitive functioning

The cornerstone of the clinical management of schizophrenia remains treatment with drugs that all have as a common feature antagonism of dopamine at the D_2 receptor. The primary goal of most clinicians in using the drugs is the reduction in 'positive' symptoms (agitation, hallucinations, delusions, etc.).

In the last 10–15 years, increasing emphasis has been placed on alleviating 'negative symptoms' (asociality, anhedonia, lack of motivation, etc.). This has been driven not only by an increased awareness that negative symptoms are related to poor outcome in schizophrenia, but also because of the advent of newer antipsychotics that may have a greater beneficial effect on negative symptoms. More recently, however, cognitive dysfunction has been identified as perhaps the primary cause of poor functional outcome in schizophrenia (Kaufman and Weinberger, 1987; Green, 1996). This has fostered a desire to improve cognitive functioning in schizophrenia and a hope that the newer, or 'atypical', antipsychotics can fulfill this need (Borison, 1996; Tollefson, 1996).

Typical antipsychotics

The effect of typical antipsychotics on cognition in schizophrenia has been reviewed elsewhere (Cassens *et al.*, 1990; Mortimer, 1997). Evidence for anything but small effects—either deleterious or salutary—of typical antipsychotics on general cognition is sparse. Even a hypothetical relationship between memory dysfunction and intrinsic anticholinergic activity of typical antipsychotic agents (e.g. as might be seen with thioridazine which has substantial *in vitro* and *in vivo* anticholinergic properties) has been difficult to demonstrate empirically. However, anticholinergic agents used to counteract symptoms of Parkinsonism induced by typical antipsychotics may disrupt cognition in schizophrenia, and memory in particular (Spohn and Strauss, 1989).

Haloperidol has virtually no antimuscarinic properties. However, it is often prescribed concomitantly with benztropine mesylate (Cogentin®, or other antiparkinsonian drugs) and thus may have as much or more net anticholinergic liability compared with, for example, thioridazine, which is much less likely to be prescribed with benztropine mesylate. This concept of intrinsic anticholinergic activity of antipsychotics and liability for extrapyramidal symptoms (EPS) was first addressed systematically by Snyder *et al.* in 1974.

Executive functioning, in the words of Mortimer (1997), "seems impervious to typical neuroleptic treatment". Part of the inability of typical antipsychotic medications to improve executive functioning, indeed even a propensity to induce additional dysfunction, may be the result of additional inhibition of frontal functioning by drugs that have prominent dopamine D_2 receptor blockade. On the other hand, substantial evidence provided by selective D_1 antagonists, such as SCH23390, indicates that this dopamine receptor subtype may be involved selectively in cognitive domains that are linked to prefrontal cortical functioning, including executive functioning and working memory (for a review, see Friedman *et al.*, 1999). This may explain why antipsychotic agents with pharmacological properties consisting largely of D_2 receptor antagonism have little impact on cognitive tasks supported by the prefrontal cortex.

Atypical antipsychotics

The definition of 'atypical' when referring to antipsychotic drugs is a matter of debate. All definitions will include a low propensity to cause EPS and, indeed, these drugs all share that property when used in appropriate dose ranges. Given this property, it would be expected that a lack of use of anticholinergic drugs to treat EPS might differentiate atypical antipsychotics from typical antipsychotics, at least with respect to memory.

Certainly indirect benefits on cognition such as diminished need for anticholinergic agents to treat drug-induced Parkinsonism exist with risperidone. For example, spatial working memory was found to be improved following treatment with risperidone as compared with haloperidol (McGurk *et al.*, 1996). This beneficial effect of risperidone was accounted for largely by differential co-administration of benztropine to the haloperidol-treated patient group. However, direct beneficial effects of risperidone have been provided by demonstrated improvement on verbal working memory that was not explained by diminished need for benztropine in the risperidone-treated patients (Green *et al.*, 1997). Additionally, risperidone has been found to improve executive functioning (Rossi *et al.*, 1996; McGurk *et al.*, 1997), verbal learning and memory (Kern *et al.*, 1999) and fine motor control (Kern *et al.*, 1998). The antagonistic properties of risperidone for 5-HT$_{2A}$ receptors may contribute to the cognitive enhancing effects demonstrated by this drug. Blocking 5-HT$_{2A}$ receptors activates dopaminergic neurons in the ventral tegmental area, which project to the frontal cortex. This resulting increase in prefrontal dopamine may enhance cognitive functioning by activating D$_1$ receptors (see Friedman *et al.*, 1999).

On the other hand, although atypical antipsychotic medications such as risperidone may be associated with improvements in some aspects of cognitive function (e.g. Green *et al.*, 1997), the intrinsic pharmacology of other atypical antipsychotics theoretically is predictive of untoward cognitive effects. For example, given that antimuscarinic agents used as treatment for neuroleptic-induced Parkinsonism in schizophrenia may impair memory (Tune *et al.*, 1982; Goldberg *et al.*, 1993a), it might be expected that clozapine, which exhibits potent antimuscarinic activity *in vitro* at a magnitude similar to that seen with benztropine (Snyder *et al.*, 1974; Bolden *et al.*, 1991, 1992), would exert a deleterious effect on memory. Such an effect is suggested by impairment in visual memory function during clozapine treatment (Hoff *et al.*, 1996). This had been suggested previously by Goldberg and Weinberger in an overview of the effects of clozapine on cognition (Goldberg and Weinberger, 1994). Other studies of the effect of clozapine on cognition have found no improvement (Classen and Laux, 1988; Goldberg *et al.*, 1993b), mixed improvement (Hagger *et al.*, 1993) or some improvement in memory and executive function (Buchanan *et al.*, 1994).

Another newer antipsychotic, olanzapine, also exhibits *in vitro* antimuscarinic activity (Bymaster *et al.*, 1996). There is also evidence of substantial *in vivo* antimuscarinic activity (Raedler *et al.*, 1998), although others, using a different paradigm, have presented data to the contrary (Basson *et al.*, 1998). Olanzapine has been shown to impair learning in rats in the Morris water maze task (Skarsfeldt, 1996), but the effect of olanzapine on cognitive function in humans has not been investigated systematically. At this time, there is little evidence for either a deleterious or beneficial effect of olanzapine on memory function in patients with schizophrenia.

Two other new antipsychotics, quetiapine and ziprasidone, both of which have demonstrated effectiveness in alleviating symptoms of schizophrenia, have yet to be investigated systematically in alleviating cognitive impairment in schizophrenia. Quetiapine, available to clinicians since 1998, has significant histamine H1-blocking properties which would be predictive of a propensity to cause sedation, which in turn may cause additional cognitive impairment. Clinically, sedation is seen in a substantial number of patients treated with quetiapine. Ziprasidone, which at the time of writing has yet to be approved for use by regulatory agencies, may have potential to improve cognitive functioning. For example, ziprasidone has a low affinity for muscarinic and histaminergic receptors and thus is unlikely to cause additional problems due to such pharmacology. In addition, it has the unique (among antipsychotics) properties of functioning as an agonist at the 5-HT_{1A} receptor and as a reuptake blocker of both serotonin and norepinephrine at the presynaptic site (Tandon *et al.*, 1997). These aspects of the pharmacology of ziprasidone might be predictive of enhancing cognitive function in schizophrenia, especially given findings of an inverse correlation of cortical levels of both serotonin and norepinephrine with cognitive function in persons with schizophrenia (Powchik *et al.*, 1998).

Table 14.2 depicts the binding affinities for the muscarinic M1 receptor of several new antipsychotics, their dose ranges and an estimated relative anticholinergic load of a daily dose of those drugs compared with a daily dose of 6 mg of benztropine mesylate. As can be seen, amongst the newer antipsychotics, risperidone and ziparsidone have the least daily anticholinergic load. The anticholinergic loads of olanzapine and clozapine are 2–4 orders of magnitude greater than that of risperidone, 1–4 orders of magnitude greater than that of ziprasidone and 0–1 orders of magnitude greater than that of benztropine.

Table 14.2 *In vitro* receptor binding

Drug	Affinity for muscarinic M1 receptors (K_i in nM)	Usual daily dose range	Anticholinergic load relative to benztropine(K_i benztropine/ K_i drug)?daily dose
Benztropine mesylate	0.125	6 mg	N/A
Haloperidol	5500	5–20 mg	<0.001
Thioridazine	2.7	50–400 mg	2–40
Clozapine	2	200–600 mg	12–37
Risperidone	>1000	2–6 mg	<0.001
Olanzapine	2	5–20 mg	0.3–1.3
Quetiapine	>1000	300–750 mg	0.03–0.1
Zipradisone	>1000	80–160 mg (anticipated)	0.01–0.02

Affinity values at K_i in nM; adapted from Larson *et al.* (1991) and Schotte *et al.* (1996).

Summary and unanswered questions

Cholinergic neurotransmission is important in many cognitive, motor and behavioral processes. Many of these processes are disrupted in schizophrenia. From a theoretical perspective, it is attractive to posit therefore that cholinergic mechanisms are involved. However, as is usually the case in biological systems, things are not so simple.

An example of this complexity is that both hyper- and hypocholinergic states have been implicated in the symptoms of schizophrenia. For example, increased cholinergic activity has been implicated in exacerbation of positive symptoms (Shiovitz *et al.*, 1996) and possibly as a root cause of negative symptoms (Tandon and Greden, 1989). These hypotheses might not be mutually exclusive, but the data are far from clear. Both positive and negative symptoms lessen during effective treatment with antipsychotic drugs, both typical and atypical and with or without concomitant use of anticholinergic drugs. On the other hand, anticholinergic drugs, in high enough doses, may induce (Woody and O'Brien, 1974) or exacerbate psychosis (Singh and Smith, 1973). The abuse of anticholinergic drugs for their euphorigenic effect (Smith, 1980) may lend some credence to a role for hypercholinergic states contributing to negative symptoms, but there does not seem to be any consistent evidence that would suggest that greater alleviation of negative symptoms occurs in patients treated with anticholinergics plus an antipsychotic drug versus the antipsychotic drug alone.

Post-mortem evidence for a cholinergic contribution to cognitive dysfunction is at best contradictory. Some authors have pointed to AD-like findings with a presumptive similar cholinergic deficit (Prohovnik *et al.*, 1993) or cholinergic deficits in the mesopontine areas of the brain (Garcia-Rill *et al.*, 1995). Others have found little or no evidence of AD-like changes (Powchik *et al.*, 1993; Purohit *et al.*, 1993) or a deficit in cholinergic function (Haroutunian *et al.*, 1994).

Sensory gating deficits, which are mediated in part by nicotinic receptor dysfunction, may contribute to cognitive deficits in schizophrenia. However, because up to 50% of first-degree relatives of persons with schizophrenia who exhibit P50 gating abnormalities exhibit the abnormality themselves but without having cognitive deficits similar to persons with schizophrenia, nicotinic receptor dysfunction may be at most a vulnerability factor for cognitive dysfunction.

The treatment of schizophrenia itself may alter cholinergic transmission and have effects on cognition, but this has not been demonstrated in a consistent way. For example, although it is known that anticholinergic drugs may exert subtle, but measurable, memory impairments (Tune *et al.*, 1982; Katz *et al.*, 1985), clozapine, which has substantial intrinsic anticholinergic activity, produces an inconsistent pattern of cognitive changes in persons with schizophrenia. Dopaminergic blockade, common to all effective antipsychotic drugs, could be expected to produce a rebound increase in variety of brain areas. This increase could be postulated to mitigate some of cognitive deficits seen in schizophrenia (e.g. via an increase in dopamine in prefrontal cortex) but, as described above, there has been no convincing pattern of improvement.

The atypical antipsychotics offer a mixed bag of findings with regard to cognition in schizophrenia. It is possible that the main cognitive benefit of the atypical antipsychotics is that because of their low liability for causing extrapyramidal symptoms, they are unlikely (or much less likely than typical antipsychotics) to be used in combination with anticholinergic drugs. Both clozapine and olanzapine have significant anticholinergic properties, but these do no seem to impart any substantial cognitive impairment although, in the case of olanzapine, it has not been studied sufficiently. Risperidone has the most evidence available for a salutary effect on cognition. Quetiapine is relatively unstudied. Ziprasidone, with its unique pharmacology, may have potential for cognitive improvement in schizophrenia, but the results of systematic studies are not yet available.

Despite the lack of consistent evidence of specific cholinergic neuropathology in post-mortem analyses in brains of schizophrenia patients, cholinergic replacement therapy in this population may still be indicated (for a review, see Friedman *et al.*, 1999). This is based on the overwhelming evidence of a selective, and often profound, deficit in memory for recent events which is quite similar to cognitive impairments produced by interruption of cholinergic transmission. It is possible that cholinergic agonists, such as anticholinesterases used in the treatment of cognitive impairment in AD, may improve memory in schizophrenia. Currently, at least one group is investigating the use of donepezil in chronic schizophrenia (K.L. Davis, personal communication).

Many questions remain unanswered. Among these are: do the newer antipsychotics offer any real benefit in terms of cognition? If cognition is enhanced with treatment, does that translate into better functional outcome? Are muscarinic or nicotinic receptors more important in cognitive impairment in schizophrenia?

The answers to these questions will only be derived by systematic study. The methodological problems that are inherent in such study are substantial, but surmountable. Among the many confounds that must be addressed are: premorbid intellectual functioning; baseline level of functioning; age of onset; length of illness; anticholinergic load of treatment; the intrinsic pharmacology of primary antipsychotic treatment including 'downstream' effects of the drug on cholinergic and other activity; drug–drug interactions; and the use of proper cognitive paradigms, to name a few. These confounds, even though some might be dealt with using statistical methods, make study design a challenge.

Another study design challenge is that translating cognitive changes that are measurable with psychometric tests into clinically meaningful outcomes often must rely on surrogate measures of functioning. The most significant outcome for a person with schizophrenia would be to achieve at least the level of social and occupational functioning that would have been predicted by their premorbid functioning. However, there are many practical and social impediments to achieving the highest level of function that might have been possible. Social stigma, loss of psychiatric health care benefits if working, and a dearth of effective rehabilitation programs that set goals for patients beyond that of entry level to low-skilled jobs are just some of the challenges that must be overcome.

With newer antipsychotics—not only those available or soon-to-be-available, but also those in the pipeline of many pharmaceutical companies—there are additional hurdles to the systematic study of cognitive function in schizophrenia. New drug development often takes years and may cost hundreds of millions of dollars to bring a new drug to market. Regulatory agencies are likely to give approval to a new drug for certain indications. In the case of schizophrenia, it is primarily psychosis that is of interest, although in the past several years negative symptoms are being recognized increasingly as a target of therapy. It may be several years more before regulatory agencies recognize cognitive impairment in schizophrenia as a viable focus of treatment. Until then, a major financial disincentive exists for pharmaceutical companies which would need to invest tens of millions of dollars investigating the cognitive effects of an antipsychotic prior to an uncertain approval for the treatment of psychosis. After a drug is approved, there is a greater likelihood that other aspects of a disease (e.g. cognition) might be investigated.

References

Adler, L.E., Pachtman, E., Franks, R., Pecevich, M., Waldo, M.C. and Freedman, R. (1982) Neurophysiological evidence for a defect in neuronal mechansims involved in sensory gating in schizophrenia. *Biological Psychiatry*, **17**, 639–654.

Adler, L.E., Hoffer, L.J., Griffith, J., Waldo, M.C. and Freedman, R. (1992) Normalization by nicotine of deficient auditory sensory gating in the relatives of schizophrenics. *Biological Psychiatry*, **32**, 607–616.

Alpern, H.P. and Marriott, J.G. (1973) Short-term memory: facilitation and disruption with cholinergic agents. *Physiology and Behavior*, **11**, 571–575.

Arnold, S.E., Franz, B.R. and Trojanowski, J.Q. (1994) Elderly patients with schizophrenia exhibit infrequent neurodegenerative lesions. *Neurobiology of Aging*, **15**, 299–303.

Bartus, R.T. and Johnson, H.R. (1976) Short-term memory in the rhesus monkey: disruption from the anti-cholinergic scopolamine. *Pharmacology, Biochemistry, and Behavior*, **5**, 39–46.

Bartus, R.T., Dean, R.L. and Flicker, C. (1987) Cholinergic psychopharmacology: an integration of human and animal research on memory. In: Meltzer, H.Y. (ed.), *Psychopharmacology: The Third Generation of Progress*. Raven Press, New York, pp.

Basson, B.R., Kennedy, J.S., Tran, P.V. *et al.* (1998) The comparative anti-muscarinic-like side effect profiles of olanzapine and risperidone treatment in patients with schizophrenia spectrum psychosis. Abstract from the 1998 meeting of the ACNP.

Beatty, W. and Bierley, R.A. (1985) Scopolamine degrades spatial working memory but spares spatial reference memory: dissimilarity of anticholinergic effect and restriction of distal visual cues. *Pharmacology, Biochemistry, and Behavior*, **23**, 1–6.

Bogerts, B. (1993) Recent advances in the neuropathology of schizophrenia. *Schizophrenia Bulletin*, **19**, 431–45.

Bolden, C., Cusack, B. and Richelson, E. (1991) Clozapine is a potent and selective muscarinic antagonist at the five cloned human muscarinic acetylcholine receptors expressed in CHO-K1 cells. *European Journal of Pharmacology*, **192**, 205–206.

Bolden, C., Cusack, B. and Richelson, E. (1992) Antagonism by antimuscarinics and neuroleptic compounds at the five cloned human muscarinic cholinergic receptors cloned on hamster ovary cells. *Journal of Pharmacology and Experimental Therapeutics*, **260**, 576–580.

Borison, R.L. (1966) The role of cognition in the risk–benefit and safety analysis of antipsychotic medication. *Acta Psychiatrica Scandinavica*, **94**, 5–11.

Bowen, D.M., Smith, C.B., White, P. and Davison, A.N. (1976) Neurotransmitter-related enzymes and indices of hypoxia in senile dementia and other abiotrophies. *Brain*, **99**, 459–496

Bowen, D.M., Benton, J.S., Spillane, J.A., Smith, C.C.T. and Allen, S.J. (1982) Choline acetyltransferase activity and histopathology of frontal neocortex from biopsies of demented patients. *Journal of Neurological Science*, **57**, 191–202.

Braff, D.L., Grillon, C. and Geyer, M.A. (1992) Gating and habituation of the startle reflex in schizophrenic patients. *Archives of General Psychiatry*, **49**, 206–215.

Brito, G.N.O., Davis, B.J., Stopp, L.C. and and Stanton, M.E. (1983) Memory and the septo-hippocampal cholinergic system in the rat. *Psychopharmacology*, **81**, 315–320.

Broks, P., Preston, G.C., Traub, M., Poppleton, P., Ward, C., Stahl, S.M. (1988) Modelling dementia: effects of scopolamine on memory and attention. *Neuropsychologia*, **26(5)**, 685–700.

Buchanan, R.W., Holstein, C. and Breier, A. (1994) The comparative efficacy and long-term effect of clozapine treatment on neuropsychological test performance. *Biological Psychiatry*, **36**, 717–725.

Bymaster, F.P., Hemrick-Luecke, S.K., Perry, K.W. and Fuller, R.W. (1996) Neurochemical evidence for antagonism by olanzapine of dopamine, serotonin, alpha 1-adrenergic and muscarinic receptors *in vivo* in rats. *Psychopharmacology*, **124**, 87–94.

Calev, A. (1983) Anti-cholinergic drugs and memory. *British Journal of Psychiatry*, **143**, 422–423.

Cassens, G., Inglis, A.K., Appelbaum, P.S. and Guthell, T,G. (1990) Neuroleptics: effects on neuropsychological function in chronic schizophrenic patients. *Schizophrenia Bulletin*, **16**, 477–499.

Classen, W. and Laux, G. (1988) Sensorimotor and cognitive performance of schizophrenic patients treated with haloperidol, flupenthixol or clozapine. *Pharmacopsychiatry*, **21**, 295–297.

Clementz, B.A., Geyer, M.A. and Braff, D.L. (1997) P50 suppression among schizophrenia and normal comparison subjects: a methodological analysis. *Biological Psychiatry*, **41**, 1035–1044.

Dalack, G.W., Healy, D.J. and Meador-Woodruff, J.H. . (1998) Nicotine dependence in schizophrenia: clinical phenomena and laboratory findings. *American Journal of Psychiatry*, **155**, 1490–1501.

Davidson, M., Harvey, P.H., Powchik, P., Parrella, M., White, L., Knobler, H.Y., Losonczy, M.F., Keefe, R.S.E., Katz, S. and Frecska, E. (1995) Severity of cognitive impairment in geriatric schizophrenic patients. *American Journal of Psychiatry*, **152**, 197–207.

Davies, P. and Maloney, A.J. (1976) Selective loss of central cholinergic neurons in Alzheimer's disease [letter]. *Lancet*, **2**, 1403.

Dawson, G.R. and Iverson, S.D. (1993) The effects of novel cholinesterase inhibitors and selective muscarinic receptor agonists in tests of reference and working memory. *Behavioral Brain Research*, **57**, 143–153.

Eckerman, D.A., Gordon, W.A., Edwards, J.D., MacPhail, R.C. and Gage, M.I. (1979) Effects of scopolamine, pentobarbital, and amphetamine on radial arm maze performance in the rat. *Pharmacology, Biochemistry, and Behavior*, **12**, 595–602.

Etienne, P., Robitaillle, Y., Wood, P., Gauthier, S., Nair, N.P.V. and Quirion, R. (1986) Nucleus basalis neuronal loss, neuritic plaques and choline acetyltransferase activity in advanced Alzheimer's disease. *Journal of Neuroscience*, **19**, 1279–1291.

Fibiger, H.C. (1986) Learning and memory deficits after ibotenate lesions of the nucleus basalis: reversal by cholinomimetics. *Canadian Journal of Neurological Sciences*, **13**, 498.

Friedman, J., Temporini, H. and Davis, K.L. (1999) Pharmacological strategies for augmenting cognitive performance in schizophrenia. *Biological Psychiatry*, **45**, 1–16.

Garcia-Rill, E., Biedermann, J.A., Chambers, T., Skinner, R.D., Mrak, R.E., Husain, and Karson, C.N. (1995) Mesopontine neurons in schizophrenia. *Neuroscience*, **66**, 321–335.

Gold, J.M. and Harvey, P.D. (1993) Cognitive deficits in schizophrenia. *Psychiatric Clinics of North American*, **16**, 295–312.

Goldberg, T.E. and Weinberger, D.R. (1994) The effects of clozapine on neurocognition: an overview. *Journal of Clinical Psychiatry*, **55** (9, Suppl. B), 88–90.

Goldberg, T.E., Torrey, E.F., Gold, J.M., Ragland, J.D., Bigelow, L.B. and Weinberger, D.R. (1993a) Learning and memory in monozygotic twins discordant for schizophrenia. *Psychological Medicine*, **23**, 71–85.

Goldberg, T.E., Greenberg, R.D. and Griffin, S.J. (1993b) The effect of clozapine on cognition and psychiatric symptoms in patients with schizophrenia. *British Journal of Psychiatry*, 162, 43–48.

Goldman-Rakic, P.S. (1994) Working memory dysfunction in schizophrenia. *Journal of Neuropsychiatry and Clinical Neurosciences*, **6**, 348–357.

Green, M.F. (1996) What are the functional consequences of neurocognitive deficits in schizophrenia? *American Journal of Psychiatry*, **153**, 321–320.

Green, M.F., Marshall, B.D., Jr, Wirshing, W.C., Ames, D., Marder, S.R., McGurk, S., Kern, R.S. and Mintz, J. (1997) Does risperidone improve verbal working memory in treatment-resistant schizophrenia? *American Journal of Psychiatry*, **154**, 799–804.

Griffith, J.M., O'Neill, J.E., Petty, F., Garver, D., Young, D. and Freedman, R. (1988) Nicotinic receptor desensitization and sensory gating deficits in schizophrenia. *Biological Psychiatry*, **44**, 98–106.

Hagger. C., *et al.* (1993) Improvement in cognitive functions and psychiatric symptoms in treatment refractory schizophrenic patients receiving clozapine. *Biological Psychiatry*, **34**, 702–712.

Haroutunian, V., Davidson, M., Kanof, P.D., Perl, D.P., Powchik, P., Losonczy, M.F., McCrystal, J., Purohit, D.P., Bierer, L. and Davis, K.L. (1994) Cortical cholinergic markers in schizophrenia. *Schizophrenia Research*, **12**, 137–144.

Haroutunian, V., Powchik, P., Purohit, P.D. *et al*. Cognitive dysfunction in the absence of cholinergic deficits: a postmortem study of 95 elderly schizophrenic patients. *Neuroscience Letters* (submitted).

Heise, G.A., Hrabrich, B., Lilie, N.L., Martin, R.A. (1975) Scopolamine effects on delayed spatial alternation in the rat. *Pharmacology Biochemistry and Behaviour*, **3(6)**, 993–1002.

Hoff, A.L., Faustman, W.O., Wieneke, M. *et al*. (1996) The effects of clozapine on symptom reduction, neurocognitive function, and clinical management in treatment-refractory state hospital schizophrenic inpatients. *Neuropsychopharmacology*, **15**, 361–369.

Katz, I.R., Greenberg, W.H., Barr, G.A., Garbarino, C., Buckley, P. and Smith, D. (1985) Screening for cognitive toxicity of anticholinergic drugs. *Journal of Clinical Psychiatry*, **46**, 323–326.

Kaufman, C.A. and Weinberger, D.R. (1987) The neurobiological basis of psychiatric disability. In: Meyerson, A.T. and Fine, T. (eds), *Psychiatric Disability: Clinical, Legal, and Administrative Dimensions*. American Psychiatric Press, Washington, DC.

Kern, R.S., Green, M.F., Marshall, B.D., Wirshing, W.C., Wirshing, D., McGurk, S.R., Marder, S.R. and Mintz, J. (1998) Risperidone vs. haloperidol on reaction time, manual dexterity, and motor learning in treatment-resistant schizophrenia patients. *Biological Psychiatry*, **44**, 762–732.

Kern, R.S., Green, M.F., Marshall, B.D., Wirshing, W.C., Wirshing, D., McGurk, S.R., Marder, S.R. and Mintz, J. (1999) Risperidone vs. haloperidol on secondary memory: can newer antipsychotic medications aid in learning? *Schizophrenia Bulletin*, **25(2)**, 223–232.

Kesner, R.P., DiMattia, B.V. and Crutcher, K.A. (1987) Evidence for neocortical involvement in reference memory. *Behavioral and Neural Biology*, **47**, 40–53.

Larson, E.W., Pfenning, M.A. and Richelson, E. (1991) Selectivity of antimuscarinic compounds for muscarinic receptors of human brain and heart. *Psychopharmacology*, **103**, 162–165.

Levin, E.D. (1990) Characterization of the cognitive effects of combined muscarinic and nicotinic blockade. *Behavioral and Neural Biology*, **53**, 103–112.

Levin, E.D. and Simon, B.B. (1998) Nicotinic involvement in cognitive function in animals. *Psychopharmacology*, **138**, 217–230.

Levin, E.D., Wilson, W., Rose, J.E. and McEvoy, J. (1996) Nicotine–haloperidol interactions and cognitive performance in schizophrenics. *Neuropsychopharmacology*, **15**, 429–436.

Levy, A., Kluge, P.B. and Elsmore, T.F. (1983) Radial arm maze performance of mice: acquisition and atropine effects. *Behavioral and Neural Biology*, **39**, 229–240.

Liljequist, R., Mattila, M.J. (1979) Effect of physostigmine and scopolamine on the memory functions of chess players. *Medicine and Biology*, **57(6)**, 402–405.

Liu, J.L. and Su, S.N. (1993) The role of acetycholine in the cognitive function of frontal neurons in monkeys. *Science China*, **36**, 1510–1517.

Lydon, R.G. and Nakajima, S. (1992) Differential effects of scopolamine on working and reference memory depend upon level of training. *Pharmacology, Biochemistry, and Behavior*, **43**, 645–650.

McGhie. A. and Chapman, S. (1961) Disorders of attention and perception in earlier schizophrenia. *British Journal of Medical Psychology*, **34**, 103–116.

McGurk, S.R. and Butcher, L.L. (1987) The medial cholinergic pathway and memory. *Federation Proceedings*, **2**, A342.

McGurk, S.R., Levin, E.D., Butcher, L.L. (1988) Cholinergic-dopaminergic interactions in radial-arm maze performance. *Behaviour and Neural Biology*, **49(2)**, 234–239.

McGurk, S.R., Levin, E.D. and Butcher, L.L. (1991) Impairment of radial-arm maze performance in rats following lesions involving the cholinergic medial pathway: reversal by arecoline and differential effects of muscarinic and nicotinic anatogonists. *Neuroscience*, **44**, 137–147.

McGurk, S.R., Green, M.F., Wirshing, W.C., Ames, D., Marshall, B.D. and Mader, S.R. (1996) The effects of risperidone vs. haloperidol on spatial working memory in treatment-resistant schizophrenia. *Fifty-first Annual Meeting of the Society of Biological Psychiatry*, New York.

McGurk, S.R., Green, M.F., Wirshing, W.C., Ames, D., Marshall, B.D., Marder, M.D. and Mintz, J. (1997) The effects of risperidone vs. haloperidol on cognitive functioning in treatment-resistant schizophrenia: the Trail Making Test. *CNS Spectrums*, **2**, 60–64.

Mesulam, M. (1995) Structure and function of cholinergic pathways in the cerebral cortex, limbic system, basal ganglia, and thalamus of the human brain. In: Bloom, F.E. and Kupfer, D.J. (eds), *Psychopharmacology: The Fourth Generation of Progress*. Raven Press, New York, pp. 135–146.

Missar, C.D., Gold, J.M., Goldberg, T.E. (1994) WAIS-R short forms in chronic schizophrenia. *Schizophrenia Research*, **12(3)**, 247–250.

Mortimer, A.M. . (1997) Cognitive function in schizophrenia—do neuroleptics make a difference? *Pharmacology, Biochemistry, and Behavior*, **56**, 789–795.

Murray, C.L. and Fibiger, H.C. (1985) Learning and memory deficits after lesions of the nucleus basalis magnocellularis: reversal by physostigmine. *Neuroscience*, **14**, 1025–1032.

Olton, D.S. and Papas, B.C. (1979) Spatial memory and hippocampal function. *Neuropsychologia*, **17**, 669–682.

Park, S. and Holzman, P. (1992) Schizophrenics show spatial working memory deficits. *Archives of General Psychiatry*, **49**, 975–982.

Penetar, D.M. and McDonough, J.H., Jr (1983) Effects of cholinergic drugs on delayed match-to-sample performance of rhesus monkeys. *Pharmacology, Biochemistry, and Behavior*, **19**, 963–967.

Perry, E.K., Perry, R.H., Blessed, G. and Tomlinson, B.E. (1977) Necropsy evidence of central cholinergic defects in senile dementia [letter]. *Lancet*, **1**, 189.

Powchik, P., Davidson, M., Haroutunian, V., Gabriel, S.M., Purohit, D.P., Perl, D.P., Harvey, P.D. and Davis, K.L. (1998) Postmortem studies in schizophrenia. *Schizophrenia Bulletin*, **24**, 325–341.

Powchik, P., Friedman, J., Haroutunian, V., Greenberg, D., Altsteil, L., Purohit, D., Perl, D. and Davidson, M. (1997) Apolipoprotein E4 in schizophrenia: a study of one hundred and sixteen cases with concomitant neuropathological examination. *Biological Psychiatry*, **42**, 296–298.

Powchik, P., Davidson, M., Nemeroff, C.B., Haroutunian, V., Losonczy, M., Bissette, G., Perl, D.P., Ghanbari, H., Miller, B. and Davis, K.L. (1993) Alzheimer's disease related protein in geriatric schizophrenic patients with cognitive impairment. *American Journal of Psychiatry*, **150**, 1726–1727.

Prohovnik, I., Dwork, A.J., Kaufman, M.A. and Willson, N. (1993) Alzheimer-type neuropathology in elderly schizophrenic patients. *Schizophrenia Bulletin*, **19**, 805–816.

Prohovnik, I., Arnold, S.E., Smith, G. and Lucas, L.R. (1997) Physostigmine reversal of scopolamine-induced hypofrontality. *Journal of Cerebral Blood Flow and Metabolism*, **17**, 220–228.

Purohit, P., Davidson, M., Perl, D.P., Powchik, P., Haroutunian, V., Bierer, L., McCrystal, J., Losonczy, M. and Davis, K.L. (1993) Severe cognitive impairment in schizophrenic patients: a clinicopathological study. *Biological Psychiatry*, **33**, 255–260.

Raedler, T.J., Knable, M.B., Lafargus, T. *et al.* (1998) *In vivo* determination of muscarinic cholinergic receptor occupancy in patients treated with olanzapine. Abstract from the 1998 meeting of the ACNP.

Reisine, T.D., Yamamura, H.I., Bird, E.D., Spokes, E. and Enna, S.J. (1978) Pre- and post-synaptic neurochemical alterations in Alzheimer's disease. *Brain Research*, **159**, 477–481.

Richter, J.A., Perry, E.K. and Tomlinson, B.E. (1980) Acetylcholine and choline levulose in postmortem human brain tissue: preliminary observations in Alzheimer's disease. *Life Science*, **26**, 1683–1689.

Ridley, R.M., Barratt, N.G. and Baker, H.F. (1984) Cholinergic learning deficits in the marmoset produced by scopolamine and ICV hemicholinium. *Psychopharmacology*, **83**, 340–345.

Ridley, R.M., Murray, T.K., Johnson, J.A. and Baker, H.F. (1986) Learning impairment following lesion of the basal nucleus of Meynert in the marmoset: modification by cholinergic drugs. *Brain Research*, **376**, 108–116.

Ridley, R.M., Baker, J.A., Baker, H.F. and Maclean, C.J. (1994) Restoration of cognitive abilities by cholinergic grafts in cortex of monkeys with lesions of the basal nucleus of Meynert. *Neuroscience*, **63**, 653–666.

Rossi, A., Mancini, F., Stratta, P., Mattei, P., Gismondi, R., Pozzi, F. and Casacchia, M. (1996) Risperidone, negative symptoms and cognitive deficit in schizophrenia: an open study. *Acta Psychiatrica Scandinavica*, **95**, 40–43

Rupniak, N.M.J., Tye, S.J. and Field, M.J. (1997) Enhanced performance of spatial and visual recognition memory tasks by the selective acetylcholinesterase inhibitor E2020 in rhesus monkeys. *Psychopharmacology*, **131**, 406–410.

Saykin, A.J., Gur, R.C., Gur, R.E., Mozley, P.D., Mozley, L.H., Resnick, S.M., Kester, B. and Stafiniak, P. (1991) Neuropsychological function in schizophrenia: selective impairment in memory and learning. *Archives of General Psychiatry*, **48**, 618–624.

Schotte, A., Janssen, P.F.M., Gommeren, W., Luyten, W., Van Grompel, P., Lesage, A.S., De Loore, K. and Leysen, J.E. (1996) Risperidone compared with new and reference antipsychotic drugs: *in vitro* and *in vivo* receptor binding. *Psychopharmacology*, **124**, 57–73.

Shiovitz, T.M., Welke, T.L., Tigel, P.D., Anand, R., Hartman, R.D., Sramek, J.J., Kurtz, N.M. and Cutler, N.R. (1996) Cholinergic rebound and rapid onset psychosis following abrupt clozapine withdrawal. *Schizophrenia Bulletin*, **22**, 591–595.

Singh, M.M. and Smith, J.M. (1973) Reversal of some therapeutic effects of an antipsychotic agent by an antiparkinsonian drug. J Nerv Ment Dis, 157, 50–58.

Skarsfeldt, T. (1996) Differential effect of antipsychotics on place navigation of rats in the Morris water maze. A comparative study between novel and reference antipsychotics. *Psychopharmacology*, **124**, 126–133.

Smith, J.M. (1980) Abuse of antiparkinsonian medications: a review of the literature. *Journal of Clinical Psychiatry*, **41**, 351–354.

Smith, Y. and Parent, A. (1986) Differential connections of caudate and putamen in the squirrel monkey (*Saimiri sciureus*). *Neuroscience*, **18**, 347–371.

Snyder, S., Greenberg, D. and Yamamura, H.I. (1974) Antischizophrenic drugs and brain cholinergic receptors: affinity for muscarinic sites predicts extrapyramidal effects. *Archives of General Psychiatry*, **31**, 58–71.

Spohn, H.E. and Strauss, M.E. (1989) Relation of neuroleptic and anticholinergic medication to cognitive functions in schizophrenia. *Journal of Abnormal Psychology*, **98**, 367–380.

Stevens, R. (1981) Scopolamine impairs spatial maze performance in rats. *Physiol Behav*, **27(2)**, 385–386.

Strauss, M.E., Reynolds, K.S., Jayaram, G. and Tune, L.E. (1990) Effects of anticholinergic medication on memory in schizophrenia. *Schizophrenia Research*, **3**, 127–129.

Tandon, R. and Greden, J.F. (1989) Cholinergic hyperactivity and negative schizophrenic symptoms: a model of cholinergic/dopaminergic interactions in schizophrenia. *Archives of General Psychiatry*, **46**, 745–753.

Tandon, R., Harrigan, E. and Zorn, S.H. (1997) Ziprasidone: a novel antipsychotic with unique pharmacology and therapeutic potential. *Journal of Serotonin Research*, **4**, 159–177.

Tollefson GD. (1996) Cognitive function in schizophrenic patients. *Journal of Clinical Psychiatry*, **57** (Suppl. 11), 31–39.

Tune, L.E., Strauss, M.E., Lew, M.F., Greitlinger, E. and Coyle, J.T. (1982) Serum levels of anticholinergic drugs and impaired recent memory in chronic schizophrenic patients. *American Journal of Psychiatry*, **139**, 1460–1462.

Vitiello, B., Martin, A., Hill, J., Mack, C., Molchan, S., Martinez, R., Murphy, D.L. and Sunderland, T. (1997) Cognitive and behavioral effects of cholinergic, dopaminergic, and serotinergic blockade in humans. *Neuropsychopharmacology*, **16**, 15–24.

Woody, G.E. and O'Brien, C.T. (1974) Anticholinergic toxic psychosis in drug abusers treated with benztropine. *Comprehensive Psychiatry*, **15**, 439–442.

15 Cognitive enhancement as a treatment strategy in schizophrenia

Tonmoy Sharma and Philip D. Harvey

Introduction

Cognitive dysfunction, a symptom of schizophrenia, is a core and enduring feature of the illness. It recently has been identified as an important measure of long-term outcome and is probably more important than the characteristic psychotic symptoms in the treatment of this disorder. Deficits in cognition are the most consistent findings in the schizophrenia literature. These deficits are pervasive, with virtually all patients affected to some degree, when compared with healthy peers or relatives. Since Kraepelin's (1919) first clinical accounts, it has been recognized that they are a prominent feature of schizophrenia. It is well established that schizophrenic patients exhibit significant pervasive cognitive impairments when compared with healthy controls. Furthermore, it would appear that a vast array of cognitive domains are affected by the disease, as outlined in Section 1 of this book. Thus, understanding of the pattern and reversibility of specific cognitive dysfunctions may provide important clues to pathophysiological processes and the mechanisms of effective treatments. This chapter focuses on neurocognitive impairments that occur in schizophrenia, with the possibility that cognitive enhancement or reversal of these deficits may have an impact on the longer term outcome of the illness.

The central role of cognitive impairment in schizophrenia

Kraepelin (1919) believed that cognitive impairment in schizophrenia was produced directly by the underlying neuropathology of the disorder, especially impairments in the functions of the frontal lobes. After a long period of neglect, cognitive impairment is again seen to be a central feature and not some epiphenomenon of other aspects of the illness or its treatment. However, in contrast to many other conditions such as dementia, general or specific cognitive deficits, unfortunately, are not part of the diagnostic criteria for schizophrenia in DSM-IV. In addition, the regulatory agencies in Europe and North America do not require demonstration of efficacy against cognitive impairments for a drug to be approved for the treatment for schizophrenia.

Considerable controversy still exists about the magnitude, pattern and course of these cognitive deficits. Poor performance on tests sensitive to nearly every cognitive function is the norm in patients with schizophrenia, with many patients scoring 2–4 standard deviations (SDs) below the normal mean (Saykin *et al.*, 1991). On tests where patients with schizophrenia underperform normative standards by 3 SDs, a level of impairment that is common to several different types of cognitive functioning, the magnitude of impairment is consistent with an IQ difference of 45 points. Patients with dementia are often found to underperform normal individuals by less than this amount.

There is a possibility that cognitive impairment may be more common than most other symptoms of the illness. On a group-mean basis, patients with schizophrenia perform neuropsycholgical tests on average at the 2nd to 15th percentile, which would be considered impaired to borderline by most standards (Heaton *et al.*, 1994). A recent study demonstrated that 85% of patients with schizophrenia were impaired on the basis of a comprehensive neuropsychological assessment, while 5% of a sample of normal comparison subjects were seen to be abnormal using the same criteria (Palmer *et al.*, 1997). The patients in this study were high-functioning out-patients living in the community, who might be expected to have less cognitive impairment than poorer outcome patients routinely seen in clinical practice. How does this compare with the prevalence of other 'common' symptoms of schizophrenia? Between 50 and 75% of patients with schizophrenia are found to have hallucinations, delusions, communication disorders and negative symptoms (WHO, 1974). 'Lack of insight' or 'unawareness of illness' is the only clinical symptom of schizophrenia that has been reported to have a higher prevalence than cognitive impairment (WHO, 1974). However, unawareness of illness may itself be a sign of cognitive dysfunction (Amador *et al.*, 1991), although this is in some dispute (Young *et al.*, 1993).

It commonly has been felt by clinicians that schizophrenia is a result of positive symptoms. Whilst it may be impossible to test patients when they are extremely psychotic, there seems to be a very poor correlation between positive symptoms (e.g. auditory hallucinations) and the severity of impairments in cognitive functioning (Perlick *et al.*, 1992; Riley *et al.*, 1999). However there is a relationship between formal thought disorder and verbal memory as well as working memory deficits (Spitzer, 1993). This may be as a result of a patient's inability to refer adequately to his/her previous verbal expressions (Harvey, 1983; Chapter 6). The lack of association between psychotic symptoms such as delusions and hallucinations and cognitive dysfunction in schizophrenia points to the fact that different brain systems may be involved in these largely independent dysfunctions. Cognitive impairments are correlated moderately with negative symptoms (McCreadie *et al.*, 1994; Roy and DeVriendt, 1994; Davidson and McGlashan, 1997). Indeed, some assessments of negative symptoms (such as lack of motivation) may be indirect assessments of cognitive function. There is a conceptual overlap between the constructs, with certain symptoms or deficits considered both negative symptoms and cognitive impairment. Thus, any measure of negative symptom severity also provides an index of cognitive impairment in an approximate way.

Cognitive impairment is present at the onset and throughout the course of the illness

Cognitive impairments can be identified in individuals who later develop schizophrenia as early as the first year in school (Crow *et al.*, 1995). Cognitive deficits of various types have been considered as markers of vulnerability to the illness, meaning that they would be expected to be stable over time even before other aspects of the illness are obvious (Asarnow and MacCrimmon, 1978; Knight *et al.*, 1979). Patients in their first episode of psychosis present with neurocognitive impairment by the time they come to the attention of the mental health services. Studies examining neurocognition in first-episode psychosis patients have found patients to perform significantly less well than normal, healthy controls on many cognitive functions including memory, attention and concentration, executive function, language skills, psychomotor speed, spatial abilities and general cortical function (Bilder *et al.*, 1992a; Hoff *et al.*, 1992; Sweeney *et al.*, 1991a, 1992; Saykin *et al.*, 1994; Censits *et al.*, 1997; Riley *et al.*, 1999). Furthermore, the overall performance deficit can be up to 1.5 SDs below that of a normal control population (Bilder *et al.*, 1995). This is clinically significant and meaningful as 1 SD in IQ below normal controls would be a difference of 15 IQ points. This could make the difference between being able to complete a college degree or not in a young person afflicted with the illness.

Many different cognitive deficits have been demonstrated to be unchanged in their magnitude after the remission of positive symptoms (Asarnow and MacCrimmon, 1978; Knight *et al.*, 1979). The stability of cognitive impairments across various follow-up intervals appears to be much greater than that of other symptoms of the illness, including negative symptoms. Thus, cognitive impairment appears to be present before, during and after cyclical episodes of psychotic symptoms. Is there evidence of progressive cognitive decline in schizophrenia? The majority of studies have employed a cross-sectional design comparing first-episode patients, chronic patients and, occasionally, normal control subjects (Bilder *et al.*, 1991, 1992a; Hoff *et al.*, 1991, 1992; Sweeney *et al.*, 1991a, 1992; Saykin *et al.*, 1994; Albus *et al.*, 1997; Censits *et al.*, 1997; Binder *et al.*, 1998; Hutton *et al.*, 1998). Most studies (Sweeney *et al.*, 1992; Saykin *et al.*, 1994) but not all (Hoff *et al.*, 1992) found no significant differences between first-episode and chronic patients. These results suggest that there may be progressive decline on some functions while others remain preserved.

However, cross-sectional studies are confounded by the possible effects of medication and institutionalization. One way of overcoming such confounds is to employ a longitudinal design. Few studies have pursued this line of investigation and the results are generally consistent with a pattern of lack of decline over the first 12–24 months after the onset of the illness (Bilder *et al.*, 1991; Hoff *et al.*, 1991; Sweeney *et al.*, 1991b). Indeed, in these studies, there is some evidence of improvements on measures of executive function, attention concentration, psychomotor speed and memory. However, Bilder *et al.* (1991) also reported non-significant declines on some measures of language and a significant decline on digit span. Could it be that digit span can distinguish between those who will go on to suffer from recurring episodes? Also, is the improvement in cognitive function a result of the decrement of clinical psychopathology? It appears that there is no relationship between the neuro-psychological difference scores and clinical change scores. These longitudinal studies have shown that cognitive dysfunction is a core and enduring feature of schizophrenia. Whilst there is little evidence of deterioration in the short term, there seems to be a cohort of patients who may be on a deteriorating course with bad outcome. Thus, cognitive dysfunction is a stable feature of the illness, is evident in remitted patients and is not due to symptom severity

The relationship between cognitive deficits and functional impairments

Most patients with schizophrenia have great difficulty with independent living and thus poor functional outcome. They have trouble navigating through life. Less than one-third of patients with schizophrenia are able to sustain even part-time employment, the rate of marriage and reproduction of patients with schizophrenia is quite low and they have problems managing their finances and maintaining a household, family relations, friendships and community ties. These impairments are often life-long and cost society 3–4 times more than does direct patient care (Gunderson *et al.*, 1975; Andrews *et al.*, 1985; Hall *et al.*, 1985). Interestingly, functional impairment has a more direct impact on the patient's life than do the psychotic symptoms of their illness.

Since the focus of clinical psychiatry has been on reduction of psychotic symptoms (perhaps due to the success in reducing these symptoms with the conventional 'typical' antipsychotics), the functional deficits have taken a back seat. However, these deficits persist even in periods of remission of positive symptoms of the illness and are predicted most strongly by the current severity of cognitive impairment, followed by the severity of negative symptoms (Green, 1996). Positive symptom severity is not correlated strongly with the level of functional deficit, even in patients with very poor outcome schizophrenia (Perlick *et al.*, 1992; Harvey *et al.*, 2000; Chapter 9). Cognitive deficits contribute to impairment in social functioning and the course of the illness in schizophrenia (Green, 1996). Thus, cognitive impairment may be an important predictor of outcome in schizophrenia.

The issue of interference or rate-limiting effects of cognitive impairment on treatment is an important one. Most rehabilitation treatments for schizophrenia, from the most basic token economy programme to the most sophisticated social problem-solving training, are learning based. Since many patients with schizophrenia have severe deficits in memory and attention, it is not surprising that these patients are often very slow to learn. As a result, the extent of cognitive impairment in schizophrenia may impact directly on the extent that non-pharmacological treatments can improve the functional status of patients with the illness.

Cognitive impairment is the best predictor of adaptive outcome

As mentioned previously, certain aspects of cognitive impairments are strongly correlated with the global severity of negative symptoms. Thus, any measure of negative symptom severity also provides an approximate index of cognitive impairment. Longitudinal research has clearly shown that cognitive and negative symptoms are correlated with each other at successive assessments, but does not show the patterns of correlation over time that suggest a causal relationship between the two factors (Harvey *et al.*, 1996). In addition, when patients are referred from long-term psychiatric care to community residences, their negative symptoms improve but their cognitive impairments remain the same (Leff *et al.*, 1994). In all studies where both negative and cognitive symptoms have been used to predict overall outcome, as well as specific measures of adaptive functioning and life skills (Breier *et al.*, 1991; Harvey *et al.*, 1997), cognitive symptoms have always been found to be associated more strongly than negative symptoms with adaptive outcome (Green, 1996). It is noteworthy that across all neurological and psychiatric conditions, premorbid and concurrent measures of cognitive functioning are associated consistently with functional outcome over the lifespan (Heaton and Drexler, 1987). Some studies have indicated that responsiveness to social skills training procedures was predicted by pre-treatment verbal memory, verbal fluency and inferential reasoning ability (Silverstein *et al.*, 1998), the same measures that have been shown to be impaired in neuroleptic-naive patients with schizophrenia (Riley *et al.*, 1999).

Patients with schizotypal personality disorder have social and emotional deficits resembling the negative symptoms of schizophrenia, but rarely have extended institutional stays or profound functional impairments resembling those seen in schizophrenia. Patients with schizotypal personality disorder repeatedly have been shown to have cognitive impairments that are much less severe than those seen in schizophrenia despite the presence of significant negative or deficit symptoms (Voglmaier *et al.*, 1997; Bergman *et al.*, 1998). Thus, the differences in overall functional outcome between patients with schizotypal personality disorder and schizophrenia are related more to differences in cognitive functioning than to similarities in negative symptoms. Neuropsychological measures administered before or early in the course of treatment generally accounted for between 15 and 32% of the variance in long-term outcome measures, acquired months or even years later. Among the most predictive measures were those assessing motor speed, executive functions and attention (Bilder and Bates, 1994). It is also important to recognize that symptoms observed during an acute psychotic episode most often show no significant relationship to long-term outcome.

The empirical literature suggests that, in fact, typical neuroleptic medication has essentially no impact on the majority of important cognitive functions in schizophrenia (Medalia *et al.*, 1988; Spohn and Strauss, 1989; Sharma, 1999). Conventional antipsychotic agents have little effect on neurocognitive function. Short-term treatment improves attention along with positive symptoms, but performance on motor tasks declines (Medalia *et al.*, 1988; Spohn and Strauss, 1989; Cassens *et al.*, 1990; King, 1990; Earle-Boyer *et al.*, 1991; see Chapter 13). Cognitive impairment is not caused by treatment with typical neuroleptic medication. Since deficits in attention are found commonly in patients in remission (Asarnow *et al.*, 1988; Harvey *et al.*, 1990) and in individuals vulnerable to schizophrenia (Asarnow *et al.*, 1978; Harvey *et al.*, 1981), they do not predict outcome of the illness. Typical neuroleptics may enhance practice effects on task that might be performed in an 'automatic' manner (Granholm *et al.*, 1996).

The generalizability of these findings directly to clinical rehabilitation settings may be limited by the relatively simple nature of the task requirements, which certainly do not parallel those of more complex occupational or social skills. Cognitive impairment is, however, worsened by anticholinergic medication that frequently is administered to treat the side effects resulting from treatment with typical neuroleptic medication. Anticholinergics have been shown to be associated with poorer performance on tests of memory (Strauss *et al.*, 1990).

Given that typical neuroleptics have very little effect on cognitive functioning, it should come as no surprise that they do not improve overall outcome in schizophrenia. According to Hegarty *et al.* (1994), approximately one-third of all patients with schizophrenia had a good outcome before the 1940s, essentially the same as today. Thus, despite the biological treatment revolution in the 1950s, the outcome of schizophrenia before the wide availability of atypical antipsychotic medication was no better than in 1898—the time when Kraepelin coined the term dementia praecox. Thus, patients with minimal cognitive impairments will, on average, have a better outcome than patients with moderate or more severe cognitive impairment, regardless of how severe their positive symptoms would be without treatment with typical neuroleptic medication.

Cognitive enhancement as a treatment strategy

Cognitive impairment is of immense importance in dementing conditions. Thus, most treatment approaches for Alzheimer's disease and related conditions have focused on cognitive enhancement. Since schizophrenia is an illness where the cognitive impairments have major functional implications, cognitive enhancement may be the preferred treatment modality which, unlike the treatment of psychotic symptoms, is highly likely to improve functional outcome.

Typical neuroleptics and cognition

None of the widely used typical antipsychotic drugs has shown superior cognitive efficacy compared with others, although there is some agreement that treatment regimens involving high anticholinergic load (either through the intrinsic actions of the compound or through the addition of adjuvant treatments for extrapyramidal symptoms) lead to impairments in learning/memory function (Strauss *et al.* 1990).

Why cognitive enhancement with atypical antipsychotics?

After 40 years of treatment that centred on drugs which mainly blocked dopamine D_2 receptors, there is hope for people with schizophrenia with the advent of the newer antipsychotics which are referred to as 'atypical' (Sharma, 1996). The (re) introduction of clozapine created the first cracks in the traditional 'dopamine hypothesis' of schizophrenia. In general, the atypical antipsychotics have significantly lower affinity for D_2 receptors with increased affinity for a broad array of other receptors (D_1, D_4, 5-HT_2, adrenergic and anticholinergic). They have a lower liability to produce extrapyramidal side effects (EPS) and tardive dyskinesia, and some of them have shown efficacy in patients who have failed to respond to typical antipsychotics. Risperidone, olanzapine, quetiapine and amisulpride currently are considered to be atypical antipsychotics.

However, given the failures of typical antipsychotics to produce any cognitive enhancement, why should the second generation antipsychotic drugs that were developed primarily to treat psychotic symptoms be expected to enhance cognition? The neurotransmitter systems affected by antipsychotic medications include (but are not limited to) cholinergic, adrenergic, serotonergic, dopaminergic and glutamatergic types. Given that the atypical antipsychotic drugs vary in their pharmacological profiles, this could result in selective effects of a specific antipsychotic drug on cognition. Alteration of adrenergic, serotonergic or histaminergic functioning may increase attentional or memory performance. Studies in primates have suggested that manipulations of these neurotransmitters improve cognitive functioning in various ways (Berridge *et al.*, 1993). In addition, the decreased need to co-prescribe anticholinergic drugs to counter neurological side effects is beneficial. It is possible that these drugs may target more specifically regions of the brain responsible for psychosis while sparing those which are responsible for EPS. This fact may also be responsible for their cognitive enhancement properties. Indeed, it has been shown recently that patients who have been switched from typical neuroleptics to risperidone show improvement of blood flow to the frontal and parietal lobes while carrying out a cognitive task involving working memory (Honey *et al.*, 1999). Drugs that increase muscarinic cholinergic, 5-HT$_{2A/2C}$ serotonergic, and α-2A adrenergic activity are also likely to improve cognitive function. It may well be the balance between multiple systems, rather than the function of one system, that is most crucial to optimal cognitive function. Thus, it is unlikely that the cognitive effects of a drug are predictable exclusively from receptor-binding studies at present, and must be determined empirically *in vivo*. Animal studies of cognitive function suggest that the effect of drugs will be altered if there are central nervous system impairments in particular neurotransmitter systems. For example, effects of α-adrenergic agonists depend on an intact prefrontal cortex. Thus, results of studies conducted with healthy human subjects may not be applicable to patients with brain diseases, such as schizophrenia.

A number of preliminary studies examining the cognitive effects of atypical neuroleptics have been performed, with a variety of encouraging findings. In these studies, patients with schizophrenia have been studied in a cognitive enhancement design. Although these studies have several methodological limitations (for a comprehensive discussion of these issues, see Harvey and Keefe, 1999; Keefe *et al.*, 1999), there is much to be learned from them. Several previously published articles have suggested that atypical neuroleptics are superior to typical drugs for cognitive enhancement. This is reviewed in detail in Sharma (1999) and Keefe *et al.* (1999). There are published reports with both clozapine and risperidone showing enhancement of cognitive function. It is important to note that the cognitive functions which improve with atypical antipsychotics are those which have been associated more strongly with outcome (e.g. verbal memory, working memory and executive function) (Green, 1996; Green *et al.*, 1997). The effects of cognitive enhancement in studies can be seen within ~6 weeks of starting treatment with an atypical antipsychotic. One might speculate that a drug that enhances cognitive functioning will improve the capacity of patients to respond to psychosocial rehabilitation. In other words, the newer drugs may help patients to recover lost skills or learn new ones in a rehabilitation setting. Thus, cognitive enhancement could help the ability to benefit from psychosocial treatment, especially interventions based on learning such as social skills training.

As reviewed by Keefe *et al.* (1999), 14 studies have been published in the literature on cognitive enhancement with novel antipsychotic medications (Goldberg *et al.*, 1993; Hagger *et al.*, 1993; Lee *et al.*, 1994; Zahn *et al.*, 1994; Gallhofer *et al.*, 1996; Hoff *et al.*, 1996; Stip and Luisier, 1996; Green *et al.*, 1997; McGurk *et al.*, 1997; Myer-Lindenberg *et al.*, 1997; Rossi *et al.*, 1997, Kern *et al.*, 1998; Serper and Chou, 1997; Kee *et al.*, 1998), and these studies utilized a wide range of test measures. Some studies examined only a few neurocognitive measures, while others conducted a more comprehensive neuropsychological assessment. Three of the four randomized, double-blind studies reported significant neurocognitive improvement on at least one measure following treatment with atypical antipsychotic medication compared with conventional antipsychotics. Seven of the nine open-label studies demonstrated improvement following treatment with atypical antipsychotics. Overall, 11 of 13 studies demonstrated improvement in some aspects of cognitive functioning compared with treatment with conventional antipsychotic medication. These studies have examined cognitive improvement following treatment with risperidone, clozapine, aripipazole and ziprasidone. Furthermore, several different medications are being evaluated in studies that are not yet published, including cognitive enhancing effects of olanzapine and quetiapine.

However, some important questions remain: do specific agents have specific cognitive profiles? To what extent can cognitive functions be normalized? Most of the studies with risperidone and clozapine have sampled treatment with refractory or partially refractory patients. While there are significant improvements compared with baseline scores, these patients still show deficits relative to normal levels. Previous studies also failed to include matched controls to address the role of repeated practice when considering the magnitude of performance improvement in patients. Furthermore, first episode patients may have less severe neurocognitive impairment and greater plasticity than chronic patients. Thus, they may be more likely to show maximum benefit from treatment with novel drugs. In addition, only short-term studies have been done to date. Determining the effects of the new treatments on cognitive function over the longer term, which may be reflected in improved social/vocational function, is of utmost importance. Another critical issue is that of functional change. If cognitive deficits are the major predictor of functional impairment, does the change in cognition associated with treatment with these newer medications have a large enough benefit to improve functional status? This issue is addressed below.

It is unclear whether there are direct effects of these compounds on cognition, or whether the improvement is mediated by a reduction in EPS and secondary negative symptoms. These novel agents have complex and sometimes paradoxical effects on multiple neurotransmitter systems which may be relevant to cognition. For example, clozapine and olanzapine have high affinity for muscarinic receptor subtypes, and thus should have anticholinergic effects which would compromise attention and memory. However, recent studies suggest that these drugs may act as agonists, rather than as antagonists at muscarinic (m4) receptors (Arnt and Skarsfeldt, 1998). Animal models have offered some clues as to which agents may selectively affect cognition. Clozapine has been shown to reverse deficits in sensory gating produced by the noncompetitive NMDA antagonist PCP in serveral, but not all studies (Arnt and

Skarsfeldt, 1998). This has been replicated in human studies of schizophrenia (Kumari *et al.* 1999).

Treatment with clozapine has been reported in several different studies to improve performance of chronic schizophrenic patients on verbal fluency tests (Goldberg *et al.*, 1993; Hagger *et al.*, 1993; Lee *et al.*, 1994; McGurk *et al.*, 1997). In addition, measures of psychomotor speed and executive functioning have also shown improvements. These improvements appear to persist over time and improve with more extended treatment with clozapine. At the same time, in short-term studies, clozapine appears to be associated with a slight worsening of performance on tests of visual memory. In studies of maze learning, clozapine was found to significantly improve speed of performance compared with conventional antipsychotic medications. However clozapine is licensed for treatment-refractory patients in North America and some parts of Europe.

Treatment with risperidone has been reported to enhance executive functioning as measured by maze learning in the same study where clozapine enhanced performance (Gallhofer *et al.*, 1996). In addition to increasing speed, risperidone was reported to increase the efficiency of performance in the maze tests. In two reports describing different cognitive measures collected on the same sample of patients (Green *et al.*, 1997; Kern *et al.*, 1998), evidence of cognitive enhancement with treatment with risperidone was found. In this study, 60 chronic schizophrenic patients with a history of failure to respond to treatment with conventional antipsychotic medications were assigned to double-blind parallel treatment with conventional antipsychotics or with risperidone. Patients treated with risperidone manifested improvement in performance on the digit span distraction test described above and also on the trail making test. These tests measure important aspects of cognitive functioning, and the improvement effect was quite large. In a subsample of this cohort, Kee *et al.* (1998) showed superior effects of risperidone compared with haloperidol on affect recognition which has implications for social cognition with this compund. A study by Stip and Lussier (1996) found that risperidone treatment normalized reaction time performance, as well as improving measures of both sustained and selective attention. Finally, a study by Rossi and colleagues (1997) found that treatment with risperidone enhanced performance on a variety of different cognitive tests, including measures of motor speed and executive functioning (i.e. the Wisconsin Card Sorting Test; WCST). Interestingly, these investigators found that the extent of improvement in WCST performance was correlated with improvement in negative symptoms, suggesting that these two domains of functioning may be linked in some important way.

In a study using the digit span distraction test and the Continuous Performance Test (CPT), Serper and Chou (1997) found that treatment with the novel antipsychotic medications ziprasidone and aripipazole were associated with improvement in speed of response and in memory span. The number of subjects who were treated with each of those two medications was very small ($n = 4$), suggesting that these results should be considered preliminary.

These data provide exciting new information regarding the possibility of treatment of cognitive impairment with novel antipsychotic medications. Since few of these studies were comprehensive and none made systematic comparisons of the effects of different novel medications, it is not yet possible to comment on the differential effectiveness of these medications in the treatment of cognitive impairment in schizophrenia. This is clearly a goal for later research. These studies are likely to be funded directly by pharmaceutical companies, so their results will deserve careful scrutiny for methodological standards and for appropriate interpretation of the results.

Special treatment strategies and neuroprotection in patients with first-episode psychosis

Longitudinal studies suggest that the most devastating clinical progression in patients with schizophrenia occurs within the first 5 years from the time of onset (McGlashan, 1988). Episodes of psychosis in the early stages of illness may reflect an active pathophysiological process that can produce enduring cognitive and functional impairment in patients and reduce their capacity to respond to treatment (Lieberman *et al.*, 1990; Loebel *et al.*, 1992). Wyatt (1991) has suggested that early intervention with neuroleptic medication may alter outcome in schizophrenia. This is of considerable importance as it is possible that some types of neurodegenerative process may be interrupted by prompt intervention with neuroleptics. It is possible that early intervention would reduce cognitive impairment as well as improve outcome. It is also possible that relapse may be accompanied by frank neurotoxicity. This model of the 'neurodegenerative' effects of psychosis in patients with schizophrenia suggests that the most debilitating effects of psychosis can best be limited by early, effective intervention (Wyatt, 1995).

It is generally accepted that 70–80% of first-episode patients satisfy objective criteria for 'response' following initial treatment (Lieberman, 1996). However these figures are based primarily on the favourable response of psychotic symptoms, and fail to capture the extent to which patients—even the 'good responders'—continue to suffer and remain functionally impaired. In this context, it needs to be appreciated that typical antipsychotics have no effective cognitive-enhancing effects and there is burgeoning evidence about the cognitive effects of newer antipsychotic treatments, with several multi-centre studies of newer drugs in first-episode psychosis currently underway.

Furthermore, since atypical neuroleptics appear to improve positive symptoms, negative symptoms and cognitive deficits even in short-term studies, it is possible that this 'neurodegenerative' process may be reversed by atypical neuroleptics (Wyatt, 1995). Thus, intervention with atypical neuroleptics in the early stages of schizophrenia may promote cognitive and functional abilities later on in the illness. In addition, it is plausible that early intervention could have the potential to reverse some of the disability associated with the illness before it has secondary effects on the patient.

Relationship of cognitive enhancement to outcome

As discussed previously, the biological treatment revolution initiated with the advent of chlorpromazine for schizophrenia 50 years ago, but treatment has had a limited impact on the overall outcome of the illness. Most studies linking neurocognitive function to longer term outcome have been conducted in patients treated with conventional agents. In the only study carried out with atypical antipsychotics that examined the relationship between cognition and social–vocational outcome in patients on clozapine, it was found that scores on executive function, attention and memory were related to employment measures in neuroleptic-resistant patients treated with clozapine for 12 months (Meltzer *et al.*, 1996). Another study found that improvement in memory function was associated with perceived quality of life at 1 year in patients treated with clozapine, but not in patients treated with haloperidol (Buchanan *et al.*, 1994). If new generation agents produce more improvement in cognition than conventional agents and cognition does in fact relate to social–vocational function, we may expect better functional outcomes for patients treated with the novel agents.

Future directions

To reiterate our earlier statements, treatment with these novel agents from the beginning of the illness should provide the maximum opportunity to demonstrate their potential benefits in preventing the long-term multidimensional morbidity which tragically affects the lives of patients and their families and results in a great economic burden to society. Historically, the treatment of schizophrenia concentrated on positive symptom decrement. In the 1980s the emphasis shifted towards a reduction in negative symptoms by pharmacological and non-pharmacological means, but by the 1990s cognitive dysfunction, a core deficit in schizo-phrenia, had been identified as an important outcome measure in the treatment of schizophrenia. A paradigm shift is now required in the conceptualization of treatment success away from symptom decrement and towards treatments which improve cognitive function in schizophrenia.

It should be clear from our arguments in this chapter that the treatment of schizophrenia is progressing gradually from rational research to clinical reality with our understanding of neurocognitive function in relation to the treatment of schizophrenia. However, major studies in first-episode psychosis are still to present their results on cognitive function, and these are eagerly awaited. The recognition of cognitive function as the holy grail of treatment success in schizophrenia has caused a paradigm shift in how we conceptualize treatment options for patients with the illness. This, coupled with the recognition that early treatment of psychosis or impending psychosis may change the trajectory of the illness, offers hope to patients with schizophrenia. For the first time, we are beginning to see rational psychopharmacology

The advent of newer brain imaging technologies allows us to use the 'brain as a dependent variable' (Bilder, 1997). Functional magnetic resonance imaging has already allowed us to map haemodynamic responses to cognitive probes and to examine the effects of newer antipsychotic compounds such as risperidone (Honey *et al.*, 1999). This technology is now enabling us to visualize the brain in action in almost real time and seek evidence of the effects of the newer drugs on brain function. We are thus moving from observing behavioural effects to direct observation of drug effects on the real time operation of complex neural systems. This allows increased understanding of effects at the level of neural systems, which carries the promise of bringing psychopharmacology beyond 'receptorology'. It is now possible to carry out a battery of functional system assessments in the scanner, which can then be used in selecting the compounds most likely to enhance the normalization of those systems, with follow-up scanning used to monitor and modulate ongoing treatment. If we can develop sufficiently sensitive and specific assessment methods, knowledge of cognitive deficits ultimately could help to guide specific psychopharmacological treatment decisions involving dosage and type of treatment instead of the hit and miss approach of yester years.

Conclusion

The recent focus on the central role that cognitive impairments play in the day to day function of patients with schizophrenia underscores the importance of finding better treatments for these symptoms. Since cognitive impairment is correlated with the majority of the disability seen in chronic schizophrenia, treatment of this condition with atypical antipsychotics appears to have the potential to reduce this disability. The next few years are likely to bring forth the results of several large well-designed studies that will go beyond the current group of preliminary studies of cognitive efficacy with atypical antipsychotics.

This will allow informed clinical decision making regarding the potential for cognitive enhancement with the new antipsychotic medications. For the first time, we may be able really to make an impact on the long-term outcome of the illness and change the word 'schizophrenia' from a life sentence to a diagnosis. Newer drugs that are being developed may be screened for cognitive enhancement potential.

References

Albus, M., Hubmann, W., Mohr, F., Scherer J., Sobizack N., Franz U., Hecht S., Borrmann M. and Wahlheim, C. (1997) Are there gender differences in neuropsychological performance in patients with first-episode schizophrenia. *Schizophrenia Research*, **28**, 39–50.

Amador, X.F., Strauss, D.H., Yale, S.A. and Gorman, J. (1991) Awareness of illness in schizophrenia. *Schizophrenia Bulletin*, **17**, 113–132.

Andrews, G., Hall, W., Goldstein, G., Lapsley, H., Bartels, R., Silove, D. (1985) The economic costs of schizophrenia. Implications for public policy. *Arch Gen Psychiatry*, **42**, 537–543.

Andrews, G. (1991) The cost of schizophrenia revisited. *Schizophrenia Bulletin*, **17**, 389-94.

Arnt, J., and Skarsfeldt, T. (1998) Do novel antipsychotics have similar pharmacological characteristics? A review of the evidence. *Neuropsychopharmacology*, **18**, 63-101.

Asarnow, R.F. and MacCrimmon, D.J. (1978) Residual performance deficit in clinically remitted schizophrenics: a marker of schizophrenia? *Journal of Abnormal Psychology*, **87**, 597–608.

Asarnow, R.F., Marder, S.R., Mintz, J., Van Putten, T., Zimmerman, K.E. (1988) Differential effect of low and conventional doses of fluphenazine on schizophrenic outpatients with good or poor information processing abilities. *Archives in General Psychiatry*, **45**, 822-6.

Bergman, A., Harvey, P.D., Mitroupolou, V., Lees-Roitman, S. and Siever, L.J. (1998) Learning and memory in patients with schizotypal personality disorder. *Schizophrenia Bulletin*, **24**, 635–641.

Berridge, C.W., Arnsten, A.F., and Foote, S.L. (1993) Noradrenergic modulation of cognitive function: clinical implications of anatomical, electrophysiological and behavioural studies in animal models. *Psychological Medicine*, **23**, 557-64.

Bilder, R.M. (1997) Neurocognitive impairment in schizophrenia and how it affects treatment options. *Canadian Journal of Psychiatry*, **42**, 255–264.

Bilder, R.M. and Bates, J. (1994) Neuropsychological prediction of neuroleptic treatment response. In: Gaebel, W. and Awad, A.G. (eds), *Prediction of Neuroleptic Treatment Outcome in Schizophrenia—Concepts and Methods*. Springer-Verlag, New York, pp. 99–110.

Bilder, R.M., Lipschutz-Broch, L., Reiter, G., Geisler, S., Mayerhoff, D., Lieberman, J.A. (1991) Neuropsychological deficits in the early course of first episode schizophrenia. *Schizophr Res.* **5**, 198–199.

Bilder, R.M., Lipschutz, L.B, Reiter, G., Geisler, S.H., Mayerhoff, D.I. and Lieberman, J.A. (1992a) Intellectual deficits in first-episode schizophrenia: evidence for progressive deterioration. *Schizophrenia Bulletin*, **18**, 437–448.

Bilder, R.M., and Bates, J. (1994) Neuropsychological prediction of neuroleptic treatment response. In: W. Gaebel, A.G. Awad (eds) *Prediction of neuroleptic treatment outcome in schizophrenia – concepts and methods*. Springer-Verlag, New York, pp.99-110.

Bilder, R.M., Bogerts, B., Ashtari, M., Wu, H., Alvir, J.M., Jody, D., Reiter, G., Bell, L. and Lieberman, J.A. (1995) Anterior hippocampal volume reductions predict 'frontal lobe' dysfunction in first episode schizophrenia. *Schizophrenia Research*, **17**, 47–58.

Binder, J., Albus, M., Hubmann, W., Scherer, J., Sobizack, N., Franz, U., Mohr, F., Hecht, S. (1998) Neuropsychological impairment and psychopathology in first-episode schizophrenic patients related to the early course of illness. *Eur Arch Psychiatry Clin Neurosci*, **248**, 70–77.

Breier, A., Schreiber, J.L., Dyer, J. and Pickar, D. (1991) National Institute of Mental Health longitudinal study of chronic schizophrenia. Prognosis and predictors of outcome. *Archives in General Psychiatry*, **48**, 239-46.

Buchanan, R.W., Holstein, C. and Brier, A. (1994) The comparative efficacy and long-term effect of clozapine treatment on neuropsychological test performance. *Biological Psychiatry*, **36**, 717–725.

Cassens, G., Inglis, A.K., Applebaum, P.S. and Gutheil, T.G. (1990) Neuroleptics: effects on neuropsychological function in chronic schizophrenic patients. *Schizophrenia Bulletin*, **16**, 477–499.

Censits, D.M., Ragland, J.D., Gur, R.C. and Gur, R.E. (1997) Neuropsychological evidence supporting a neurodevelopmental model of schizophrenia: a longitudinal study. *Schizophrenia Research*, **24**, 289–298.

Crow, T.J., Done, D.J. and Sacker, A. (1995) Childhood precursors of psychosis as clues to its evolutionary origins. *European Archives in Psychiatry and Clinical Neuroscience*, **245**, 61–9.

Davidson, M. and McGlashan, T.H. (1997) The varied outcomes of schizophrenia. *Canadian Journal of Psychiatry*, **42**, 34-43.

Earle-Boyer, E.A., Serper, M.R., Davidson, M. and Harvey, P.D. (1991) Auditory and visual continuous performance tests in medicated and unmedicated schizophrenic patients: clinical and motoric correlates. *Psychiatry Research*, **37**, 47–56.

Gallhofer, B., Bauer, U., Lis, S., Krieger, S. and Gruppe, H. (1996) Cognitive dysfunction in schizophrenia: comparison of treatment with atypical antipsychotic agents and conventional neuroleptic drugs. *European Neuropsychopharmacology*, **6** (Suppl. 2), 13–20. .

Goldberg, T.E., Greenberg, R.D., Griffin, S.J., Gold, J.M., Kleinman, J.E., Pickar, D., Schulz, S.C. and Weinberger, D.R. (1993) The effect of clozapine on cognition and psychiatric symptoms in patients with schizophrenia. *British Journal of Psychiatry*, **162**, 43–48.

Granholm, E., Asarnow, R.F. and Marder, S.R. (1996) Dual task performance operating characteristics, resource limitations, and automatic processing in schizophrenia. *Neuropsychology*, **10**, 3–11.

Green, M.F. (1996) What are the functional consequences of neurocognitive deficits in schizophrenia? *American Journal of Psychiatry*, **153,** 321-30.

Green, M.F., Marshall, B.D., Wirshing, W.C., Ames, D., Marder, S.R., McGurk, S., Kern, R.S. and Mintz, J. (1997) Does risperidone improve verbal working memory in treatment-resistant schizophrenia? *American Journal of Psychiatry*, **154**, 799–804.

Gunderson, J.G. and Mosher, L.R. (1975) The cost of schizophrenia. *American Journal of Psychiatry*, **132**, 901-6.

Hagger, C., Buckley, P., Kenny, J.T., Friedman, L., Ubogy, D. and Meltzer, H.Y. (1993) Improvement in cognitive functions and psychiatric symptoms in treatment-refractory schizophrenic patients receiving clozapine. *Biological Psychiatry*, **34**, 702–712.

Hall, W., Andrews, G., and Goldstein, G. (1985) The costs of schizophrenia. *Australian and New Zealand Journal of Psychiatry*, **19**, 3-5.

Hall, W., Goldstein, G., Andrews, G., Lapsley, H., Bartels, R., Silove, D. (1985) Estimating the economic costs of schizophrenia. *Schizophr Bull*, **11**, 598–610.

Harvey, P.D. (1983) Speech competence in manic and schizophrenic psychoses: The association between clinically rated thought disorder and cohesion and reference performance. *J Abnorm Psychology*, **92**, 368–377.

Harvey, P.D. and Keefe, R.S.E. (1999) Standards for the assessment of cognitive change in schizophrenia treatment studies. *American Journal of Psychiatry* (in press).

Harvey, P.D., Docherty, N.M., Serper, M.R. and Rasmussen, M. (1990) Cognitive deficits and thought disorder: II. An eight-month follow up study. *Schizophrenia Bulletin*, **16**, 147–156.

Harvey, P.D., Jacobsen, H., Mancini, D., Parrella, M., White, L., Haroutunian, V., Davis, K.L. (2000) Clinical, cognitive and functional characteristics of long-stay patients with schizophrenia: a comparison of VA and state hospital patients. *Schizophr Res*, **43**, 3–9.

Harvey, P.D., Lombardi, J., Leibman, M., White, L., Parrella, M., Powchik, P. and Davidson, M. (1996) Cognitive impairment and negative symptoms in geriatric chronic schizophrenic patients: a follow-up study. *Schizophrenia Research*, **22**, 223–231.

Harvey, P.D., Sukhodolsky, D., Parrella, M., White, L., and Davidson, M. (1997) The association between adaptive and cognitive deficits in geriatric chronic schizophrenic patients. *Schizophrenic Research*, **27**, 211-18.

Harvey, P.D., Winters, K, Weintraub, S. and Neale, J.M. (1981) Distractibilty in children vulnerable to psychopathology. *Journal of Abnormal Psychology*, **90**, 298-304.

Harvey, P.D., and Neale, J.M. (1983) The specifity of thought disorder to schizophrenia: research methods in their historical perspective. *Progress in Experimental Pers Research*, **12**, 153-80.

Heaton, R.K. and Drexler, M. (1987) Clinical neuropsychological findings in schizophrenia and aging. In: Miller, N.E., and Cohen, G.D. (eds) *Schizophrenia and aging*. Gulford Press, New York, pp. 145-61.

Heaton,R., Paulsen, J.S., McAdams, L.A., Kuck, J., Zisook, S., Braff, D., Harris, M.J. and Jeste, D.V. (1994) Neuropsychological deficits in schizophrenics: relationship to age, chronicity, and dementia. *Archives of General Psychiatry*, **51**, 469–476.

Hegarty, J.D., Baldessarini, R.J. and Tohen, M. (1994) One hundred years of schizophrenia: a meta-analysis of the outcome literature. *American Journal of Psychiatry*, **151**, 1409–1416.

Hoff, A., Riordan, M.A., O'Donnell, D.W., Morris, L. and De Lisi, L.E. (1992) Neuropsychological functioning of first episode schizophreniform patients. *American Journal of Psychiatry*, **149**, 898–903.

Hoff, A.L., Faustman, W.O., Wieneke, M., Espinoza, S., Costa, M., Wolkowitz, O. and Csernansky, J.G. (1996) The effects of clozapine on symptom reduction, neurocognitive function, and clinical management in treatment-refractory state hospital schizophrenic inpatients. *Neuropsychopharmacology*, **15**, 361–369.

Hoff, A.L., Riordan, H., O'Donnell, D.W., and DeLisi, L.E. (1991) Cross-sectional and longitudinal neuropsychological test findings in first episode schizophrenic patients. *Schizophrenic Research*, **5**, 197-8.

Honey, G.D., Bullmore, E.T., Soni, W., Varatheesan, M., Williams, S.C.R. and Sharma, T. (1999) Differences in frontal cortical activation by a working memory task following substitution of risperidone for typical antipsychotic drugs in patients with schizophrenia, *Proceedings of the National Academy of Sciences of the United States of America*, **96**, 13432–13437.

Kee, K.S., Kern, R.S., Marshall, B.D., Jr and Green, M.F. (1998) Risperidone versus haloperidol for perception of emotion in treatment-resistant schizophrenia: preliminary findings. *Schizophrenia Research*, **31**, 159–165.

Keefe, R.S.E., Silva, S., Perkins, D. *et al.* (1999) The effects of atypical antipsychotic drugs on neurocognitive impairment in schizophrenia. *Schizophrenia Bulletin*, **25**, 201–222.

Kern, R.S., Green, M.F., Marshall, B.D., Jr, Wirshing, W.C., Wirshing, D., McGurk, S., Marder, S.R. and Mintz, J. (1998) Risperidone vs. haloperidol on reaction time, manual dexterity, and motor learning in treatment-resistant schizophrenia patients. *Biological Psychiatry*, **44**, 726–732.

King, D.J. (1990) The effect of neuroleptics on cognitive and psychomotor function. *British Journal of Psychiatry*, **157**, 799–811.

Knight, R.A., Roff, J.D, Barrnet, J. and Moss, L. (1979) Concurrent and predictive validity of thought disorder and affectivity: a 22 year followup of acute schizophrenics. *Journal of Abnormal Psychology*, **88**, 1–12.

Kumari, V., Soni, W. and Sharma, T. (1999) Normalization of information processing deficits in schizophrenia with clozapine. *American Journal of Psychiatry*, **156**, 1046–1051

Lee, M.A., Thompson, P.A. and Meltzer, H.Y. (1994) Effects of clozapine on cognitive function in schizophrenia. *Journal of Clinical Psychiatry*, **55** (Suppl. B), 82–87.

Leff, J.P., Thornicroft, G., Coxhead, N. and Trieman, N (1994) The TAPS Project. 22: a five-year follow-up of long stay psychiatric patients discharged to the community. *British Journal of Psychiatry*, **165** (Suppl. 25), 13–17.

Lieberman, J.A. (1999) Is schizophrenia a neurodegenerative disorder? A clinical and neurobiological perspective. *Biology and Psychiatry*, **46**, 729-39.

Lieberman, J.A., Alvir, J.M., Koreen, A., Geisler, S., Chakos, M., Sheitman, B., Woerner, M. (1996) Psychobiologic correlates of treatment response in schizophrenia. *Neuropsychopharmacology*, **14**, 13S–21S.

Loebel, A.D., Lieberman, J.A., Alvir, J.M., Mayerhoff, D.I., Deisler, S.H. and Szymanski, S.R. (1992) Duration of psychosis and outcome in first episode schizophrenia. *American Journal of Psychiatry*, **149**, 1183–1188.

McCreadie, R.G., Connolly, M.A., Williamson, D.J., Athawes, R.W. and Tilak-Singh, D. (1994) The Nithsdale Schizophrenia Surveys. XII. 'Neurodevelopmental' schizophrenia: a search for clinical correlates and putative aetiological factors. *British Journal of Psychiatry*, **165**, 340–346.

McGlashan, T.H. (1988) A selective review of recent North American long-term follow-up studies of schizophrenia. *Schizophrenia Bulletin*, **14**, 515–542.

McGurk, S.R., Green, M.F., Wirshing, W.C., Ames, D., Marshall, B.D., Jr, Marder, A.R. and Mintz, J. (1997) The effects of resperidone vs haloperidol on cognitive functioning in treatment-resistant schizophrenia: the Trail Making Test. *CNS Spectrums*, **2**, 60–64.

Medallia, A., Gold, J. and Merriam A. (1988) The effects of neuroleptics on neuropsychological test results of schizophrenics. *Archives of Clinical Neuropsychology*, **3**, 249–271.

Meltzer, H.Y., Thompson, P.A., Lee, M.A., Ranjan, R. (1996) Neuropsychologic deficits in schizophrenia: relation to social function and effect of antipsychotic drug treatment. *Neuropsychopharmacology*, **14**, 27S–33S.

Myer-Lindenberg, A., Gruppe, H., Bauer, U., Lis, S.,Krieger S. and Galhoffer, B. (1997) Improvement of cognitive function in schizophrenic patients receiving clozapine or zotepine: results from a double-blind study. *Pharmacopsychiatry,* **30**, 35–42.

Palmer, B.W., Heaton, R.K., Paulsen, J.S. *et al.* (1997) Is it possible to be schizophrenic and neuropsychologically normal? *Neuropsychology*, **11**, 437–447.

Perlick, D., Stastny, P., Mattis, S. and Teresi, J. (1992) Contribution of family, cognitive, and clinical dimensions to long-term outcome in schizophrenia. *Schizophrenia Research*, **6**, 257–265.

Riley, E.M., McGovern, D., Mockler, D., Doku, V., O'Cealleigh, S., Fannon, D.G., Tennakoon, L., Santamaria, M., Soni, W., Morris, R.G. and Sharma, T. (1999) Neuro-psychological functioning in first-episode psychosis—evidence of specific deficits. *Schizophrenia Research*, **43(1)**, 47–55.

Rossi, A., Mancini, F., Stratta, P., Mattei, P., Gismondi, R., Pozzi, F. and Casacchia, M. (1997) Risperidone, negative symptoms and cognitive deficit in schizophrenia: an open study. *Acta Psychiatrica Scandinavica*, **95**, 40–43.

Roy, M.A., DeVriendt, X. (1994) Positive and negative symptoms in schizophrenia: a current overview. *Can J Psychiatry*, **39**, 407–414.

Saykin, A.J., Gur, R.C., Gur, R.E., Mozeley, D., Mozeley, L.H., Resnick, S.M. *et al.* (1991)

Neuropsychological function in schizophrenia: selective impairment in memory and learning. *Archives of General Psychiatry*, **48**, 618–623.

Saykin, A.J., Shtasel, D.L., Gur, R.E., Kester, D.B., Mozley, L.H., Stafniack, P. and Gur, R.C. (1994) Neuropsychological deficits in neuroleptic naïve patients with first-episode schizophrenia. *Archives of General Psychiatry*, **51**, 124–131.

Serper, M.R. and Chou, J.C.Y. (1997) Novel neuroleptics improve attentional functioning in schizophrenic patients: ziprasidone and aripiprazole. *CNS Spectrums*, **2**, 56–59.

Sharma, T. (1996) Schizophrenia: recent advances in psychopharmacology. *British Journal of Hospital Medicine*, **55**, 194–198.

Sharma, T. (1999) The cognitive effects of conventional and atypical antipsychotics in schizophrenia. *British Journal of Psychiatry*, **174** (Suppl. 38), 23–30.

Spitzer, M. (1993) The psychopathology, neuropsychology, and neurobiology of associative and working memory in schizophrenia. *European Archives of Psychiatry and Clinical Neuroscience*, **243**, 57–70.

Spohn, H.E. and Strauss, M.E. (1989) Relation of neuroleptic and anticholinergic medication to cognitive functions in schizophrenia. *Journal of Abnormal Psychology*, **98**, 478–486.

Stip, E. and Lussier, I. (1996) The effect of risperidone on cognition in patients with schizophrenia. *Canadian Journal of Psychiatry*, **41** (Suppl. 2), 35–40.

Strauss, M.E., Reynolds, K.S., Jayaram, G. and Tune, L.E. (1990) Effects of anticholinergic medication on memory in schizophrenia. *Schizophrenia Research*, **3**, 127–129.

Sweeney, J.A., Haas, G.L., Keilp, J.G. and Long, M. (1991a) Evaluation of the stability of neuropsychological functioning after acute episodes of schizophrenia: a one year follow-up study. *Psychiatry Research*, **38**, 63–76

Sweeney, J.A., Keilp, J.G., Haas, G.L., Hill, J. and Weiden, P.J. (1991b) Relationships between medication treatments and neuropsychological test performance in schizophrenia. *Psychiatry Research*, **37**, 297–308.

Sweeney, J.A., Haas, G.L. and Shuhua, L. (1992) Neuropsychological and eye movement abnormalities in first-episode and chronic schizophrenia. *Schizophrenia Bulletin*, **18**, 283–293.

Voglmaier, M.M., Seidman, L.J., Salisbury, D. and McCarley, R.W. (1997) Neuropsychological dysfunction in schizotypal personality disorder: a profile analysis. *Biological Psychiatry*, **41**, 530–540.

World Health Organization (1974) *The International Pilot Study of Schizophrenia*. Geneva.

Wyatt, R.J. (1991) Neuroleptics and the natural course of schizophrenia. *Schizophrenia Bulletin*, **17**, 325–351.

Wyatt, R.J. (1995) Early intervention for schizophrenia: can the course of illness be altered? *Biological Psychiatry*, **38**, 1–3.

Young, D.A, Davila, R. and Scher, H. (1993) Unawareness of illness and neuropsychological performance in schizophrenia. *Schizophrenia Research*, **10**, 117–124.

Zahn, T.P., Pickar, D., and Haier, R.J. (1994) Effects of clozapine, flufenazine, and placebo on reaction time measures of attention and sensory dominance in schizophrenia. *Schizophrenia Research*, **13**, 133–144.

16 Specific cognitive enhancers

Joseph I. Friedman

Introduction

Although typical neuroleptics are effective in the management of positive symptoms associated with schizophrenia, they do not address the cognitive dysfunction (Cleghorn *et al.*, 1990; Seidman *et al.*, 1993; Verdoux *et al.*, 1995). Most patients experience cognitive deficits despite having achieved remission of positive symptoms (Nuechterlein and Dawson, 1984; Bilder *et al.*, 1992), Therefore, cognitive symptoms have emerged as an independent feature of schizophrenia that needs to be targeted for remediation independently of positive symptoms.

There is a great deal of evidence implicating the prefrontal cortex (PFC) in cognitive functions relevant to schizophrenia (Goldman-Rakic, 1987). The PFC has rich cate-cholaminergic innervation (Lewis, 1992) so that dysfunction of this brain region probably could involve disruption of normal dopaminergic and noradrenergic functioning. Therefore, pharmacological remediation of cognitive symptoms through manipulations of these neuro-transmitter systems merits investigation. In addition, evidence implicating the involvement of acetylcholine and glutamate in cognitive processes relevant to schizophrenia provides potential for remediation strategies by manipulations of these neurotransmitters.

This review will be limited to the dopamine (DA), norepinephrine (NE), acetylcholine (ACh) and glutamate (Glu) neurotransmitter systems for a few reasons. First, animal models demonstrate that enhancement of these neurotransmitter systems improves cognitive function, especially those relevant to schizophrenia. Second, there is direct evidence from human studies that dysfunction of these neurotransmitter systems correlates with the cognitive dysfunction in schizophrenia. Lastly, drugs targeting these neurotransmitter systems are available for clinical trials in schizophrenic patients and have already demonstrated cognitive-enhancing potential in human subjects.

Given the evidence supporting risperidone's ability to improve the performance of schizophrenic patients on tasks of verbal working memory (Green *et al.*, 1997) and executive function (McGurk *et al.*, 1997), there is a growing interest in examining the potential of atypical neuroleptics as drugs which can remediate the cognitive dysfunction of schizophrenia. The proposed mechanism of this beneficial effect on cognition is antagonism of serotonin 5-HT$_{2A}$ receptors, which in turn activates dopaminergic neurons which project to the PFC, thereby increasing DA neurotransmission in the PFC. However, pharmaco-logical studies of 5-HT$_2$ receptor antagonists administered alone have demonstrated that these drugs either impair or have no effect on the performance of animals and humans on tests of learning, memory or attention (Danjou *et al.*, 1992; Harvey, 1996; Routsalainen *et al.*, 1997; Vitiello *et al.*, 1997; Welsh *et al.*, 1998). Therefore, references to the effects of atypical neuroleptics on cognition in relation to 5-HT$_2$ receptors will be reviewed in the section on dopamine given that these effects are mediated through cortical dopaminergic neurotransmission.

Based on the data that will be presented, the following recommendations are offered for manipulating the DA, NE, ACh and Glu neurotransmitter systems with the goal of enhancing the therapeutics of schizophrenia by remediating some of the cognitive deficits. These represent testable hypotheses only and require controlled clinical trials to test the therapeutic legitimacy of these approaches.

(i)   Drugs which increase dopamine in the PFC, within a limited concentration range, such as atypical neuroleptics, may improve prefrontal cognitive deficits, such as working memory and executive functions, in schizophrenic patients (Friedman *et al.*, 1999).

(ii) Drugs which activate D$_1$ receptors in the PFC, within a limited concentration range, may improve prefrontal cognitive deficits, such as working memory and executive functions, in schizophrenic patients (Friedman *et al.*, 1999).

(iii) Drugs which activate postsynaptic α-2 adrenergic receptors in the PFC may improve serial learning, working memory and attention in schizophrenic patients (Friedman *et al.*, 1999).

(iv) Drugs which increase cortical cholinergic activity, such as acetylcholinesterase (AChE) inhibitors and M1/M4 muscarinic agonists, may improve memory, language use and constructional praxis in schizophrenic patients (Friedman *et al.*, 1999).

(v)   Drugs which enhance the activity of α-amino-3-hydroxy-5-methyl-4-isoxazole proprionic acid (AMPA)-type glutamate receptors may enhance verbal and visual learning in schizophrenic patients.

Dopamine

Role of dopamine in cognition

The PFC plays a critical role in the organization of higher order behavior which utilizes working memory. The cellular basis of working memory involves a group of neurons found in the PFC whose firing creates an internal representation of a visual target. These cells are characterized by increased firing when the animals must retain the location of the target during a delay period between target presentation and time of response. Different neurons encode different target locations. When these neurons fail to maintain their activity during the delay period, performance on the task worsens (Williams and Goldman-Rakic, 1995).

Measurement of DA concentration in the PFC of monkeys before and during performance of a delayed response task (a task which measures working memory) shows a significant increase in the DA levels while the animals are engaged in the test (Watanabe *et al.*, 1997). Experimental manipulations of DA in the PFC significantly alter working memory performance. When dopaminergic neurons projecting to the PFC from the ventral tegmental area in the rat are destroyed by injection of 6-hydroxydopamine (6-OHDA), DA concentration in the PFC falls to levels significantly below baseline, and performance on the delayed response task becomes severely impaired (Simon *et al.*, 1980). The same impairment in delayed alternation tasks is observed when the 6-OHDA injection is applied directly to the PFC.

Role of the dopamine D_1 receptor in cognition

Dopamine's actions at D_1 receptors in the PFC are of paramount importance in mediating working memory processes. This is highlighted by the administration of selective dopaminergic D_1 receptor antagonists, such as SCH2330, which worsens performance on the delayed response paradigm (Didriksen, 1995). In contrast, neither D_2 selective antagonists such as sulpiride, nor the D_2/D_3 antagonist raclopride impair working memory functions, suggesting that the observed deficits are specific to D_1 receptor blockade (Sawaguchi and Goldman-Rakic, 1991, 1994).

This is consistent with anatomical data indicating that the D_1 receptor is the most abundant dopaminergic receptor in the mammalian PFC (Cortes *et al.*, 1989; Goldman-Rakic *et al.*, 1990) and, therefore, is most likely to be involved in the cognitive processes mediated by DA in the PFC.

Since the organization of the cortical DA system in both the human and primate PFC is comparatively similar (Goldman-Rakic *et al.*, 1992), information generated from pharmacological studies in monkeys can be extrapolated validly to humans. DA depletion in the monkey PFC, induced by 6-OHDA injection, produces a performance deficit in the delayed alternation task which can be reversed to pre-depletion performance by intraperitoneal administration of either L-DOPA or apomorphine (Brozoski *et al.*, 1979). Furthermore, more precise iontophoretic application of DA to the PFC of animals performing a delayed response task induces an increase in neuronal firing during the delay period (Sawaguchi *et al.*, 1988) which constitutes the basis for the previously described task improvements observed after L-DOPA and apomorphine administration.

It should be clarified that the facilitative effects of DA in the PFC occur only within a certain limited concentration range beyond which it can become excessive for optimal working memory function, and below which deficits are also encountered. An increase in extracellular DA concentration in the PFC can be detrimental for working memory if it is above basal levels. Such an increase, equivalent to the one seen under mild stress (Thierry *et al.*, 1976), can be achieved experimentally via administration of the anxiogenic β-carboline FG7142 (Tam and Roth, 1985) producing performance deficits in working memory tasks in both rats and monkeys. This impairment is correlated positively with DA turnover (i.e. more DA induces more impairment) and can be reversed by the D_1 selective antagonist SCH23390, the D_1/D_2 antagonist haloperidol or the atypical neuroleptic clozapine (Murphy *et al.*, 1996). An equivalent result can be seen with administration of the D_1 selective agonists A77636 and SKF81297. At low doses, there is improved performance in working memory tasks, but, when the dose is increased, the result can be impairment (Cai and Arnsten, 1997).

Implications for schizophrenia

Pharmacological studies with phencyclidine (PCP) demonstrate the relevance of these findings to schizophrenia because the PCP-induced glutamatergic dysfunction is believed to best mimic the symptoms of schizophrenia (Luby *et al.*, 1959; Davies and Beach, 1960; Rosenbaum *et al.*, 1959). Chronic administration of PCP, a non-competitive *N*-methyl-D-aspartate (NMDA) receptor antagonist, induces a decrease in basal and stress-related DA levels in the PFC of mammals that continues after cessation of PCP administration. Consistent with the dopaminergic model of frontal cognitive dysfunction, this decrease translates as behavioral deficits in working memory tasks in the monkey (Jentsch *et al.*, 1997). This impairment can be corrected by administration of the atypical neuroleptic clozapine, which increases extracellular DA in the PFC of monkeys (Youngren *et al.*, 1994).

Poor visuospatial working memory performance in schizophrenic patients has been demonstrated with a human analog of the monkey's delayed response task (Park and Holtzman, 1992). There is evidence that this working memory deficit is already present at the time of the first episode (Hoff *et al.*, 1992) and that this deficit is independent of medication (Carter *et al.*, 1996; Fleming *et al.*, 1997). In addition, verbal working memory, as measured by the Brown–Peterson paradigm or the digit span test, is also defective in schizophrenia (Fleming *et al.*, 1995; Green *et al.*, 1997) and may also be responsive to pharmacological strategies which enhance dopaminergic function.

The revised dopaminergic hypothesis of schizophrenia posits the co-existence of a hyperdopaminergic state in the mesolimbic pathway along with hypodopaminergia in the mesocortical tract. Positive symptoms are induced by elevation of DA in the limbic system, while negative and cognitive symptoms are due to decreased DA prefrontal function (Davis *et al.*, 1991). The degree to which decreased cortical DA is related to the cognitive impairment of schizophrenia (Kahn *et al.*, 1994) is worth investigating because of the potential strategies for improving the cognitive deficits of schizophrenia that this work uncovers.

PFC concentrations of the DA metabolite homovanillic acid (HVA) show a direct correlation with cerebrospinal fluid (CSF) HVA concentrations (Elsworth *et al.*, 1987; Wester *et al.*, 1990). Consequently, changes in mesocortical DA in schizophrenia can be measured via CSF levels of HVA. It is not surprising, therefore, that CSF HVA correlates with performance on neuropsychological measures in schizophrenic patients. A low CSF concentration of HVA predicts poor performance in visuospatial recall tasks, attention in verbal tasks and executive function measured by the Wisconsin Card Sorting Test (WCST), in schizophrenic patients (Berman *et al.*, 1988; Kahn *et al.*, 1994).

A consistent pattern of decreased PFC blood flow in schizophrenia has been demonstrated by functional imaging studies (Ingvar and Franzen, 1974; Berman and Weinberger, 1991). Moreover, tasks that normally produce increases in blood flow to the PFC, such as the WCST, fail to have such an effect in schizophrenic patients (Weinberger *et al.*, 1986, 1988). It is well recognized that schizophrenics perform poorly on the WCST (Goldberg *et al.*, 1987; Elliott *et al.*, 1995) related to deficits in working memory. Based on these data, it can be hypothesized that enhancing working memory via manipulation of DA in the PFC should result in improved WCST performance. Indeed, administration of amphetamine (elevating PFC DA) during the

WCST induces an increase in PFC blood flow, which correlates with the improvement seen in task performance (Daniel *et al.*, 1991).

However, the PFC cognitive dysfunction associated with schizophrenia is not simply a consequence of decreased PFC DA concentrations. The number of prefrontal D_1 receptors is decreased in schizophrenic patients, irrespective of medication status. Moreover, there is a direct correlation between D_1 receptor number in the PFC and WCST performance (Okubo *et al.*, 1997), suggesting that decreased numbers of PFC D_1 receptors in addition to decreased dopaminergic turnover in the PFC produce impairments in executive function seen in schizophrenia.

As mentioned earlier, typical neuroleptics have demonstrated no ability to affect executive function and working memory in schizophrenia. However, it is surprising that typical neuroleptics do not worsen pre-existing working memory functions further in schizophrenic patients. Typical neuroleptics, such as haloperidol, a mixed D_2/D_1 antagonist, induce decreases in neuronal firing in the delay period of the delayed response task which does not translate into a behavioral deficit in humans (Sawaguchi and Goldman-Rakic, 1991). In addition, chronic administration (6 months) of neuroleptics decreases the amount of D_1 receptors in the PFC of monkeys (Lidow and Goldman-Rakic, 1994; Lidow *et al.*, 1997). Perhaps neuroleptics do not worsen executive performance in schizophrenia, as could be expected by the reduction in D_1 receptors, because there is decreased D_1 receptor activity prior to treatment, and chronic treatment induces little further decreases in PFC D_1 receptor density of schizophrenic patients.

Specific treatments

Drugs which increase dopamine concentration in the PFC

Atypical neuroleptics provide an option for improving PFC-mediated cognitive deficits in schizophrenia by increasing concentrations of DA in the PFC. This mechanism involves the antagonism of serotonin 5-HT_{2A} receptors located on the soma of dopaminergic neurons in the ventral segmental area (VTA), increasing dopaminergic release by these neurons and their projections to the PFC. Indeed, systemic administration of low doses of 5-HT_{2A} blockers, such as ritanserin, or atypical neuroleptics with 5-HT_{2A}-blocking properties, such as risperidone or ziprasidone, selectively increases firing of VTA neurons, with a consequent increase in PFC DA turnover.

The ability of atypical neuroleptics to remediate PFC-dependent cognitive deficits in schizophrenia has been demonstrated in several recent clinical trials. In a 4 week trial comparing risperidone and haloperidol, risperidone demonstrated a greater beneficial effect on verbal working memory across both distraction and non-distraction conditions (Green *et al.*, 1997). Similar beneficial effects on digit span distraction test performance have also been seen with ziprasidone and aripiprazole (Serper and Chou, 1997). Other comparisons of risperidone and haloperidol have found risperidone to be superior in enhancing executive function as measured by the Trails B test (McGurk *et al.*, 1997). Despite these improvements seen with atypical neuroleptics, overall performance of the schizophrenic patients in these studies was not normalized and remained clinically impaired. Therefore, it is uncertain if these improvements are of sufficient magnitude to translate into gains in overall functional status.

Long-term follow-up studies are necessary to determine whether the observed improvements in executive function and working memory lead to improvements in illness outcome.

Clozapine, another member of the atypical class of neuroleptics, also induces an increase in extracellular concentration of DA in the PFC. This increase is seen both as a response to a challenge dose, as an increase in basal DA turnover after subchronic (21 day) administration (Youngren *et al.*, 1994), and is sufficient to ameliorate acutely the cognitive deficits induced by chronic PCP administration in the monkey. However, long-term (12–15 months) administration of clozapine to schizophrenic patients does not appear to improve executive function (Goldberg *et al.*, 1993; Hagger *et al.*, 1993; Buchanan *et al.*, 1994; Hoff *et al.*, 1996) despite improvement in other areas of cognition such as verbal fluency or digit coding. One possible explanation is clozapine's interaction with other transmitter systems, such as its potent anticholinergic effects. Another possibility is the development of tolerance to the actions of clozapine on PFC DA. However, there are no data on basal DA measures after long-term clozapine administration. It is also possible that the induced increase in PFC DA is beyond the optimal range which would improve working memory.

Drugs which stimulate dopamine D_1 receptors in the PFC

An alternative approach targeting the DA system to remediate cognitive dysfunction in schizophrenia involves the direct stimulation of D_1 receptors in the PFC. D_1 receptor agonists are still in experimental phases. However, at present, one treatment trial with a selective partial D_1 agonist, SKF-38393, has been conducted with schizophrenic patients (Davidson *et al.*, 1990). This trial had modest results on the WCST, but the study used acute doses of drug within a narrow dose range. The full D_1 agonist, dihydrexidine, being developed for the treatment of Parkinson's disease, has demonstrated cognitive-enhancing properties, particularly in delayed response performance, in animal studies (Schneider *et al.*, 1994; Steele *et al.*, 1996). However, testing in humans has demonstrated considerable dose-limiting adverse effects, including flushing, hypotension and tachycardia, in all cases (Blanchet *et al.*, 1998). These findings suggest a marginal therapeutic window for this drug, making clinical applications to the treatment of cognitive dysfunction in schizophrenia impractical. Other full D_1 agonists are under development, some of which may prove more practical for this purpose.

Norepinephrine

Role of norepinephrine in cognition

Although the significance of dopaminergic inputs to the PFC with relation to PFC-mediated cognitive functions is undoubted (Brozoski *et al.*, 1979; Goldman-Rakic *et al.*, 1992; Arnsten *et al.*, 1994), noradrenergic inputs from the locus ceruleus (LC) also have an importance influence (Arnsten *et al.*, 1996) Therefore, noradrenergic influences on PFC cognitive functions serve as another point of intervention for remediating cognitive impairment in schizophrenia. Furthermore, this projection may be reciprocal, such that the PFC may supply cortical afferents to the LC (Arnsten and Golman-Rakic, 1984; Sara and Herve-Minvielle,

1995). Therefore, PFC dysfunction may impair regulation of the LC, a notion that is supported by direct evidence from rodent studies where lesions of the PFC disinhibit firing of the LC (Sara and Herve-Minvielle, 1995). Consequently, schizophrenic patients may experience cognitive dysfunction related to LC dysregulation in addition to the cognitive impairments associated with PFC dysfunction.

The central noradrenergic system has two distinct projections: those originating from the ventrolateral tegmental noradrenergic cells which are associated mainly with sexual and feeding behaviors, and those originating from the LC cells which are associated with certain cognitive functions (Crow, 1968; Mason and Iversen, 1979), including those dependent upon an intact PFC to which it projects (Arnsten and Goldman Rakic, 1985). It is hypothesized that the LC is activated with the presentation of novel stimuli, which then attenuate the influence of distracting stimuli, thereby focusing attention on task-relevant behaviors (Coull, 1994). By modulating distractibility in response to novel stimuli, LC functioning can influence diverse cognitive tasks associated with the presentation of novel stimuli, such as new learning, distractibility and vigilance, cognitive functions severely impaired in schizophrenic patients (Harvey and Keefe, 1997). Also, since the PFC is rich in noradrenergic terminal fields from the LC, and the PFC is involved in cognitive functions relevant to schizophrenia (Goldman-Rakic, 1987), dysfunction of noradrenergic receptors in the PFC could contribute significantly to the cognitive dysfunction of schizophrenia.

A variety of cognitive deficits, relevant to patients with schizophrenia, can be produced in animals with lesions of the LC noradrenergic system. These include deficits in sustained attention (Carli et al., 1983, Cole and Robbins, 1992) and shifting attention (Devauges and Sara, 1990). In addition, rats with lesions of the LC demonstrate impaired learning directly associated with decreased levels of cortical NE (Anlezark et al., 1973). These deficits are reversible by the administration of drugs which enhance noradrenergic neurotransmission. For example, the administration of diethyldithiocarbamate (DDC), an inhibitor of the enzyme dopamine-β-hydroxylase (DBH), to rats depletes NE stores in the brain and produces complete retention failure of passive avoidance learning (Hamburg and Cohen, 1973; Stein et al., 1975). Subsequently, normal learning of the passive avoidance task is restored in DDC-treated rats with a single intraventricular dose of NE (Stein et al., 1975). Puromycin also induces amnesia of maze learning in rats through reductions of NE (Roberts et al., 1970). Subsequently, this amnesia is reversed by the administration of drugs increasing noradrenergic activity, such as imipramine, tranylcypromine and D-amphetamine (Roberts et al., 1970).

Role of the α-2 adrenergic receptor in cognition

NE acts at four different adrenergic receptor families: α-1, α-2, β-1 and β-2, each of which has further subtypes identified. Studies indicate that NE's beneficial actions in the PFC result from stimulation of post-junctional α-2 receptors. Furthermore, a high density of α-2 receptors has been observed in the area of the principal sulcus of the PFC (Goldman-Rakic et al., 1990). Therefore, pharmacological studies of PFC NE influences on cognition in non-human primates have utilized drugs selective for the α-2 receptor. α-2 agonists, such as the antihypertensive drug clonidine, have been the drugs of choice in studies of non-human primates. The delayed response task has been utilized extensively in these investigations because performance on this task is known to depend on the integrity of frontal lobe function. This is relevant to the understanding of PFC-dependent cognitive dysfunction in schizophrenia because poor performance on a delayed response task is characteristic of the working memory abnormality of schizophrenia.

Young monkeys with localized 6-OHDA lesions to the PFC are rendered unable to perform a delayed response task. Subsequently, the α-2 adrenergic agonist clonidine improves performance on the spatially delayed response task (Arnsten and Goldman-Rakic, 1985), presumably at postsynaptic sites in the PFC. Improvements in spatial delay response tasks in aged non-human primates is also achieved with clonidine as well with as another α-2 agonist, guanfacine (Arnsten et al., 1988). Guanfacine was found to be ~25 times more potent than clonidine in enhancing delayed response performance, 10 times less potent in lowering blood pressure and much less likely to cause sedation (Arnsten et al., 1988). This differential response profile produced by these two α-2 agonists is attributed to the existence of three α-2 receptor subtypes, which have been cloned in humans; α-2A, α-2B and α-2C (Kobilka et al., 1987; Regan et al., 1988; Lomasney et al., 1990). The regional distribution of α-2 receptor messenger RNA (mRNA) in the rat brain shows that mRNA for the α-2B receptor is found exclusively in the thalamus (Nicholas et al., 1993; Scheinin et al., 1994), the site of α-2 agonists' sedative actions (Buzsaki et al., 1991), and α-2A and α-2C mRNA in the nucleus tractus solitarius (Nicholas et al., 1993; Scheinin et al., 1994), the site of α-2 agonists' hypotensive effects (Reis et al., 1984). Immunocytochemical studies in the monkey brain have revealed that the α-2A subtype is densest in the PFC (Aoki et al., 1994). Therefore, the adverse effects of α-2 agonists may be dissociated from their beneficial effects according to their relative affinities for each receptor subtype. The ability of guanfacine to improve PFC function without significant adverse effects corresponds to its selectivity for the α-2A site (Uhlen et al., 1995).

Implications for schizophrenia

NE has been implicated in the etiology of symptoms of schizophrenia. Such hypotheses have been in existence for almost three decades since Stein and Wise (1971) first proposed that schizophrenia was due to a "progressive deterioration of central noradrenergic pathways leading to anhedonia and loss of drive." However, the results of studies measuring NE activity in schizophrenic patients have been conflicting. CSF studies of NE initially identified generalized NE increases in chronic schizophrenic patients compared with age-matched normal controls (Lake et al., 1980; Kemali et al., 1982). When medication and symptom status were factored into the analysis, medication-free relapsing patients demonstrated significantly higher levels of NE and 3-methoxy-4-hydroxyphenylglycol (MHPG) in CSF (van Kammen et al., 1989a, 1990). In addition, post-mortem studies identified increases in NE levels in the nucleus accumbens of patients with paranoid schizophrenia (Bird et al., 1974; Farley et al., 1978; Crow et al., 1979). These data implicate a role for NE in the mediation of acute psychoses, and appear contrary to the model being proposed for decreased cortical noradrenergic functioning mediating the cognitive symptoms of schizophrenia. However, a relationship was not sought between cognitive status and NE parameters in these studies. Furthermore, the nature of noradrenergic dysregulation in schizophrenia may not be homogenous throughout the central nervous system (CNS) owing to the distribution pattern of pre- and post-junctional α-2 receptors in the brain. When NE acts at pre-junctional α-2 autoreceptors, its release is inhibited, whereas NE has agonist effects at post-junctional α-2 receptors. Therefore, abnormal activity at both pre- and post-junctional α-2 receptors in different regions of the schizophrenic brain may provide an explanation for the co-existence of low and high NE states mediating different symptom clusters in schizophrenia. Support for this hypothesis is demonstrated by clonidine-induced reductions in CSF NE and MHPG being associated with better antipsychotic response (van Kammen *et al.*, 1989b) and clonidine's ability to reverse impaired cognitive performance induced by NE-depleting lesions in the frontal cortex (Arnsten and Goldman-Rakic, 1985). A similar pattern is demonstrated in patients with Alzheimer's disease (AD), where cognitive impairment is the hallmark feature. Post-mortem findings demonstrate measures of decreased NE function in AD, whereas *in vivo* CSF measures of NE are elevated in AD (Raskind *et al.*, 1984).

When ante-mortem cognitive functioning was correlated with central catecholamine function in schizophrenic patients, Bridge and associates (1985) demonstrated significant decreases in noradrenergic function at post-mortem examination. Those schizophrenic subjects classified as demented [Mini Mental Status Examination (MMSE; Folstein *et al.*, 1975) score <20] had significantly decreased concentrations of NE in the nucleus accumbens and hypothalamus at post-mortem examination compared with those schizophrenic patients not classified as demented (MMSE >20). Similar findings were encountered in a post-mortem examination of schizophrenic brain tissue conducted by Powchick and colleagues (1998). In that study, NE was found to be significantly reduced in frontal cortex of cognitively impaired schizophrenic subjects in Brodmann areas 8, 32 and 44 compared with the schizophrenic subjects without such impairment. Since noradrenergic deficits can be age related, it is important to note that age was not significantly different in the two groups.

Specific treatments

Drugs which stimulate postsynaptic α-2 receptors in the PFC

The ability of α-2 agonists to improve cognitive performance in monkeys with lesions of the PFC has also been demonstrated in humans with psychiatric disorders associated with PFC dysfunction, such as attention deficit hyperactivity disorder (ADHD) and Korsakoff's syndrome, in addition to schizophrenia (Arnsten *et al.*, 1996). Studies of α-2 agonists in these clinical populations has demonstrated that these drugs can improve PFC-mediated cognitive functions in humans as well as they have in animals. For example, clonidine improves PFC-mediated cognitive tasks, such as verbal fluency and the Stroop test, in patients with Korsakoff's syndrome (Mair and McEntee, 1986; Moffoot *et al.*, 1994). To support a PFC mechanism mediating clonidine's beneficial effects on verbal fluency test performance, Moffoot and associates (1994) demonstrated that improved performance correlated with increased frontal cortical function by single-photon emission computed tomography imaging. Extrapolating these findings to patients with schizophrenia, Fields and associates (1988) demonstrated clonidine's ability to improve performance of schizophrenic patients significantly on the Trails B task, a task linked, in part, to the PFC. In addition, performance on tests of learning and delayed recall was also significantly improved by clonidine (Fields *et al.*,

1988), although this is inconsistent with animal data demonstrating that α-2 agonists do not improve cognitive functions associated with parietal and temporal lobe functions

Even though clonidine has demonstrated cognitive-enhancing ability in schizophrenic patients, it may not be the optimal choice for this purpose. Given the results of animal studies, it might be expected that guanfacine will have more beneficial effects on cognition in schizophrenic patients while producing fewer undesirable effects because of its selectivity for the putative R_1 site. In a double-blinded comparison of the differences in performance produced by guanfacine and clonidine in healthy subjects, Kugler and associates (1980) demonstrated guanfacine's superiority as a cognitive-enhancing agent, consistent with the findings of Arnsten and associates (1988) in aged non-human primates. Mental activity was less suppressed on electroencephalography (EEG) with guanfacine than clonidine, and performance on tests of information processing and reaction time was better with guanfacine than with clonidine (Kugler *et al.*, 1980).

Drugs which stimulate β-adrenergic receptors

Evidence suggests that the amygdala modulates functions of the hippocampus which are required for memory formation. Electrophysiological studies have shown that stimulation of the basolateral amygdala (BLA) facilitates the induction of hippocampal long-term potentiation (LTP) (Ikegaya *et al.*, 1996), a form of synaptic plasticity that may underlie learning and memory. Furthermore, the modulatory effects of the BLA on hippocampal LTP are mediated by the activity of β-adrenergic receptors in the BLA (Ikegaya *et al.*, 1997). Infusion of β-adrenoreceptor antagonists into the BLA significantly impairs LTP formation in the hippocampus (Ikegaya *et al.*, 1997) and therefore memory formation (Izquierdo *et al.*, 1998). Moreover, the administration of β-adrenergic agonists reverses the memory deficits induced by neurotoxic depletions of NE in animal models (Crowe and Shaw, 1997). However, animal models also demonstrate that amygdala-modulated memory processing in the hippocampus is activated by emotional arousal. Indeed, pharmacological studies in humans have demonstrated that endogenous levels of β-adrenergic receptor activation selectively enhance memory associated with emotional arousal. In humans, β-adrenergic receptor antagonists cause impairments in memory for emotionally arousing stimuli (Cahill *et al.*, 1994; van Stegeren *et al.*, 1998), but have no effect on memory for more emotionally neutral stimuli (Greenblatt *et al.*, 1993; Cahill *et al.*, 1994; van Stegeren *et al.*, 1998). Since it is not known if enhancement of memory associated with emotional experiences in schizophrenic patients would have any therapeutic value for improving illness outcome, it is difficult to make recommendations for the use of β-adrenergic receptor agonists to enhance cognition in schizophrenia. In addition, β-adrenergic receptor agonists have a significant side effect profile, including reflex tachycardia, other arrhythmias and angina, which would limit their use as cognitive-enhancing agents in humans.

Drugs which non-specifically increase noradrenergic activity

Finally, other drugs which will increase noradrenergic activity non-specifically, such as tricyclic antidepressants, monoamine oxidase inhibitors, amphetamines and specific norepinephrine reuptake inhibitors such as reboxetine, should be considered for enhancing cognition based on the animal data of Roberts and colleagues (1970). However, these drugs lack specificity for stimulating those noradrenergic receptors which are beneficial to cognitive functions. Furthermore, increased levels of NE activity at some receptors have a deleterious effect on cognition. For example, high levels of α-1 adrenoreceptor stimulation in the PFC impairs prefrontal cortical cognitive function (Arnsten et al., 1999).

Acetylcholine

Role of acetylcholine in cognition

Central cholinergic function is impaired in a number of diseases associated with cognitive dysfunction, such as dementia of the Alzheimer's type and Parkinson's disease. These patients experience cognitive deficits that include disturbances of mnemonic function and language usage. Schizophrenic patients also show impairments of mnemonic function that affect both verbal and episodic long-term memory and language use (Goldberg et al., 1989; Tamlyn et al., 1992; Saykin et al., 1994; Davidson et al., 1996), and therefore may be cholinergically mediated as well. Although post-mortem studies of schizophrenic patients have not identified gross abnormalities of the cholinergic system, as is found in patients with AD, subtle changes in cholinergic function in the more cognitively impaired schizophrenic patients may provide a rationale for enhancing cholinergic neurotransmission to improve cognitive performance in these patients.

The relationship between memory and ACh has been studied in animals using directed lesions and behavioral pharmacology. The basal cholinergic complex sends afferents to the entire non-striatal telencephalon with two projections: the septo-hippocampal and the nucleus basalis of Meynart (nbM)–cortical pathways (Woolf and Butcher, 1989). The correlation between lesions in these pathways and subsequent memory deficits indicates the involvement of these pathways in memory processes (Miyamoto et al., 1987). Lesions of the septo-hippocampal pathway decrease performance in the delayed non-match to position paradigm in rats (Aggleton et al., 1992; McAlonan et al., 1995), whereas lesions of the nbM produce deficits in passive avoidance conditioned responses, radial arm maze and water maze performance (Page et al., 1991; Winkler et al., 1995). Taken together, these findings demonstrate that the septo-hippocampal pathway is associated with working memory processes through hippocampal storage of intermediate-term memory (Brito et al., 1983; Eichenbaum et al., 1994; Fadda et al., 1996), and that the nbM–cortical pathway is involved in reference memory through long-term information storage in the neocortex (Dunnett, 1985; Meek et al., 1987). The memory deficits caused by the above lesions are ameliorated by administration of AChE inhibitors, such as physostigmine (Mandel et al., 1989). Also, the grafting of ACh-producing cells into the brains of lesioned rats improves performance levels on memory tasks, such as the water maze (Dunnett, 1985; Winkler et al., 1995).

Further insight into the importance of ACh in memory and learning comes from pharmacological studies of behavior. Administration of scopolamine or atropine induces memory dysfunction in rats, primates and humans (Blozovski et al., 1977; Drachman, 1977; Aigner et al., 1986). This drug-induced impairment subsequently is reversed after displacement of the blocking agent (Dawson *et al.*, 1992), and by the use of AChE inhibitors. These drugs act by preventing the breakdown of ACh in the synaptic cleft. The administration of physostigmine to both young and aged monkeys produces an overall improvement of mnemonic processes in both groups (Bartus and Uehara, 1979). Tacrine and donepezil, two AChE inhibitors, can reverse the deficits induced by scopolamine in T-maze and passive avoidance tests in rats (Nielsen *et al.*, 1989; Wanibuchi *et al.*, 1994) and induced deficits in memory in monkeys (Rupniak *et al.*, 1997). This supports the notion that memory function can be improved by increasing synaptic ACh, and specifically by AChE inhibition.

A role for ACh in the processes of attention has been demonstrated in rats. Performance on the five-choice serial reaction task is impaired following basal forebrain lesions (Robbins *et al.*, 1989). Furthermore, both the systemic administration of physostigmine and the transplant of cholinergic embryonic cells into the brains of rats with basal forebrain lesions improves the visual attentional impairments (Muir *et al.*, 1992). The role of ACh in attentional processes has also been described in monkeys. Continuous intraventricular injections of scopolamine during a Continuous Performance Task requiring localization of briefly presented visual stimuli results in a decrease in the number of responses. This effect becomes more apparent when the stimulus presentation is shortened and towards the end of the testing session (Callahan *et al.*, 1993).

Implications for schizophrenia

Although the size and number of cells in the nbM of schizophrenic patients are not significantly different from those of normal controls (El-Mallack *et al.*, 1991), a correlation does exist between the degree of cognitive impairment in schizophrenic patients and measures of cortical choline acetyl transferase (ChAT) activity (Haroutunian *et al.*, submitted). The activity of ChAT, a marker of cholinergic function, was not significantly reduced in the parietal cortex of the schizophrenic subjects compared with normal elderly controls; nevertheless, ChAT activity did significantly correlate with Clinical Dementia Rating (CDR) scores in the schizophrenic cohort (Haroutunian *et al.*, submitted). These findings suggest that although the activity of ChAT in the parietal cortex of schizophrenic patients is not significantly reduced in comparison with normal elderly controls, its relative activity may nevertheless contribute to cognitive dysfunction. Indeed, normal subjects, presumably with an intact cholinergic system, who recall a smaller number of words during a serial learning task under drug-free conditions are most sensitive to the enhancing or impairing properties of cholinomimetics (Sitaram *et al.*, 1978). This finding is particularly relevant to schizophrenic patients since it is the norm for schizophrenic patients to perform 2–3 SDs below normal performance on tests of serial learning (Harvey and Keefe, 1997).

Specific treatments

Drugs which increase cholinergic transmission

Physostigmine, when given intravenously to normal volunteers, significantly improves new learning (Davis *et al.*, 1978). However, intravenous physostigmine is quite short acting and would not be a viable long-term treatment strategy. Other agents, such as the AChE inhibitors donepezil and tacrine, represent additional choices for the purpose of cognitive enhancement. Donepezil use is associated with a lower incidence of gastrointestinal and hepatotoxic effects than tacrine, making donepezil the better choice of AChE inhibitor for use to enhance cognition in patients with schizophrenia (Summers *et al.*, 1986; Rogers *et al.*, 1996). In addition, administration to patients is considerably easier with donepezil than tacrine given that donepezil is administered only once daily. A daily dose of 5 mg has an incidence of side effects similar to that of placebo. Also, its ability to improve cognitive function has been demonstrated in controlled trials (Rogers *et al.*, 1996). Patients with AD demonstrate enhanced cognition, as measured by improvement on the cognitive subscale of the Alzheimer's Disease Assessment Scale (ADAS-cog), with the use of donepezil (Rogers *et al.*, 1996).

Drugs which stimulate M1 and M4 muscarinic receptors

Another approach is the use of selective muscarinic agonists. From the five muscarinic receptors, M1 has been identified as a potential site for cognitive-enhancing drugs because of its postsynaptic localization and dense distribution in the hippocampus and cerebral cortex (Levey *et al.*, 1991; Flynn *et al.*, 1995). M4 receptors have a similar anatomical distribution, in addition to sites in the substantia nigra and striatum (Yasuda *et al.*, 1993). Since a high density of M1 and M4 receptors are located in the cortex, where cholinergic activity correlates with CDR scores in schizophrenic patients (Haroutunian *et al.*, 1999), use of an M1/M4 agonist, such as xanomeline, may also improve deficits in mnemonic functioning associated with schizophrenia. Xanomeline has been developed as a potential treatment for cognitive dysfunction associated with AD (Bymaster *et al.*, 1994). Clinical trials in AD have demonstrated treatment with xanomeline to improve scores on the ADAS-cog. Specific improvements were noted on tests of constructional praxis, orientation, spoken language ability and word-finding difficulty in spontaneous speech (Bodick *et al.*, 1997). Since schizophrenic patients perform even more poorly than AD patients on tests of naming and constructional praxis (Davidson *et al.*, 1996), xanomeline may be particularly useful in schizophrenia given its ability specifically to improve these two cognitive measures in AD patients. However, xanomeline, orally administered, has a dose-dependent side effect profile, which includes nausea, dyspepsia and diaphoresis, and leads to a high rate of drug discontinuation. Cognitive improvements are also dose dependent and are observed predominately in the high dose group, limiting the use of this particular muscarinic agonist for cognitive remediation in schizophrenics. Therefore, development of a muscarinic agonist which can produce improvements in cognitive performance without producing side effects is warranted, and may prove useful in treating the cognitive deficits associated with schizophrenia.

Glutamate

Role of glutamate in cognition

The amino acid glutamate is the major excitatory neurotransmitter in the CNS. Evidence suggests that the Glu system is involved in fast synaptic transmission, plasticity and higher cognitive functions. Glu receptors are divided into the ionotropic and metabotropic receptor families. Ionotropic Glu receptors can be distinguished pharmacologically by binding of specific agonists including NMDA, kainic acid (KA) and AMPA. NMDA receptor activity is regulated via several allosteric regulatory binding sites on the receptor–channel complex. Facilitation of glutamatergic transmission promotes the formation of long-term potentiation (LTP) (Arai and Lynch, 1992), a type of synaptic plasticity hypothesized to be involved in the encoding of memory (Bliss and Lomo, 1973).

NMDA receptors usually co-exist with either AMPA or KA receptors at synapses and are thought to be involved in the amplification of the Glu signal. At rest, NMDA channels are blocked by Mg^{2+}, requiring sufficient depolarization of the postsynaptic neuronal membrane to relieve the Mg^{2+} block and allow the NMDA channel to contribute to the electrical response of the cell. This level of depolarization depends on AMPA or KA activation and/or other modulatory postsynaptic signals. Precise modulation of NMDA channel activity is required for normal neuronal function. There are several regulatory sites on the NMDA receptor–channel complex which control NMDA-mediated activity further. Among these is a glycine-binding site through which glycine binding increases the frequency of agonist-induced channel opening. In addition, there is a polyamine-binding site which, when activated, potentiates the NMDA current. The NMDA receptor–channel complex can also be inhibited via a Zn^{2+}-binding site and a distinct site within the channel that binds MK-801 and PCP. Therefore, there is capacity for several different mechanisms for positive and negative control of NMDA channel function.

Role of the glutamate NMDA receptor in cognition

NMDA receptor activation is linked to facilitation of LTP, an integral process of learning and memory. NMDA antagonists have been shown to disrupt learning in laboratory animals (Packard and Teather, 1997; Escobar *et al.*, 1998), and these impairments are reversed by the administration of drugs which augment NMDA receptor activation (Kawabe *et al.*, 1998; Meyer *et al.*, 1998). Since direct Glu administration leads to seizures and excitotoxicity by its actions at both NMDA and non-NMDA receptors (Olney, 1989), this strategy does not present a viable clinical option. Therefore, studies examining the effects of augmenting NMDA receptor activation on cognitive deficits have employed drugs acting at the glycine site on the NMDA receptor, which augment receptor function without reaching excessive levels of activation. One strategy involves direct treatment with glycine. Treatment with glycine restored normal learning in rats with disruption of temporal glutamatergic systems (Myhrer *et al.*, 1993). In addition, treatment with the glycine pro-drug milacemide enhanced learning in normal mice (Finkelstein, 1994). Another strategy involves the use of the antituberculous drug D-cycloserine (DCS), a partial agonist at the NMDA glycine-binding site. Both intra-hippocampal (Kawabe *et al.*, 1998) and systemic administration of DCS (Meyer *et al.*, 1998) were effective in reversing NMDA receptor blockade-induced learning deficits in rats.

Role of the glutamate AMPA receptor in cognition

More recently, the facilitatory effect of AMPA receptor modulation on the induction of LTP has been a focus of investigations aiding in the development of drugs which are likely to enhance LTP and therefore the encoding of new information. Subsequently, a new class of drugs, referred to as 'ampakines' has been developed, which increase AMPA-type Glu receptor-gated currents (Arai *et al.*, 1994), thereby increasing the size of excitatory synaptic responses (Isaacson and Nicoll, 1991; Vyklicky *et al.*, 1991) and reduce the amount of afferent activity needed to induce LTP (Staubli *et al.*, 1994a). Either effect could promote the encoding of memory. Ampakines readily cross the blood–brain barrier (Staubli *et al.*, 1994b) and in a number of animal studies have been shown to improve the encoding of memory. Behavioral studies in rats indicate that ampakines improve retention in tasks involving spatial cues (Staubli *et al.*, 1994b), facilitate olfactory learning (Larson *et al.*, 1995) and the acquisition of a conditioned response (Shors *et al.*, 1994), and reverse age-associated memory impairments (Granger *et al.*, 1996). The ability of ampakines to produce significant effects across this variety of paradigms suggested a generalized effect on plasticity mechanisms that enhance learning and memory.

Implications for schizophrenia

Hypofunction of the Glu transmitter system was first proposed as a causal mechanism in schizophrenia by Kim and colleagues (1980) based on their findings of low concentrations of Glu in the CSF of schizophrenic patients. Subsequently other markers of Glu dysfunction in the schizophrenic brain have been identified (Tsai *et al.*, 1995), including alterations in Glu receptor composition and density (Breese *et al.*, 1995; Eastwood *et al.*, 1997a,b). The observation that PCP, a non-competitive inhibitor of the NMDA receptor, can induce a psychotic state that closely mimics schizophrenia has contributed further to the hypothesis of Glu hypofunction at the NMDA receptor as a causal factor in schizophrenia. When PCP is given to normal human subjects, it can produce a variety of schizophrenic symptoms including positive symptoms, negative symptoms and cognitive impairment (Rosenbaum *et al.*, 1959; Luby *et al.*, 1959; Davies and Beach, 1960). Moreover, when ketamine, another non-competitive NMDA receptor antagonist, is administered to neuroleptic-free schizo-phrenic patients, exacerbations of positive and negative symptoms is observed in addition to decrements in cognitive performance (Malhotra *et al.*, 1997).

Specific treatments

NMDA receptor partial agonists

The data supporting the contribution of Glu/NMDA receptor hypofunction to the positive, negative and cognitive symptomatology of schizophrenia have given rise to new treatment strategies to reverse these deficits pharmacologically. Current efforts to treat schizophrenic patients with Glu agonists are based on this principle. The administration of the NMDA partial agonist DCS and the glycine pro-drug milacemide to normal volunteers significantly improves memory performance (Jones *et al.*, 1991; Schwartz *et al.*, 1991). However, the results of studies using these drugs to reverse cognitive impairment in schizophrenic patients have been inconclusive. Some studies have shown glycine to reduce negative symptoms significantly in schizophrenic patients (Javitt *et al.*, 1994; Heresco-Levy *et al.*, 1996, 1999), but others have not (Rosse *et al.*, 1989, 1991; Potkin *et al.*, 1992). Furthermore, these studies generally did not evaluate the effects of glycine on cognition. The exception is the study of Heresco-Levy *et al.* (1999); however, the effect on cognition was measured by the Positive and Negative Syndrome Scale (PANSS) cognitive factor score and not by specific cognitive measures. Similar conflicting results on negative symptoms have been demonstrated in clinical trials with DCS (Cascella *et al.*, 1994; Goff *et al.*, 1996, 1999). Furthermore, positive effects of DCS on specific cognitive measures could not be replicated (Goff *et al.*, 1995, 1999). Based on these data, no specific recommendations for the use of NMDA agonists to enhance cognition in schizophrenia can be made. More thorough investigations of glycine and DCS are required using specific cognitive measures to evaluate their efficacy.

Ampakines

The ability of ampakines to produce a generalized effect on plasticity mechanisms which enhance learning and memory in animal models presents an alternative glutamatergic approach to the treatment of cognitive impairment in schizophrenia. CX516, the ampakine compound most frequently used thus far in behavioral studies, enhances the encoding of various forms of memory in normal humans (Lynch *et al.*, 1996, 1997; Ingvar *et al.*, 1997). Preliminary results from an ongoing trial of CX516 in schizophrenic patients demonstrates the potential for this drug as a cognitive enhancer for these patients (Goff *et al.*, 1998). Six schizophrenic patients receiving clozapine were entered into a placebo-controlled dose escalation trial of CX516 and were assessed over a 4 week period. Subjects receiving CX516 demonstrated improvements in measures of verbal learning and memory, sentence comprehension and attention. Although these results are promising, they are preliminary and require corroboration from future controlled trials.

References

Aggleton, J., Keith, A., Rawlins, J., Hunt, P. and Sahgal, A. (1992) Removal of the hippocampus and transection of the fornix produce comparable deficits on delayed non-match to position by rats. *Behavioral Brain Research*, **52**, 61–71.

Aigner, T. and Mishkin, M. (1986) The effects of physostigmine and scopolamine on recognition memory in monkeys. *Behavioral and Neural Biology*, **45**, 81–87.

Aoki, C., Go, C.G., Venkatesan, C. and Kurose, H. (1994) Perikaryal and synaptic localization of α-2A adrenergic receptor like immunoreactivity. *Brain Research*, **650**,181–204.

Anlezark, G.M., Crow, T.J. and Greenway, A.P. (1973) Impaired learning and decreased cortical norepinephrine after bilateral locus coeruleus lesions. *Science*, **181**, 682–684.

Arai, A. and Lynch, G. (1992) Factors regulating the magnitude of LTP induced by theta pattern stimulation. *Brain Research*, **598**, 173–184.

Arai, A., Kessler, M., Xaio, P., Ambros-Ingerson, J., Rogers, G. and Lynch, G. (1994) A centrally active drug that modulates AMPA receptor gated currents. *Brain Research*, **638**, 343–346.

Arnsten, A.F.T. and Goldman-Rakic, P.S. (1984) Selective prefrontal cortical projections to the region of the locus ceruleus and raphe nuclei in the Rhesus monkey. *Brain Research*, **306**, 9–18.

Arnsten, A.F.T. and Goldman-Rakic, P.S. (1985) Alpha-2 adrenergic mechanisms in prefromtal cortex associated with cognitive decline in aged nonhuman primates. *Science*, **230**, 1273–1276.

Arnsten, A.F.T., Cai, J.X. and Goldman-Rakic, P.S. (1988) The alpha-2 adrenergic agonist guanfacine improves memory in aged monkeys without sedative or hypotensive side effects: evidence for alpha-2 receptor subtypes. *Journal of Neuroscience*, **8**, 4287–4297.

Arnsten, A.F.T., Cai, J.X., Murphy, B.L. and Goldman-Rakic, P.S. (1994) Dopamine D1 receptor mechanisms in the cognitive performance of young adult and aged monkeys. *Psychopharmacology*, **116**, 143–151.

Arnsten, A.F.T., Steere, J.C. and Hunt, R.D. (1996) The contribution of alpha-2 noradrenergic mechanisms to prefrontal cortical cognitive function. *Archives of General Psychiatry*, **53**, 448–455.

Arnsten, A.F.T., Mathew, R., Ubriani, R., Taylor, J.R. and Li, B.-M. (1999) α-1 noradrenergic receptor stimulation impairs prefrontal cortical cognitive function. *Biological Psychiatry*, **45**, 26–31.

Bartus, R. and Uehara, Y. (1979) Physostigmine and recent memory: effects in young and aged nonhuman primates. *Science*, **206**, 1085–1087.

Berman, K.F. and Weinberger, D.R. (1991) Functional localization in the brain in schizophrenia. In: Tasman, A. and Goldfinger, S.M. (eds), *American Psychiatric Press Review of Psychiatry*. American Psychiatric Press, Washington, Vol. 10, pp. 24–59.

Berman, K.F., Illowsky, B.P. and Weinberger, D.R. (1988) Physiological dysfunction of dorsolateral prefrontal cortex in schizophrenia: IV. Further evidence for regional and behavioral specificity. *Archives of General Psychiatry*, **45**, 616–622.

Bilder, R., Lipshitz-Broch, L., Reiter, G., Geisler, S., Mayerhoff, D. and Lieberman, J. (1992) Intellectual deficit in first episode schizophrenia, evidence for progressive deterioration. *Schizophrenia Bulletin*, **18**, 437–448.

Bird, E.D., Spokes, E.G. and Iversen, L.L. (1974) Brain norepinephrine and dopamine in schizophrenia. *Science*, **204**, 93–94.

Blanchet, P.J., Fang, J., Gillespie, M., Sabounjian, L., Locke, K.W., Gammans, R., Mouradian, M.M. and Chase, T.N. (1998) Effects of the full D1 receptor agonist dihydrexidine in Parkinson's disease. *Clinical Neuropharmacology*, **21**, 339–343.

Bliss, T.V. and Lomo, T. (1973) Long-lasting potentiation of synaptic transmission in the dentate area of the anaesthetized rabbit following stimulation of the perforant path. *Journal of Physiology*, **232**, 331–356.

Blozovski, D., Cudennec, A. and Garrigou, D. (1977) Deficits in passive avoidance learning following atropine in the developing rat. *Psychopharmacology*, **54**, 139–144.

Bodick, N.C., Offen, W.W., Levey, A.I., Cutler, N.R., Gauthier, S.G., Satlin, A., Shannon, H.E., Tollefson, G.D., Ramussen, K., Bymaster, F.P., Hurley, D.J., Potter, W.Z. and Paul, S.M. (1997) Effects of xanomeline, a selective muscarinic receptor agonist, on cognitive function and behavioral symptoms in Alzheimer disease. *Archives of Neurology*, **54**, 465–473.

Breese, C.R., Freedman, R. and Leonard, S.S. (1995) Glutamate receptor subtype expression in human postmortem brain tissue from schizophrenics and alcohol abusers. *Brain Research*, **674**, 82–90.

Bridge, T.P., Kleinman, J.E., Karoum, F. and Wyatt, R.J. (1985) Postmortem central catecholamines and ante mortem cognitive impairment in elderly schizophrenics and controls. *Biological Psychiatry*, **14**, 57–61.

Brito, G., Davis, B., Stopp, L. and Stanton, M. (1983) Memory and the septohippocampal cholinergic system in the rat. *Psychopharmacology*, **81**, 315–320.

Brozoski, T., Brown, R., Rosvold, H. and Goldman, P. (1979) Cognitive deficit caused by regional depletion of dopamine in prefrontal cortex of rhesus monkeys. *Science*, **205**, 929–932.

Buchanan, R.W., Holstein, C. and Breier, A. (1994) The comparative efficacy and long term effect of clozapine treatment on neuropsychological test performance. *Biological Psychiatry*, **36**, 717–725.

Buzsaki, G., Kennedy, B., Solt, V.B. and Ziegler, M. (1991) Noradrenergic control of thalamic oscillation: the role of alpha-2 receptors. *European Journal of Pharmacology*, **3**, 222–229.

Bymaster, F.P., Wong, D.T., Mitch, C.H., Ward, J.S., Calligaro, D.O., Schoepp, D.D., Shannon, H.E., Sheardown, M.J., Olesen, P.H., Suzdak, P.D. *et al.* (1994) Neurochemical effects of the MI muscarinic agonist xanomeline. *Journal of Pharmacology and Experiemental Theraputics*, **269**, 282–289.

Cahill, L., Prins, B., Weber, M. and McGaugh, J.L. (1994) Beta-adrenergic activation and memory for emotional events. *Nature*, **371**, 702–704.

Cai, J.X. and Arnsten, A.F. (1997) Dose dependent effects of the dopamine D1 receptor agonists A77636 or SKF81297 on spatial working memory in aged monkeys. *Journal of Pharmacology and Experimental Therapeutics*, **283**, 183–189.

Callahan, M., Kinsora, J., Harbaugh, R., Reeder, T. and Davis, R. (1993) Continuous icv infusion of scopolamine impairs sustained attention of rhesus monkeys. *Neurobiology of Aging*, **14**, 147–151.

Carli, M., Robbins, T.W., Evenden, J.L. and Everitt, B.J. (1983) Effects of lesions to ascending noradrenergic neurons on performance of a 5-choice serial reaction task in rats. Implications for theories of dorsal noradrenergic bundle functions based on selective attention and arousal. *Behavioral Brain Research*, **9**, 361–380.

Carter, C., Robertson, L., Nordahl, T., Chaderjian, M., Kraft, L. and O'Shora-Celaya, L (1996) Spatial working memory deficits and their relationship to negative symptoms in unmedicated schizophrenia patients. *Biological Psychiatry*, **40**, 930–932.

Cascella, N.G., Macciareli, P., Cavallini, C. and Smeraldi, E. (1994) D-Cycloserine adjuvant therapy to conventional neuroleptic treatment in schizophrenia: an open label study. *Journal of Neural Transmission*, **95**, 105–111.

Cleghorn, J., Kaplan, R., Szechtman, B., Szechtman, M. and Brown, G. (1990) Neuroleptic drug effects on cognitive function in schizophrenia. *Schizophrenia Research*, **3**, 211–219.

Cole, B.J. and Robbins, T.W. (1992) Forebrain norepinephrine: role in controlled information processing in the rat. *Neuropsychopharmacology*, **7**, 129–141.

Cortes, R., Gueye, B., Pazos, A., Probs, A. and Palacios, J.M. (1989) Dopamine receptors in the human brain: autoradiographic distribution of D1 sites. *Neuroscience*, **28**, 263–273.

Coull, J.T. (1994) Pharmacological manipulations of the alpha 2-noradrenergic system. Effects on cognition. *Drugs and Aging*, **5**, 116–126.

Crow, T.J. (1968) Cortical synapses and reinforcement. *Nature*, **219**, 736–737.

Crow, T.J., Baker, H.F., Cross, A.J., Joseph, M.H,, Lofthouse, R., Longden, A. *et al*. (1979) Monoamine mechanisms in chronic schizophrenia: post-mortem neurochemical findings *British Journal of Psychiatry*, **134**, 249–256.

Crowe, S.F. and Shaw, S. (1997) Salbutamol overcomes the effect of the noradrenergic neurotoxin DSP-4 on memory function in the day old chick. *Behavioral Pharmacology*, **8**, 216–222.

Daniel, D.G., Weinberger, D.R., Jones, D.W., Zigun, J.R., Cippola, R., Handel, S. *et al*. (1991) The effect of amphetamine on regional cerebral blood flow during cognitive activation in schizophrenia. *Journal of Neuroscience*, **11**, 1907–1917.

Danjou, P., Warot, D., Hergueta, T., Lacomblez, Bouhours, P. and Puech, A.J. (1992) Comparative study of the psychomotor and antistress effects of ritanserin, alprazolam and diazepam in healthy subjects: some trait anxiety-independent responses. *International Clinical Psychopharmacology*, **7**, 73–79.

Davidson, M., Harvey, P., Bergman, R., Powchik, P., Kaminsky, R., Losonczy, M. and Davis, K.L. (1990) Effects of the D1 agonist SKF-39393 combined with haloperidol in schizophrenic patients [letter]. *Archives of General Psychiatry*, **47**, 190–191.

Davidson, M., Harvey, P.D., Welsh, K.A., Powchik, P., Putnam, K.M. and Mohs, R.C. (1996) Cognitive functioning in late-life schizophrenia: a comparison of elderly schizophrenic patients with Alzheimer's disease. *American Journal of Psychiatry*, **153**, 1274–1279.

Davies, B.M. and Beach, H.L (1960) The effect of 1-arylcyclohexylamine (sernyl) on twelve normal volunteers. *Journal of Mental Science*, **106**, 912–924.

Davis, K.L., Mohs, R., Tinklenberg, J., Pfefferbaum, A., Hollister, L. and Kopell, B. (1978) Physostigmine: improvement of long-term memory in normal humans. *Science*, **201**, 272–274.

Davis, K.L., Kahn, R.S., Ko, G. and Davidson, M. (1991) Dopamine in schizophrenia: a review and reconceptualization. *American Journal of Psychiatry*, **148**, 1474–1486.

Dawson, G., Heyes, C. and Iversen, S. (1992) Pharmacological mechanisms and animal models of cognition. *Behavioral Pharmacology*, **3**, 285–297.

Devauges, V. and Sara, S.J. (1990) Activation of the noradrenergic system facilitates an attention shift in the rat. *Behavioral Brain Research*, **39**, 19–29.

Didriksen, M. (1995) Effects of antipsychotics on cognitive behavior in rats using the delayed non-match to position paradigm. *European Journal of Pharmacology*, **281**, 241–250.

Drachman, D. (1977) Memory and cognitive function in man. Does the cholinergic system have a specific role? *Neurology*, **27**, 783–790.

Dunnett, S. (1985) Comparative effects of cholinergic drugs and lesions of the nucleus basalis or fimbria-fornix on delayed-matching in rats. *Psychopharmacology*, **87**, 357–363.

Eastwood, S.L., Kerwin, R.W. and Harrison, P.J. (1997a) Immunoautoradiographic evidence for a loss of alpha-amino-3-hydroxy-5-methyl-4-isoxazole proprionate-preferring non-*N*-methyl-D-aspartate glutamate receptors within the medial temporal lobe in schizophrenia. *Biological Psychiatry*, **41**, 636–643.

Eastwood, S.L., Burnet, P.W. and Harrison, P.J. (1997b) GluR2 glutamate receptor subunit flip and flop isoforms are decreased in the hippocampal formation in schizophrenia: a reverse transcriptase–polymerase chain reaction (RT–PCR) study. *Brain Research*, **44**, 92–98.

Eichenbaum, H., Otto, T. and Cohen, N. (1994) Two functional components of the hippocampal memory system. *Behavioral Brain Science*, **17**, 449–518.

Elliott, R., McKenna, P.J., Robbins, T,W. and Sahakian, B.J. (1995) Neuropsychological evidence for frontostriatal dysfunction in schizophrenia. *Psychological Medicine*, **25**, 619–630.

El-Mallack, R., Kirch, D., Shelton, R., Fan, K., Pezeshkpour, G., Kanhouwa, S. *et al.* (1991) The nucleus basalis of Meynert, senile plaques, and intellectual impairment in schizophrenia. *Journal of Neuropsychiatry and Clinical Neurosciences*, **3**, 383–386.

Elsworth, J., Leahy, D., Roth, R. and Redmond, D. (1987) Homovanillic acid concentration in brain, CSF and plasma as indicators of central dopamine function in primates. *Journal of Neural Transmission*, **68**, 51–62.

Escobar, M.L., Alcocer, I. and Chao, V. (1998) The NMDA receptor antagonist CPP impairs conditioned taste aversion and insular cortex long-term potentiation *in vivo*. *Brain Research*, **812**, 246–251.

Fadda, F., Melis, F. and Stancampiano, R (1996) Increased hippocampal acetylcholine release during a working memory task. *European Journal of Pharmacology*, **307**, R1–R2.

Farley, I.J., Price, K.S., McCullouough, E., Deck, J.H.N., Hordynsky, W. and Hornykiewicz, O. (1978) Norepinephrine in chronic paranoid schizophrenia: above-normal levels in limbic forebrain. *Science*, **200**, 456–457.

Fields, R.B., van Kammen, D.P., Peters, J.L., Rosen, J., van Kammen, W.B., Nugent, A., Stipetic, M. and Linnoila, M. (1988) Clonidine improves memory function in schizophrenia independently from changes in psychosis: preliminary findings. *Schizophrenia Research*, **1**, 417–423.

Finkelstein, J.E., Hengemihle, J.E., Ingram, D.K. and Petri, H.L. (1994) Milacemide treatment in mice enhances acquisition of a Morris-type water maze task. *Pharmacology, Biochemistry and Behavior*, **49**, 707–710.

Fleming, K., Goldberg, T., Gold, J. and Weinberger, D. (1995) Verbal working memory dysfunction in schizophrenia: use of a Brown–Peterson paradigm. *Psychiatry Research*, **56**, 155–161.

Fleming, K., Goldberg, T., Binks, S., Randolph, C., Gold, J. and Weinberger, D. (1997) Visuospatial working memory in patients with schizophrenia. *Biological Psychiatry*, **41**, 43–43.

Flynn, D., Ferrari-DiLeo, G., Mash, D. and Levey, A. (1995) Differential regulation of molecular subtypes of muscarinic receptors in Alzheimer's disease. *Journal of Neurochemistry*, **64**, 1888–1891.

Folstein, M.F., Folstein, S.E. and McHugh, P.R (1975) Mini-mental state. *Journal of Psychiatric Research*, **12**, 189–198.

Friedman, J.I., Temporini, H. and Davis, K.L. (1999) Pharmacologic strategies for augmenting cognitive performance in schizophrenia. *Biological Psychiatry*, **45**, 1–16.

Goff, D.C., Tsai, G., Manoach, D.S. and Coyle, J.T. (1995) Dose finding trial of D-cycloserine added to neuroleptics for negative symptoms in schizophrenia. *American Journal of Psychiatry*, **152**, 1213–1215.

Goff, D.C., Tsai, G., Manoach, D.S., Flood, J., Darby, D.G. and Coyle, J.T. (1996) D-

Cycloserine added to clozapine for patients with schizophrenia. *American Journal of Psychiatry*, **153**, 1628–1630.

Goff, D.C., Berman, I., Posever, T., Herz, L., Leahy, L.F. and Lynch, G. (1998) Ampakine (CX516) added to clozapine in schizophrenia: preliminary safety and efficacy data. *Presented at The 37th Annual Meeting of The American College of Neuropsychopharmacology*. Las Croabas, Puerto Rico.

Goff, D.C., Tsai, G., Levitt, J., Amico, E., Manoach, D., Schoenfeld, D.A., Hayden, D.L., McCarley, R. and Coyle, J.T (1999) A placebo-controlled trial of D-cycloserine added to conventional neuroleptics in patients with schizophrenia. *Archives of General Psychiatry*, **56**, 21–27.

Goldberg, T.E., Weinberger, D.R., Berman, K.F., Pliskin, N.H. and Podd, M.H. (1987) Further evidence for a dementia of cortical type in schizophrenia? A controlled study of teaching the WCST. *Archives of General Psychiatry*, **44**, 1008–1014.

Goldberg, T., Weinberger, D., Pliskin, N., Berman, K. and Podd, M. (1989) Recall memory deficit in schizophrenia: a possible manifestation of prefrontal dysfunction. *Schizophrenia Research*, **2**, 251–257

Goldberg, T., Greenberg, R., Griffin, S., Gold, J., Kleinman, J., Pickar, D., Schulz, S. and Weinberger, D. (1993) The effect of clozapine on cognition and psychiatric symptoms in patients with schizophrenia. *British Journal of Psychiatry*, **162**, 43–48.

Goldman-Rakic, P.S. (1987) Circuitry of the primate prefrontal cortex and the regulation of behavior by representational memory. In: Plum, F. (ed.), *Handbook of Physiology: The Nervous System, Higher Function of the Brain*. American Physiological Society, Bethesda, MD, pp. 373–417.

Goldman-Rakic, P.S., Lidow, M.S. and Gallager, D.W (1990) Overlap of dopaminergic, adrenergic and serotoninergic receptors and complementarity of their subtypes in primate prefrontal cortex. *Journal of Neuroscience*, **10**, 2125–2138.

Goldman-Rakic, P.S., Lidow, M.S., Smiley, J.F. and Williams, M.S. (1992) The anatomy of dopamine in monkey and human prefrontal cortex. *Journal of Neural Transmission*, **36** (Suppl.), 163–177.

Granger, R., Deadwyler, S., Davis, M., Moskovitz, B., Kessler, M., Rogers, G. and Lynch, G. (1996) Facilitation of glutamate receptors reverses an age associated memory impairment in rats. *Synapse*, **22**, 332–337.

Green, M., Marshall, B., Wirshing, W., Ames, D., Marder, S., McGurk, S. *et al.* (1997) Does risperidone improve verbal working memory in treatment resistant schizophrenia? *American Journal of Psychiatry*, **154**, 799–804.

Greenblatt, D.J., Scavone, J.M., Harmatz, J.S., Engelhardt, N. and Shader, R.I. (1993) Cognitive effects of beta-adrenergic antagonists after single doses; pharmacokinetics and pharmacodynamics of propranolol, atenolol, lorazepam and placebo. *Clinical Pharmacology and Therapeutics*, **53**, 577–584.

Hagger, C., Buckley, P., Kenny, J.T., Friedman, L., Ubogy, D. and Meltzer, H. (1993) Improvement in cognitive function and psychiatric symptoms in schizophrenic patients receiving clozapine. *Biological Psychiatry*, **34**, 702–712.

Hamburg, M.D. and Cohen, R.P. (1973) Memory access pathway: role of adrenergic versus cholinergic neurons. *Pharmacology Biochemistry and Behavior*, **1**, 295–300.

Haroutunian, V., Powchik, P., Purohit, D.P., Davidson, M., McCrystal, J., Perl, D.P. and Davis, K.L. (1999) Cognitive deficits without a cholinergic cause: choline acetyltransferase activity in the parietal cortex of 95 elderly schizophrenics. *Neuroscience Letters* (submitted).

Harvey, J.A. (1996) Serotonergic regulation of associative learning. *Behavioral Brain Research*, **73**, 47–50.

Harvey, P. and Keefe, R. (1997) Cognitive impairment in schizophrenia and implications of atypical neuroleptic treatment. *CNS Spectrums*, **2**, 41–55.

Heresco-Levy, U., Javitt, D.C., Ermilov, M., Mordel, C., Horowitz, A. and Kelly, D. (1996) Double-blind, placebo-controlled, crossover trial of glycine adjuvant therapy for treatment-resistant schizophrenia. *British Journal of Psychiatry*, **169**, 610–617.

Heresco-Levy, U., Javitt, D.C., Ermilov, E., Mordel, C., Silipo, G. and Lichtenstein, M. (1999) Efficacy of high-dose glycine in the treatment of enduring negative symptoms of schizophrenia. *Archives of General Psychiatry*, **56**, 29–36.

Hoff, A.I., Riordan, H., O'Donnell, D.W., Morris, L. and DeLisi, L.E. (1992) Neuro-psychological functioning of first-episode schizophreniform patients? *American Journal of Psychiatry*, **149**, 898–903.

Hoff, A., Faustman, W., Wieneke, M., Espinoza, S., Costa, M., Wolkowitz, O. and Csernansky, J. (1996) The effect of clozapine on symptom reduction, neurocognitive function and clinical management in treatment refractory state hospital schizophrenic inpatients. *Neuropsychopharmacology*, **15**, 361–369.

Ikegaya, Y., Saito, H. and Abe, K. (1996) The basomedial and basolateral amygdaloid nuclei contribute to the induction of long-term potentiation in the dentate gyrus *in vivo*. *European Journal of Neuroscience*, **8**, 1833–1839.

Ikegaya, Y., Nakanishi, K., Saito, H. and Abe, K. (1997) Amygdala β-noradrenergic influence on hippocampal long-term potentiation *in vivo*. *NeuroReport*, **8**, 3143–3146.

Ingvar, D.H. and Franzen, G. (1974) Abnormalities in cerebral blood flow distribution in patients with chronic schizophrenia. *Acta Psychiatrica Scandinavica*, **50**, 425–462.

Ingvar, M., Ingerson, J., Davis, M., Granger, R., Kessler, M., Rogers, G.A., Schehr, R.S. and Lynch, G. (1997) Enhancement by an AMPAkine of memory encoding in humans. *Experimental Neurology*, **146**, 553–559.

Isaacson, J.S. and Nicoll, R.A. (1991) Aniracetam reduces glutamate receptor desensitization and slows the decay of fast excitatory synaptic currents in the hippocampus. *Proceedings of the National Academy of Sciences of the United States of America*, **88**, 10936–10940.

Izquierdo, I., Medina, J.H., Izquierdo, L.A., Barros, D.M., de-Souza, M.M. and Melo-e-Souza, T. (1998) Short and long-term memory are differentially regulated by mono-aminergic systems in the rat brain. *Neurobiology of Learning and Memory*, **69**, 219–224.

Javitt, D.C., Zylberman, I., Zukin, S.R., Heresco-Levy, U. and Lindenmayer, J.P. (1994) Amelioration of negative symptoms in schizophrenia by glycine? *American Journal of Psychiatry*, **151**, 1234–1236.

Jentsch, J., Redmond, D., Elsworth, J., Taylor, J., Youngren, K. and Roth, R. (1997) Enduring cognitive deficits and cortical dopamine dysfunction in monkeys after long term administration of phencyclidine. *Science*, **277**, 953–955.

Jones, R.W., Wesnes, K.A. and Kirby, J. (1991) Effects of NMDA modulation in scopolamine dementia. *Annals of the New York Academy of Science*, **640**, 241–244.

Kahn, R., Harvey, P., Davidson, M., Keefe, R., Apter, S., Neale, J. *et al.* (1994) Neuropsychological correlates of central monoamine function in chronic schizophrenia: relationship between CSF metabolites and cognitive function. *Schizophrenia Research*, **11**, 217–224.

Kawabe, K., Yoshihara, T., Ichitani, Y. and Iwasaki, T. (1998) Intrahippocampal D-cycloserine improves MK-801-induced memory deficits: radial arm maze performance in rats. *Brain Research*, **814**, 226–230.

Kemali, D., Del-Vecchio, M. and Maj, M. (1982) Increased noradrenaline levels in CSF and plasma of schizophrenic patients. *Biological Psychiatry*, **17**, 711–717.

Kim, J.S., Kornhuber, H.H., Schmid-Burgk, W. and Holzmuller, B. (1980) Low cerebrospinal fluid glutamate in schizophrenic patients and a new hypothesis on schizophrenia. *Neuroscience Letters*, **20**, 379–382.

Kobilka, B.K., Matsui, H., Kobilka, T.S., Yang-Feng, T.L., Caron, M.G., Lefkowitz, R.J. and Regan, J.W. (1987) Cloning and sequencing, and expression of the gene coding for the human platelet alpha-2 adrenergic receptor. *Science*, **238**, 650–656.

Kugler, J., Krauskoff, R., Seus, R., Brecht, H.M. and Raschig, A. (1980) Differences in psychic performance with guanfacine and clonidine in normotensive subjects. *Journal of Clinical Pharmacology*, **10**, 715–805.

Lake, C.R., Sternberg, D.E., van Kammen, D.P., Ballenger, J.C., Ziegler, M.G., Post, R.M., Kopin, I.J. and Bunney, W.E. (1980) Schizophrenia: elevated cerebrospinal fluid norepinephrine. *Science*, **207**, 331–333.

Larson, J., Lieu, T., Petchpradub, V., LeDuc, B., Ngo, H., Rogers, G.A. and Lynch, G. (1995) Facilitation of olfactory learning by a modulator of AMPA receptors. *Journal of Neuroscience*, **15**, 8023–8030.

Levey, A., Kitt, C., Simonds, W., Price, D. and Brann, M. (1991) Identification and localization of muscarinic acetylcholine receptor proteins in brain with subtype specific antibodies. *Journal of Neuroscience*, **11**, 3218–3226.

Lewis, D.A. (1992) The catecholaminergic innervation of primate prefrontal cortex. *Journal of Neural Transmission*, **36** (Suppl.), 179–200.

Lidow, M. and Goldman-Rakic, P. (1994) A common action of clozapine, haloperidol and remoxipride on D1 and D2 dopaminergic receptors in the primate cerebral cortex. *Proceedings of the National Academy of Sciences of the United States of America*, **91**, 4353–4356.

Lidow, M., Elsworth, J. and Goldman-Rakic, P. (1997) Down regulation of the D1 and D5 dopamine receptors in the primate PFC by chronic treatment with antipsychotic drugs. *Journal of Pharmacology and Experimental Therapeutics*, **281**, 597–603.

Lomasney, J.W., Lorenz, W., Allen, L.F., King, K., Regan, J.W., Yang-Feng, T.L., Caron, M., Lefkowitz, R.J. and Fremeau, R.T. (1990) Expansion of the α-2 adrenergic family: cloning and characterization of human α-2 adrenergic receptor subtype, the gene for which is located on chromosone 2. *Proceedings of the National Academy of Sciences of the United States of America*, **87**, 5094–5098.

Luby, E.D., Cohen, B.D., Rosenbaum, G., Gottlieb, J.S. and Kelley, R. (1959) Study of a new schizophrenomimetic drug—sernyl. *Archives of Neurological Psychiatry*, **81**, 363–369.

Lynch, G., Kessler, M., Rogers, G., Ambros-Ingerson, J., Granger, R. and Schehr, R.S. (1996)

Psychological effects of a drug that facilitates brain AMPA receptors. *International Clinical Psychopharmacology*, **11**, 13–19.

Lynch, G., Granger, R., Ambros-Ingerson, J., Davis, C.M., Kessler, M. and Schehr, R. (1997) Evidence that a positive modulator of AMPA-type glutamate receptors improves delayed recall in aged humans. *Experimental Neurology*, **145**, 89–92.

Mair, R.G. and McEntee, W.J. (1986) Cognitive enhancement in Korsakoff's psychosis by clonidine: a comparison with L-Dopa and ephedrine. *Psychopharmacology*, **88**, 374–380.

Malhotra, A.K., Pinals, D.A., Adler, C.M., Elman, I., Clifton, A., Pickar, D. and Breier, A. (1997) Ketamine-induced exacerbation of psychotic symptoms and cognitive impairment in neuroleptic-free schizophrenics. *Neuropsychopharmacology*, **17**, 141–150.

Mandel, R., Chen, A., Connor, D. and Thal, L. (1989) Continuous physostigmine infusion in rats with excitotoxic lesions of the nucleus basalis magnocellularis: effects on performance in the water maze task and cortical cholinergic markers. *Journal of Pharmacology and Experimental Therapeutics*, **251**, 612–619.

Mason, S.T. and Iversen, S.D. (1979) Theories of dorsal bundle extinction effects. *Brain Research Review*, **1**, 107–137.

McAlonan, G., Wilkinson, L., Robbins, T. and Everitt, B. (1995) The effects of AMPA-induced lesions of the septohippocampal cholinergic projection on aversive conditioning to explicit and contextual cues and spatial learning in the water maze. *European Journal of Neuroscience*, **7**, 281–292.

McGurk, S., Green, M., Wirshing, W., Ames, D., Marshall, B., Marder, S. *et al.* (1997) The effects of risperidol vs haloperidol in treatment-resistant schizophrenia: the trail making test. *CNS Spectrums*, **2**, 60–64.

Meek, W., Chuch, R., Wenk, G. and Olton, D. (1987) Nucleus basalis magnocellularis and medial septal area lesions differentially impair temporal memory. *Journal of Neuroscience*, **7**, 3505–3511.

Meyer, R.C., Knox, J., Purwin, D.A., Spangler, E.L. and Ingram, D.K. (1998) Combined stimulation of the glycine and polyamine sites of the NMDA receptor attenuates NMDA blockade-induced learning deficits of rats in a 14 unit T-maze. *Psychopharmacology (Berlin)*, **135**, 290–295.

Moffoot, A., O'Carroll, R.E., Murray, C., Dougall, N., Ebmeier, K. and Goodwin, G.M. (1994) Clonidine infusion increases uptake of 99mTc-exametazime in anterior cingulate cortex in Korsakoff's psychosis. *Pschological Medicine*, **24**, 53–61.

Miyamoto, M., Kato, J., Narumi, S. and Nagaoka, A. (1987) Characteristics in memory impairment following lesioning of the basal forebrain and septal nucleus in rats. *Brain Research*, **419**, 19–31.

Muir, J., Dunnett, S., Robbins, T. and Everitt, B. (1992) Attentional functions of the forebrain cholinergic systems: effects of intraventricular hemicholinium, physostigmine, basal cortical lesions and intracortical grafts on a multiple choice serial reaction time task. *Experimental Brain Research*, **89**, 611–622.

Murphy, B.L., Arnsten, A.F.T., Goldman-Rakic, P.S. and Roth, R.H. (1996) Increased dopamine turnover in the prefrontal cortex impairs spatial working memory performance in rats and monkeys. *Proceedings of the National Academy of Sciences of the United States of America*, **93**, 1325–1329.

Myhrer, T., Johannesen, T.S. and Spikkerud, E. (1993) Restoration of mnemonic function in rats with glutamatergic temporal systems disruption: dose and time of glycine injections. *Pharmacology, Biochemistry and Behavior*, **45**, 519–525.

Nuechterlein, K.H. and Dawson, M.E. (1984) Information processing and attentional functioning in the developmental course of schizophrenic disorders. *Schizophrenia Bulletin*, **10**, 160–200.

Nicholas, A.P., Pieribone, V. and Hokfelt, T. (1993) Distribution of mRNAs for α-2 adrenergic receptor subtypes in rat brain: an *in situ* hybridization study. *Journal of Comparative Neurology*, **328**, 575–594.

Nielsen, J., Mena, A., Williams, I., Nocerini, M. and Liston, D. (1989) Correlation of brain levels of 9-amino-1,2,3,4-tetrahydroacridine (THA) with neurochemical and behavioral changes. *European Journal of Pharmacology*, **173**, 53–64.

Okubo, Y., Suhara, T., Suzuki, K., Kobayashi, K., Inoue, O., Terasaki, O. *et al.* (1997) Decreased prefrontal dopamine D1 receptors in schizophrenia revealed by PET. *Nature*, **385**, 634–636.

Olney, J.W. (1989) Excitatory amino acids and neuropsychiatric disorders. *Biological Psychiatry*, **26**, 505–525.

Packard, M.G. and Teather, L.A. (1997) Posttraining injections of MK-801 produce a time-dependent impairment of memory in two water maze tasks. *Neurobiology of Learning and Memory*, **68**, 42–50.

Page, K., Everitt, B., Robbins, T., Marston, H. and Wilkinson, L. (1991) Dissociable effects on spatial maze and passive avoidance acquisition and retention following AMPA- and ibotenic acid-induced excitotoxic lesions of the basal forebrain in rats: diffrential dependence on cholinergic neuronal loss. *Neuroscience*, **43**, 457–472.

Park, S. and Holtzman, P. (1992) Schizophrenics show spatial working memory deficits. *Archives of General Psychiatry*, **49**, 975–982.

Potkin, S.G., Costa, J., Roy, S., Sramek, J., Jin, Y. and Gulasekaram, B. (1992) Glycine in the treatment of schizophrenia: theory and preliminary results, In: Meltzer, H.Y. (ed.), *Novel Antipsychotic Drugs*. Raven Press, New York, pp. 179–188.

Powchik, P., Davidson, M., Haroutunian, V., Gabriel, S.M., Purohit, D.P., Perl, D.P., Harvey, P.D. and Davis, K.L. (1998) Postmortem studies in schizophrenia. *Schizophrenia Bulletin*, **24**, 325–341.

Raskind, M.A., Peskind, E.R., Halter, J.B. and Jimerson, D.C. (1984) Norepinephrine and MHPG levels in CSF and plasma in Alzheimer's disease. *Archives of General Psychiatry*, **4**, 343–344.

Regan, J.W., Kobilka, T.S., Yang-Feng, T.L., Caron, M.G., Lefkowitz, R.J. and Kobilka, B.K. (1988) Cloning and expression of a human kidney cDNA for an α-2 adrenergic receptor subtype. *Proceedings of the National Academy of Sciences of the United States of America*, **85**, 6301–6305.

Reis, D.J., Granata, A.R., Joh, T.H., Ross, C.A., Ruggiero, D.A. and Park, D.H. (1984) Brain stem catecholamine mechanisms in tonic and reflex control of blood pressure. *Hypertension*, **6**, 7–15.

Robbins, T., Everitt, B., Marston, H., Wilkinson, J., Jones, G. and Page, K. (1989) Comparative effects of ibotenic acid and quisqualic acid-induced lesions of the substantia innominata on attentional function in the rat: further implications for the role of the cholinergic neurons of the nucleus basalis in cognitive processes. *Behavioral Brain Research*, **35**, 221–240.

Roberts, R.B., Flexner, J.B. and Flexner, L.B. (1970) Some evidence for the involvement of adrenergic sites in the memory trace. *Proceedings of the National Academy of Sciences of the United States of America*, **66**, 310–313.

Rogers, S., Doody, R. and Mohs, R. (1996) E2020 produces both clinical global and cognitive test improvement in patients with mild to moderately severe Alzheimer's disease: results of a 30 week phase III trial [abstract]. *Neurology*, **46** (Suppl.), A217.

Rosenbaum, G., Cohen, B.D., Luby, E.D., Gottlieb, J.S. and Yelen, D. (1959) Comparison of sernyl with other drugs: simulation of schizophrenic performance with sernyl, LSD-25, and amobarital (amytal), I: attention, motor function, and proprioception. *Archives of General Psychiatry*, **1**, 651–656.

Rosse, R.B., Thuet, S.K. and Banay-Schwartz, M. (1989) Glycine adjuvant therapy to conventional neuroleptic treatment in schizophrenia: an open label pilot study *Clinical Neuropharmacology*, **12**, 416–424.

Rosse, R.B., Schwartz, B.L., Davis, R.E. and Deutsch, S.I. (1991) An NMDA intervention strategy in schizophrenia with 'low dose' milacemide. *Clinical Neuropharmacology*, **14**, 268–272.

Routsalainen, S., Sirvio, J., Jakala, P., Puumala, T., MacDonald, E. and Riekkinen, P., Sr (1997) Differential effects of three 5HT receptor antagonists on the performance of rats in attentional and working memory tasks. *European Neuropsychopharmacology*, **7**, 99–108.

Rupniak, N., Spencer, T. and Field, M. (1997) Enhanced performance of spatial and visual memory tasks by the selective acetylcholinesterase inhibitor E2020 in rhesus monkeys. *Psychopharmacology*, **131**, 406–410.

Sara, S.J. and Herve-Minvielle, A. (1995) Inhibitory influence of frontal cortex on locus coeruleus. *Proceedings of the National Academy of Sciences of the United States of America*, **92**, 6032–6036.

Sawaguchi, T. and Goldman-Rakic, P.S. (1991) D1 dopamine receptors in prefrontal cortex: involvement in working memory. *Science*, **251**, 947–950.

Sawaguchi, T. and Goldman-Rakic, P.S. (1994) The role of D1-dopamine receptor in working memory: local injections of dopamine antagonists into the prefrontal cortex of rhesus monkeys performing an oculomotor delayed-response task. *Journal of Neurophysiology*, **71**, 515–528.

Sawaguchi, T., Matsumura, M. and Kubota, K. (1988) Dopamine enhances the neuronal activity of spatial short term memory task in the primate prefrontal cortex. *Neuroscience Research*, **5**, 465–473.

Saykin, A., Shtasel, D., Gur, R., Kester, D., Mozley, L., Stafiniak, P. *et al.* (1994) Neuropsycholoigcal deficits in neuroleptic naïve patients with first-episode schizophrenia. *Archives of General Psychiatry*, **51**, 124–131.

Scheinin, M., Lomasney, J.W., Hayden-Hixson, D.M., Schambra, U.B., Caron, M.G., Lefkowitz, R.J. and Fremeau, R.T. (1994) Distribution of α-2 adrenergic receptor subtype gene expression in rat brain. *Molecular Brain Research*, **21**, 133–149.

Schneider, J.S., Sun, Z.Q. and Roeltgen, D.P. (1994) Effects of dihydrexidine, a full dopamine receptor D-1 receptor agonist, on delayed response performance in chronic low dose MPTP-treated monkeys. *Brain Research*, **663**, 140–144.

Schwartz, B.L., Hashtroudi, S., Herting, R.L., Handerson, H. and Deutsch, S.I. (1991) Glycine prodrug facilitates memory retrieval in humans. *Neurology*, **41**, 1341–1343.

Seidman, L., Pepple, J., Faraone, S. *et al.* (1993) Neuropsychological performance in chronic schizophrenia in response to neuroleptic dose reduction. *Biological Psychiatry*, **33**, 575–584.

Serper, M.R. and Chou, J.C. (1997) Novel neuroleptics improve attentional functioning in schizophrenic patients: ziprasidone and aripiprazole. *CNS Spectrums*, **2**, 56–59.

Shors, T.J., Sefvatius, R.J., Thonpson, R.F., Rogers, G. and Lynch, G. (1994) Facilitation of classical conditioning through enhanced glutamatergic transmission. *Neuroscience Letters*, **186**, 1–4.

Simon, H., Scatton, B. and LeMoal, M. (1980) Dopaminergic A10 neurones are involved in cognitive functions. *Nature*, **286**, 150–151.

Sitaram, N., Weingarten, H. and Gillin, J. (1978) Human serial learning: enhancement with arecholine and choline and impairment with scopolamine. *Science*, **201**, 274–276.

Staubli, U., Perez, Y., Xu, F.B., Rogers, G., Ingvar, M., Stone-Elander, S. and Lynch, G. (1994a) Centrally active modulators of glutamate receptors facilitate the induction of long-term potentiation *in vivo*. *Proceedings of the National Academy of Sciences of the United States of America*, **91**, 11158–11162.

Staubli, U., Rogers, G. and Lynch, G. (1994b) Facilitation of glutamate receptors enhances memory. *Proceedings of the National Academy of Sciences of the United States of America*, **91**, 777–781.

Steele, T., Hodges, D., Levesque, T., Locke, K. and Sandage, B. (1996) The D1 agonist dihydrexidine releases acetylcholine and improves cognition in rats. *Annals of the New York Academy of Sciences*, **777**, 427–430.

Stein, L. and Wise, C.D. (1971) Possible etiology of schizophrenia: progressive damage to the noradrenergic reward system by 5-hydroxydopamine. *Science*, **171**, 1032–1036.

Stein, L., Belluzzi, J.D. and Wise, C.D. (1975) Memory enhancement by central administration of norepinephrine. *Brain Research*, **84**, 329–335.

Summers, W., Majovski, L., Marsh, G., Tachiki, K. and Kling, A. (1986) Oral tetrahydro-aminoacridine in long term treatment of senile dementia Alzheimer type. *New England Journal of Medicine*, **315**, 1241–1245.

Tam, S.-Y. and Roth, R. (1985) Selective increases in dopamine metabolism in the prefrontal cortex by the anxiogenic β-carboline FG7142. *Biochemical Pharmacology*, **34**, 1595–1598.

Tamlyn, D., McKenna, P.J., Mortimer, A., Lund, C., Hammond, S. and Beddeley, A. (1992) Memory impairment in schizophrenia: its extent, affiliations and neuropsychological character. *Psychological Medicine*, **12**, 564–571.

Thierry, A.M., Tassin, J.P., Glanc, G. and Glowinski, J. (1976) Selective activation of the mesocortical DA system by stress. *Nature*, **263**, 242–244.

Tsai, G., Passani, L.A., Slusher, B.S., Carter, L., Baer, L., Kleinman, J.E. and Coyle, J.T. (1995) Abnormal excitatory neurotransmitter metabolism in schizophrenic brains. *Archives of General Psychiatry*, **52**, 829–836.

Uhlen, S., Muceniece, R., Rangel, N., Tiger, G. and Wikberg, J. (1995) Comparison of the binding activities of some drugs on α-2A, α-2B, and α-2C-adrenoreceptors and non-adrenergic imidazoline sites in the guinea pig. *Pharmacology and Toxicology*, **76**, 353–364.

van Kammen, D.P., Peters, J., van Kammen, W.B., Nugent, A., Goetz, K.L., Yao, J. and Linnoila, M. (1989a) CSF norepinephrine in schizophrenia is elevated prior to relapse after haloperidol withdrawal. *Biological Psychiatry*, **26**, 176–188.

van Kammen, D.P., Peters, J.L., van Kammen, W.B., Rosen, J., Yao, J.K., McAdam, D. and Linnoila, M, (1989b) Clonidine treatment of schizophrenia: can we predict treatment response? *Psychiatry Research*, **27**, 297–311.

van Kammen, D.P., Peters, J., Yao, J., van Kammen, W.B., Neylan, T., Shaw, D. and Linnoala, M. (1990) Norepinephrine in acute exacerbations of chronic schizophrenia. *Archives of General Psychiatry*, **47**, 161–168.

van Stegeren, A.H., Everaerd, W., Cahill, L., McGaugh, J.L. and Gooren, L.J. (1998) Memory for emotional events: differential effects of centrally versus peripherally acting beta-blocking agents. *Psychopharmacvology (Berlin)*, **138**, 305–310.

Verdoux, H., Magnin, E. and Bourgeois. M. (1995) Neuroleptic effect on neuropsychological test performance in schizophrenia. *Schizophrenia Research*, **14**, 133–139.

Vitiello, B., Martin, A., Hill, J., Mack, C., Molchan, S., Martinez, R., Murphy, D.L. and Sunderland, T. (1997) Cognitive and behavioral effects of cholinergic, dopaminergic, and serotonergic blockade in humans. *Neuropsychopharmacology*, **16**, 15–24.

Vyklicky, L., Jr, Patneau, D.K. and Mayer, M.L. (1991) Modulation of excitatory synaptic transmission by drugs that reduce desensitization of AMPA/kainate receptors. *Neuron*, **7**, 971–984.

Wanibuchi, F., Nishida, T., Yamashita, H., Hikada, K., Koshiya, K., Tsukamoto, S. *et al.* (1994) Characterization of a novel muscarinic receptor agonist, YM796: comparison with cholinesterase inhibitors in *in-vivo* pharmacological studies. *European Journal of Pharmacology*, **265**, 151–158.

Watanabe, M., Kodama, T. and Hikosaka, K. (1997) Increase in extracellular dopamine in the primate prefrontal cortex during a working memory task. *Journal of Neurophysiology*, **78**, 2795–2798.

Weinberger, D.R., Berman, K.F. and Zec, R.F. (1986) Physiologic dysfunction of dorsolateral prefrontal cortex in schizophrenia. I. Regional cerebral blood flow evidence. *Archives of General Psychiatry*, **43**, 114–124.

Weinberger, D.R., Berman, K,F. and Illowsky, B.P. (1988) Physiologic dysfunction of dorsolateral prefrontal cortex in schizophrenia. II. A new cohort and evidence for a monoaminergic mechanism. *Archives of General Psychiatry*, **45**, 609–615.

Welsh, S.E., Romano, A.G. and Harvey, J.A. (1998) Effect of serotonin 5HT(2A/2C) antagonists on associative learning in the rat. *Psychopharmacology*, **137**, 157–163.

Wester, P., Bengstrom, U., Eriksson, A., Gezelius, C., Hardy, J. and Winblod, B. (1990) Ventricular CSF monoamine transmitter and metabolite concentrations reflect human brain neurochemistry in autopsy cases. *Journal of Neurochemistry*, **54**, 1148–1156.

Williams, G.V. and Goldman-Rakic, P.S. (1995) Modulation of memory fields by dopamine D1 receptors in prefrontal cortex. *Nature*, **376**, 572–575.

Winkler, J., Suhr, S., Gage, F., Thal, L. and Fisher, L. (1995) Essential role of neocortical acetylcholine in spatial memory. *Nature*, **375**, 484–487.

Woolf, N. and Butcher, L. (1989) Cholinergic systems: synopsis of anatomy and overview of physiology and pathology. In: *The Biological Substrates of Alzheimer's Disease*. Academic Press, New York, pp. 73–86.

Yasuda, R., Ciesla, W., Flores, L., Wall, S., Li, M., Satkus, S. *et al*. (1993) Development of antisera selective for m4 and m5 muscarinic cholinergic receptors: distribution of m4 and m5 receptors in the rat brain. *Molecular Pharmacology*, **43**, 149–157.

Youngren, K., Moghaddam, B., Bunney, B. and Roth, R. (1994) Preferential activation of dopamine overflow in prefrontal cortex produced by chronic clozapine treatment. *Neuroscience Letters*, **165**, 41–44.

17 Cognitive rehabilitation and remediation in schizophrenia

Til Wykes

Every man is born with a live computer of limitless possibilities but without the instruction manual. The most important job of science today is to draw up that manual. Machado (1980)

Introduction

The whole of this book is devoted to persuading its readership of the importance of problems of cognition to the disorder of schizophrenia. Not only is cognitive deficit part of current definitions of the disorder, but its severity is also predictive of future service use. Our patients also consider cognition as important. They describe problems with concentrating on simple everyday tasks not only at the time of an acute exacerbation of the illness but also between episodes. These problems may be so severe that they affect every aspect of their life. However, only recently has the focus of treatment development been on changing the cognitive disability itself rather than reducing the symptoms of schizophrenia, although in the UK these too are being changed through cognitive behavioral approaches (Wykes *et al.*, 1998)

There is also a wealth of evidence on the influence of these deficits on current and future social functioning (Wykes and Dunn, 1992; Green, 1996) and in treatment outcome (Mueser *et al.*, 1991). They also have a role in vulnerability–stress models in the prediction of both the onset and recurrence of the disorder (Nuechterlein *et al.*, 1994). Recently, Michael Green has suggested that neurocognitive deficits, unlike symptoms, are directly related to functioning outcomes. This accounts for the paucity of predictive relationships between the symptoms of psychosis and future outcome, particularly in the more chronic populations of patients (Green, 1998). If the deficits could be reduced, there are obvious benefits to both the patients and the psychiatric services. For patients, there is the likelihood of an increase in quality of life both through the direct effect of improved cognition and also because of the chance of making faster and more advantageous gains via other psychological treatments such as social skills training. For the psychiatric services, there is the likelihood that reductions in deficits could reduce relapse rates and the need for expensive and continuing psychiatric support. However, as will be seen from this chapter, the research program on the direct effects of psychological rehabilitation on cognition is in its infancy. There are few examples of well controlled clinical trials but plenty of laboratory studies which show optimistic results. The chapter will concentrate only on psychological programs and is organized into four sections which deal with issues of importance to cognitive remediation research and outcomes. These are:

- Which deficits should be the targets of intervention?
- What is cognitive remediation or rehabilitation?
- How successful are current remediation programs?
- What factors should be considered for the next set of remediation studies?

Which deficits should be the targets of intervention?

This is clearly the key to success. If the target is the reduction of positive symptoms, then we would try to change those cognitive processes which are thought to be linked to symptoms. These can be direct links, where the cognitive deficit 'causes' symptoms, as in Chris Frith's formulation (Frith, 1992). Alternatively, there may be indirect links via the attributional style of our patients which can be altered so that the severity of delusional beliefs and the interpretation of abnormal perceptual experiences change (e.g. Kuipers *et al.*, 1997). There is also a link in terms of vulnerability indicators for symptoms in the vulnerability–stress model (Nuechterlein and Dawson, 1984). In this formulation, the cognitive deficits which are of most interest are those which are predictive of symptom onset or exacerbation (mediating or stable factors), rather than ones which are only deficient within an episode (episodic factors). If the key outcome is positive symptom reduction, then stable and/or mediating factors should be the targets. Stable factors in the vulnerability–stress model of schizophrenia are those deficits which are present probably pre-onset of the disorder. Despite this, they are not necessarily immutable but may need special sorts of remediation programs.

In addition to these more direct effects of cognitive deficits, there are indirect effects via other processes such as treatment adherence and models of illness. Cognitive deficits have been reported to be related to insight, with the majority of studies showing that people with better skills have more insight (e.g. Lysaker and Bell, 1994). However, there is an intriguing study reported by Startup (1996) which suggests that there is a curvilinear relationship, with both high and low functioning patients showing poor insight. Insight is associated with treatment adherence, so cognitive deficits can affect symptoms indirectly.

An alternative strategy would be to choose those cognitive deficits which are clearly linked to poor outcome, as suggested by Green (1993, 1996). The focus of attention would then be on the disability produced by the disorder. However, the deficits which predict outcome have only recently become the focus of attention and are not well described in the literature. There are several explanations of the route of the predictive link. Cognitive deficits may interfere with learning so that patients have difficulty in taking part in traditional rehabilitation procedures (e.g. Mueser *et al.*, 1991; Wykes, 1994). Cognitive deficits could also interfere directly with social perception and so reduce the effectiveness of communication and action (Penn *et al.*, 1996; Bryson *et al.*, 1997).

Cognitive disabilities which contribute to functional outcomes would at least impact on independent living and quality of life and also the cost of care. They may also be outcomes which are measurable in the short term. The effects of improved cognitive capacities on symptoms may be too distant, i.e. they may increase the survival time before a relapse which is only measurable after several years. The evidence on the specific deficits associated with functional outcomes is relatively weak as studies have generally tested few cognitive variables and there are few replications of positive findings (Green, 1996). Because the majority of studies only use a single measure of any deficit, it is also not yet clear whether it is the measure or the underlying putative cognitive operation which is important in the predictive relationship. Clearly there is a need for more longitudinal research, but, in the meantime, one approach to targeting is to combine the predictive data with information on the pattern of deficits found in people with schizophrenia. The most commonly reported are the executive functions, most of which are reduced often in the context of average IQ in many patients (e.g. Evans *et al.*, 1997). Executive functioning describes the way in which information is controlled and processed (Shallice, 1988). These abilities are essential in controlling action in a number of different situations, for example in planning and decision making, error correction and for novel responses. The three main areas which have come under scrutiny are working memory, planning and cognitive flexibility. Descriptions of these deficits are given in Chapters 2, 3 and 4 of this volume and so will not be described in detail here. However, as an illustration of their pervasiveness, Morice and Delahunty (1996) in a small study of a group of remitted patients living in the community found that 94% had a deficit in at least one of the three components of executive function. The reason for suggesting that these deficits are targeted is threefold: (i) they are prevalent within groups of patients across the spectrum of severity and chronicity; (ii) they have been linked to functioning outcomes (Jaeger and Douglas, 1992); and (iii) they appear to be cognitive capacities with high face validity for performing everyday tasks.

What is cognitive remediation or rehabilitation?

The term remediate has been confusing in the literature. The *Oxford Dictionary* defines it as 'to make good' or 'to rectify'. In other words, it means to correct an underlying impairment. However, this does not determine the underlying process by which the impairment is 'corrected'. The following categorization is based on a distinction made by Spaulding *et al.* (1998). Remediation follows from: (i) developing new skills which replace or compensate for lost ones; (ii) impaired processes undergoing repair during therapy; and (iii) facilitating a naturally occurring recovery process. All three possibilities imply a durability of improvements, particularly for categories (ii) and (iii). The word 'rehabilitation' has different meanings from remediation in the field of psychiatry. The best definition is that we aim to provide the 'minimum level of support for our patients which achieves the maximum level of independence'. This may mean providing high levels of supervision continuously, in other words the aim is not necessarily to produce a cure. Cognitive remediation programs could also be devised to train or re-train cognitive capacities in general or specific skills.

So where the focus of a service is the remediation and rehabilitation of cognitive deficits, the goal would be to produce both lasting improvement in the deficits themselves and support in the areas of continuing weakness. This might mean continued treatment analogous to drug treatment for psychosis. In addition, this implies that rehabilitation programs should be devised which build on an individual's cognitive strengths not their weaknesses.

How successful are current remediation programs?

Cognitive remediation has been investigated sporadically over a number of years. Steffy and Galbraith (1980) found that monetary reward and verbal encouragement were effective in improving reaction time. Adams *et al.* (1981) in a single case study showed improvements in attention after a graduated program of distraction training, and Koh and Peterson (1978) showed that when patients with schizophrenia were provided with an encoding strategy their memory improved. However, only recently has there been a persistent effort to investigate the process and success of remediation techniques. There are two main ways in which they have been tested. The first group of studies were those in the laboratory where the aim of the remediation was to improve performance on individual tests and to test the durability of the training procedure. The second set of studies were performed in clinical settings where the aim was to improve performance across a number of different tests which was not only durable but which also generalized to everyday performance.

Laboratory studies

The studies appearing under this heading concentrate on the rehabilitation of a single task or component of a task and they are never integrated into general rehabilitation services. The studies are useful because they identify features which are important in the teaching of new skills. Unfortunately, many studies combine several features in one intervention and so it is difficult to untangle the key processes involved, but by a process of iteration we may be able to describe those that have potential for future programs.

The majority (but not all) of the studies reviewed in this section have focused on a single task, the Wisconsin Card Sorting Test (WCST). One of the reasons for this was that it had been proposed that the performance of patients with schizophrenia on this task was not amenable to change as a result of a fundamental deficit in the frontal lobe (e.g. Goldberg *et al.*, 1987). The challenge for researchers was therefore to test this proposition by inventing novel ways to improve performance.

In the WCST, cards containing stimuli which differ in a number of conceptual categories are sorted. Participants have to sort according to a rule which they have to guess from the feedback they are given from the test administrator. During the test, the sorting rule is also changed and the participants then have to detect the new rule. Again the only information they have is the responses of the test administrator which are in the form of 'correct' or 'incorrect'. Several different cognitive operations are thought to be involved in the performance of the test. Participants have to remember the initial task instructions, be able to perceive the differences between the conceptual categories, initiate a particular strategy and monitor their performance on this strategy and be able to modify their plan using feedback from the administrator. Patients with schizophrenia seem to have problems in all these areas of cognition. Their performance is often poor because they take a large number of trials before reaching their first category. They also perseverate on particular responses despite feedback that their behavior is incorrect. In addition, they fail to generate categories on which they score 10 correct responses.

The other tasks briefly reviewed in this section include ones involving memory (O'Carroll *et al.*, 1999) and attention training (Benedict *et al.*, 1994; Medalia *et al.*, 1998). The aim of this section was to provide a brief overview of the types of programs that have been used; therefore, the papers cited are illustrations rather than a complete literature search. The list below is a description of the sorts of training used in these studies. Again this is not an exhaustive list but contains what the current author considers to be the key interventions.

Card by card instruction

The learning support for participants using this technique is total. Patients are first told the rules of the task and then they are given didactic instructions on every trial. These take the form of reminding the learner of the category which is being sorted, telling them that they must ignore other categories, describing the card to be sorted in terms of the matching rule and then allowing the learner to respond. The learner is then given feedback on the correctness of the sort on that trial and error correction.

Didactic training

In didactic training, the learner is told the rules underlying the task with examples of each of the rules. The learner is then asked to complete some trials with each of the rules and the instructor provides prompting, feedback and error correction. The learner is reminded of the rules again at specific times during the task. This process differs from card by card instruction because it only occurs at specific time points and there are more practice trials during instruction which receive error correction.

Monetary reinforcement

The basis for promoting tangible reinforcement is that the motivation of patients with schizophrenia to take part in rehabilitation programs is poor (although who can blame them when they are being asked to sort packs of cards endlessly). Tangible reinforcers are thought to be more powerful than social reinforcers and may therefore aid patients to attend to the task throughout the procedures. The complication of this sort of reinforcer as pointed out by Vollema *et al.* (1995) is that patients may be distracted by the monetary reinforcement or have difficulty with information overload when it is coupled with other interventions such as didactic training.

Verbalization action criteria

The main aid used in these tasks has been the overt verbalization of the task instructions and/or the specific rule being followed for each trial. This is an extension of the pioneering work carried out by Meichenbaum and Cameron (1973). These authors improved non-delusional speech and increased activities by a simple program. The therapist repeated the instructions then the learner repeated the same instructions overtly and finally the learner repeated them covertly. It may be that this process aids patients in two separate ways. First, it provides memory support for those patients who experience explicit memory difficulties by increasing rehearsal strategies. However, secondly, some patients have problems in the initiation of tasks either because they are initiated without a clear plan (Morris *et al.*, 1995) or because patients have problems in error detection and self-monitoring. Both these problems are reduced when the task is paced (i.e. the response is not initiated until the plan is explicit), and errors can be detected prior to response execution.

Simplifying the task

It was thought that reducing the complexity of the task would aid the learning of task components. It was a modification generally used in conjunction with scaffolding instruction.

Scaffolding and errorless learning

Scaffolding is a form of instruction derived from Vygotsky (1962) in the 1930s. It is based on the instructor extending the learner's ability on a task by providing aid only on those aspects where the learner has difficulty but allowing the learner to use competencies which have already been achieved. The complexity of the problems facing the learner is carefully controlled so that he or she has a high potential for solving the problem. This means of instruction is also focused on the individual and their own rate of progress through a task. The instructor's role is to draw the learner's attention to key task features and through Socratic dialog to help the learner to generate solutions to the problems. The instructor also helps the learner to monitor performance and to attribute gains to their own efforts.

Scaffolding is similar to errorless learning, which was derived from work on teaching pigeons what for them is an extremely difficult discrimination, i.e. to peck only when faced with a red light not a green light. Terrace (1963) achieved this by teaching pigeons to peck on a red light and then over time faded the light into green but prevented the pigeon from making the error of pressing when the wrong light was illuminated. This technique has been used with people who have severe learning disabilities where it is often referred to as backward chaining. A similar technique has been suggested by Baddeley and Wilson (1994) to teach patients with severe memory problems following brain injury. They suggest that errorless approaches may be effective because errors are remembered implicitly and interfere with the target items to be remembered. The effectiveness of the technique was thought to depend on implicit rather than explicit memory, but recent evidence from Hunkin *et al.* (1998) has attributed improvements not to intact implicit memory but to residual explicit memory functioning. However, for whatever reasons, errorless learning does seem to work with patients who have poor memory ability.

The difference between scaffolding and errorless learning is the emphasis on the subject's own attempts to solve the problem. This is likely to improve self-esteem and enhance self-efficacy which are all helpful to the learning process and may also be the key factors which allow generalization of learning to other tasks (see discussion below on the role of self-esteem).

Table 17.1 shows a brief review of the main studies in this area, with a breakdown of the techniques used. In order to simplify the table, only broad categories of interventions are cited and there may be differences in the specific regimes adopted by studies falling into the same instructional column. Several studies also adopted a number of different techniques and, to make matters more confusing, some studies employed more than one type of instruction within a single remediation program and more rarely as a comparison group. The only study to investigate several different techniques in comparison with each other was carried out by Rossell and David (1997) but there were only three subjects in each condition, making it difficult to draw generalizable conclusions from their results. The list of differences between study samples is also long, but, despite these differences, a success rate was calculated as the proportion of studies producing a successful outcome with a particular technique. This at least gives a rough estimate of the usefulness of each technique for future clinical programs.

As can be seen from Table 17.1, there are some successes for all types of training, although the success for the most highly supportive instruction, card by card training, may be achieved only when given in conjunction with monetary reinforcement. The most promising studies seem to be those involving errorless learning, scaffolding and verbalization techniques, although none of these have been tested in many studies. However, this effect has some face validity because both errorless learning and scaffolding involve some 'learning effort' by the participants, which is known to aid learning (Wood, 1998). Verbalization techniques as well as reducing verbal memory requirements also aid monitoring of continued strategy use. You cannot verbalize a strategy unless you have first deduced it.

Few of the studies test the durable effects of training or the generalization of the training effects to other tasks, so it is not clear whether any of the concepts required for completing the WCST are actually being taught (Goldberg and Weinberger, 1994; Keefe, 1995). However, there are some studies which do show durability of learning, and this is extremely important for cognitive remediation. Patients with schizophrenia in these studies have not acted like those with brain injuries. It has been possible to maintain improvements over a follow-up period, whereas in many studies of the brain-injured once the support is removed performance returns to baseline.

Clinical studies

In contrast to the laboratory studies of instruction, in this set of studies a wide range of tasks or component cognitive skills are taught. The key idea is that changes in cognitive performance not only will lead to improved cognitive ability but will also lead to improvements in social functioning. This is an eminently sensible aim as improvements on the WCST alone have little face validity to our patients. Training elements from the laboratory studies are often involved in these more comprehensive programs, although there is also an emphasis on the practice and rehearsal of specific cognitive abilities. All the programs consist of a number of different types of training tools including paper and pencil activities, computerized activities

Table 17.1 Types of instruction used in recent laboratory studies of cognitive remediation

	Card by card instruction	Didactic teaching	Monetary reward	Simplify task	Verbalize action criteria	Errorless learning	Scaffolding	Practice on similar tests
Goldberg et al. (1987)								
Benedict and Harris (1989)								
Bellack et al. (1990)		*						
Summerfelt et al. (1991)			*					
Green et al. (1992)	*							
Goldman et al. (1992)		*						
Metz et al. (1994)		**						
Benedict et al. (1994)								
Kern et al. (1996)						**		
Bellack et al. (1996)		*						
Green et al. (1997??)					*			
Stratta et al. (1994)								
Vollema et al. (1995)		**						
Young and Freyslinger (1995)							**	
Field et al. (1997)								
Medalia et al. (1998)								*
O'Carroll et al. (1999)				*	*	*	*	
Rossell and David (1997)							*	
Proportion successful	1/3	6/7	1/5	1/2	2/2	2/2	3/3	1/4

*Some training effect shown on withdrawal of instructional technique.

**Training effect and some evidence of durability of training over the following days or weeks.

Table 17.2 Characteristics of clinical programs

	Group or individual treatment	Computerized	Scaffolding or didactic	Integration into rehabilitation programs	Errorless
Brenner et al. (1994)	Group	No	Didactic	Yes	No
Van der Gaag (1992)	Individual	No	Didactic	No	No
Hermanutz and Gestrich (1991)	Individual	Computer assisted	?	No	No
Olbrich and Mussgay (1990)	Individual	No	?	No	No
Delahunty et al. (1993)	Individual	No	Scaffolding	No	Yes
Spaulding et al. (1998)	Group	No	Didactic	Yes	No
Wykes et al. (1999)	Individual	No	Scaffolding	No	Yes

and group activities. Table 17.2 gives a brief overview of the more common programs with their main instructional elements.

One of the first clinical programs was developed by Hans Brenner in Bern and is called Integrated Psychological Therapy (IPT; Brenner *et al.*, 1994). IPT involves a number of different sub-programs only one of which focuses on cognitive abilities. Activities are run in a group format where training is didactic. Controlled studies of this approach have produced variable results, but most do show improvements in cognitive functioning although there is little support for the subsequent effects on social skills (Brenner *et al.*, 1994). In fact, more recent evaluations have suggested that it is not possible to conclude that cognitive improvements are specific to the cognitive sub-program rather than the remaining psychosocial sub-programs (Hodel and Brenner, 1994).

In a tightly controlled study, Spaulding and colleagues in Nebraska have addressed the problem of the specificity of cognitive interventions and have tried to tease out the specific effects of the sub-program. Their results do suggest a specific effect of the cognitive sub-program on improvements in social skills, although improvements in cognitive functioning seem to result from non-specific effects of the therapy (Spaulding *et al.*, 1998). More recent analyses have suggested a direct effect of improvements in social competence with improvements on card sorting and that improvements in verbal memory were associated with improved psychosocial skill acquisition (Spaulding *et al.*, 1999). Van der Gaag (1992) also tested a program derived from the work of Brenner and colleagues, but with a stronger dependence on experimental research, on the deficits of people with schizophrenia and individual training. He found some improvements, but only in those patients who had a predominantly negative symptom picture who learned to process information more elaborately.

Many other programs have used training materials, some of which are presented on a computer, which are derived from the rehabilitation of people with acquired brain injury. It is not clear what instructional method is the basis of these programs, apart from the restoration of function by practice. The results are mixed, although there are reports of improvements on both elementary and more complex processing (Olbrich and Mussgay, 1990; Hermanutz and Gestrich, 1991).

A third program was derived from a theoretical analysis of the deficits of people with schizophrenia in a similar way to the training tasks devised by Van der Gaag (1992). The program consists of three separate modules, cognitive flexibility, working memory and planning, although some of the tasks are similar across modules (Delahunty and Morice, 1993). The program is implemented on an individual basis, with the main instructional technique being scaffolding, but other techniques were also included such as practice on tasks, instruction on mnemonic techniques and encouragement of self-monitoring of errors. In addition, an errorless approach was adopted as much as possible. The tasks mostly use paper and pencils which are very easy at the outset but are graded so that they introduce complexity very slowly. The program is set at the learner's own pace. Reinforcement is given throughout in the form of praise or the instructor drawing the learner's attention to task improvements and individual efficacy. The tasks in the cognitive flexibility module provide patients with practice in engagement, disengagement and re-engagement activities for a particular cognitive set. For instance, they are given a page with a set of numbers on it and are asked to cross off the odd or even numbers. This requires them to maintain a set but also to shift set when requested. The Working Memory module requires the person to maintain two sets of information simultaneously and to carry out transformations on a held information set. There is an emphasis here on categorizing and chunking information as well as some self-instructional training in the use of mnemonic strategies. The Planning module consists of tasks in which the participant has to plan a sequence of moves in order to acquire a goal. The emphasis in this module is to organize information and to create and use sub-goals. The role of the therapist is to encourage the person to think of their own strategies for solving the task, but they may provide options if necessary. The therapist might also demonstrate the task, but the goal is for the patients to carry them out using previously acquired information processing strategies.

The first module in the program, cognitive flexibility, was investigated by Delahunty *et al.* (1993) who found that there were improvements in the WCST performance post-treatment which were maintained at 6 month follow-up. There were also improvements in social functioning and symptom measures. A further trial of the whole program from the same laboratory also showed modest improvements on a range of test scores, with many people achieving normal performance following treatment. However, social functioning was not measured in this study and so it is not clear whether these improvements generalized to other tasks (A. Delahunty and R. Morice, personal communication). Recently, a randomized control trial of the program was completed at an independent laboratory in which the cognitive remediation program was tested against a condition where patients received an attention control therapy with high face validity. This design allows the specificity of the deficits to be assessed as in the Nebraska trial. The patients entering the trial were highly symptomatic but also had social and cognitive disability. The results were very encouraging. At post-treatment, there were differential improvements in test scores in favor of cognitive remediation. For tests within the domains of memory and cognitive flexibility, there were also generalized improvements. When they reached a threshold (>50% of tests improved), there were concomitant improvements in social functioning (Wykes *et al.*, 1999). The program also had a direct effect on improving self-esteem in the experimental group, whereas the other therapy produced no change.

These studies clearly support the need for an extended research program, as the results do seem to have promise for improving aspects of a patient's life which have validity for both the patients and the services. They also support the theoretical relationship between cognitive deficits and social functioning as suggested by Green (1998). More importantly, however, these results emphasize the need for integrated studies of cognitive and psychosocial rehabilitation programs. This is particularly important in offsetting the costs of treatment. There may be also be effects of remediation on future symptom recurrence (Nuechterlein and Subotnik, 1998) which are likely to be long-term outcomes only measurable over years rather than the few months of the current studies. This is particularly problematical if what remediation is changing is mediating vulnerability indicators, as the effects of these changes are unlikely to be noticed unless the information processing system is stressed in some way. Substantial and measurable increases in these irregular stressors in the environment make it unlikely that the effects would be obvious for a number of years.

What factors should be considered for the next set of remediation studies?

What form(s) of remediation should we adopt?

One problem in the teaching of 'thinking' has been the lack of a model of what activities should be taught and how. One useful model has been expounded by Baron (1985, 1994). He suggested that there are two main components of thinking: cognitive capacities and thinking dispositions. Cognitive capacities are "ability parameters. . . . . .which affect success at tasks and which cannot be improved by instruction" (Baron, 1985, p. 14). They include perceptual speed, working memory capacity and response inhibition, and are not thought to be very malleable although they might be affected by practice. In contrast, thinking dispositions are those factors "which affect success in psychological tasks and that *are* subject to control by instruction" (Baron, 1985 p. 15, italics in the original). These parameters affect the amount of time someone will spend on a task, the willingness to switch perspectives and the disposition to weigh evidence against a personally held belief, etc. These dispositions are learnt tendencies to behave in certain ways.

According to Baron's conception, cognitive capacities cannot be affected by anything other than practice, whereas thinking dispositions can be affected by instruction. The remediation studies reviewed above certainly support this distinction. Improved performance on neuropsychological tasks has been found with extended practice but does not generalize to other similar tasks (e.g. Benedict *et al.*, 1994; Wexler *et al.*, 1997). Practice in itself, of course, may be important to a specific task. It is widely assumed that practice reduces effort on a task or sub-task, and with sufficient practice a sub-task may be performed with virtually no conscious effort at all. Practice may also reduce the need for controlled processing and, therefore, tasks become more automatic. The more sub-tasks that become automatic the more skillful performance becomes. However, practice in the discrimination of Hindi script is not likely to have a carryover effect to the reading of this chapter, despite the fact that both tasks require the visual discrimination of letters. The data on the specificity of practice effects have changed little since Thorndike and Woodworth reported it in 1901. One of the most dramatic replications was a mnemonist who, by practice, increased his digit span from seven to 79 digits after months of training. However, even after all this training, his span for remembering letters had not changed at all (Ericsson *et al.*, 1980). The role of practice in cognitive rehabilitation must be re-evaluated. It clearly has a place in all programs but not a central role if the object of training is the transfer of skills.

Thinking dispositions in Baron's (1985) theory could be extended to the disposition to adopt certain strategies for processing information, such as chunking information or using mnemonic techniques. It is clear that when instructed to use strategies, patients with schizophrenia can improve their performance. Therefore, it is possible for them to use strategies effectively. In order to get any transfer of the use of the technique, not only do educators need to teach these strategies but the learner must also understand the relevance of the strategy to new situations (Brown *et al.*, 1979). This transfer may therefore by affected by the familiarity of the material and the ability to distinguish relevant factors across different task situations. Normal individual variation in the use of strategies has only been appreciated recently by researchers in the field of neuropsychological rehabilitation. For instance, Della Sala and Logie (1997) review the well-known phonological similarity and word length effects in short-term verbal memory and show that they depend on the type of mnemonic technique used in the task. They report that in the normal population there is variability in the use of mnemonic techniques not only between individuals in the same task but within individuals across several similar tasks. So participants in memory tests who have been drawn from the normal population may evaluate the goal, and the best means to achieve the goal, very differently from each other and between different test situations. This normative information is vital in the development of more sophisticated 'thinking' rehabilitation programs as it emphasizes the need for variability and not prescription in the teaching of techniques.

The criticism of the remediation approaches so far is based mainly on how little impact information on the techniques of teaching 'thinking' has had on the design of the interventions. A further example of this is another well-replicated result, that extrinsic reinforcement is not helpful in educational settings (Amabile *et al.*, 1986). For example, children given a set of new felt tip pens who were told that they might get a certificate for a well produced picture were less likely to play with the pens at a later date than those who were not told but actually did receive a certificate (Lepper and Greene, 1978). The children in this experiment seemed to have concentrated on the extrinsic reward which weakened their belief that they played with the pens because of intrinsic reward. Therefore, the motivation for drawing out of intrinsic interest was also reduced. Despite these kinds of studies, several investigators have used monetary reward as a motivator. They too generally have found that when reinforcement was removed there was little evidence of learning transfer. Most poorly paid academics would agree that external reward is not the sole motivating factor for effort and, in situations where mental effort is required to learn a rule-governed test, it may in fact be a distractor. Rehabilitation practitioners need to make the process of cognitive remediation intrinsically rewarding to patients if they are to make gains which are durable.

The only system of teaching thinking which is supported by educational and cognitive psychology research is scaffolding (Wood, 1998). This technique encourages the learner to take an active role in the learning process but maintains a high level of intrinsic reward because tasks are pitched just above current achievement. This type of teaching may also aid thinking dispositions because it gives the learner the opportunity to investigate success following a re-evaluation of a goal or following a more detailed search of alternative responses. As patients with schizophrenia often respond impulsively, a change in 'thinking disposition' might aid reflection, which would improve performance. Programs based on this type of teaching have also proved to be very successful.

The role of self-esteem

In the teaching of thinking skills, the effects on self-efficacy and self-esteem are vital because they will affect several of the thinking dispositions. For example, improved self-efficacy may encourage a person to spend a little more time on a task and to examine more alternative hypotheses which may achieve better performance. However, few studies have tested the effects of remediation on self-esteem. It has been noticed anecdotally that in attention training, patients' self-esteem and social status seemed to be improved as they boasted of their involvement in the program to other staff and patients (Medalia *et al.*, 1998). Another study which measured the effects directly and quantitatively also showed that self-esteem was improved in the remediation group compared with the control therapy group which also had high face validity (Wykes *et al.*, 1999). The effect in this latter study is likely to result from patients receiving ongoing positive feedback not only from the therapist but from their inspection of their own performance throughout the task. Future studies should measure directly the effects of cognitive remediation on self-esteem using qualitative measures. This effect may be as important as the effect on neuropsychological performance if there is to be a transfer of training to new tasks.

Individual variation effects

A number of issues of individual variation need to be investigated in the next generation of studies.

Patterning of impairments

The pattern of disabilities in schizophrenia, although showing some general trends (Shallice *et al.*, 1991), can also show some individual variation particularly in executive functions (Evans *et al.*, 1997). These patterns can affect the results of remediation studies. For instance, performance on the WCST could be affected by the inability to learn new concepts, to deal with novel situations, to plan and initiate a strategy for test performance, poor working memory or poor response inhibition and cognitive flexibility. Variable results from laboratory studies could be explained purely on differences in the patterning of deficits in different samples. The power of most of the laboratory or clinical studies does not allow any stratification of the samples, but it is possible to employ a case study approach (cf. Laws *et al.*, 1998) which could suggest hypotheses for further study.

Effectiveness of instruction

The variable responding of patients to the IPT group treatment has sometimes been attributed to an individual's responses at different stages of the sub-program (Spaulding *et al.*, 1998). It may be difficult to provide an optimal learning environment in a group setting when patients differ in their abilities and when they may require more practice on some parts of a program than others. Individual treatment is, however, expensive, and so the effects of treatment must outweigh the added expense of providing more intense therapy.

Different instructional tools may be relevant for different aspects of task performance and this will make the interpretation of results more complex. For example, Rossell and David (1997) found that when their patients learnt to manipulate categories in the WCST they still had high perseverative error rates following training. Here it seems that the training was specific—training in categorization had effects only on categorization. Perhaps scaffolded training on categories, in addition to training to prevent perseveration such as verbalization of the action pattern required for a response, would improve performance overall.

Other studies too report some differences in the level of gains made on the tasks through training. Stratta *et al.* (1994) report three general patterns of performance: (i) those who were reasonably good on the pre-test then improved further with training, and this improvement was maintained at follow-up; (ii) some who were poor on the pre-test did improve with training, but these patients did not retain these training effects; and finally (iii) a minority who were poor on the pre-test and did not change their performance with training. These last patients were characterized by longer duration of illness and more negative symptoms. The effects of training therefore only appear durable for patients with the least deficit initially. This does not mean that patients with larger deficits cannot learn but that this particular program does not produce durable gains for this group. Information on lack of gains is vital to the development of more effective programs. Most remediation studies report gains via parametric analyses, but few investigate whether the statistically significant pattern is evident in the majority of patients. Therefore, variable responding is not obvious. Researchers should bear in mind that statistically significant improvements can be found with only half the patients in a cohort actually showing an improvement in test performance, with the other half being impervious to change.

It is still unclear what aspects of task performance remediation are actually changing, and this may of course differ between individuals. For example, Wykes (1998) illustrated this problem with a description of two patients who had participated in a cognitive remediation program and who also had SPECT brain image scans. Both patients improved their scores on the verbal fluency test from pre- to post-test; however, they achieved their improved scores in different ways. At post-test, the first participant increased his output but, despite increasing his errors (repetitions, non-words, etc.), he still achieved an overall increase in score. This person increased his output but was not self-monitoring prior to response selection. The second participant decreased his overall verbal output but he also decreased the number of errors, and so again increased his overall score. So, in contrast to the first man, he had increased his monitoring. The blood flow changes in the SPECT scans mirrored these two different strategies. They were also exhibited in other tests. Performance changes on the Tower of London showed a proportional decrease in planning time for the person who monitored less and a proportional increase in planning time for the person who was monitoring more. There was another difference between these two patients—their symptoms. The person who decreased his monitoring showed many positive symptoms at entry to the trial, whereas the second person showed mainly negative symptoms, i.e. the patients differed in their behavioral output even prior to the start of the trial. So what seemed to be changed by the cognitive remediation program was an accentuation of a strategy which had already been adopted. Both strategies clearly have their limitations if they are to be translated into everyday life.

Future prospects

From the evidence provided in this chapter, it is clear that cognitive remediation, in the sense of improvement in neuropsychological test performance, is possible with psychological interventions. These techniques, however, have not been popular. Chapters 12 to 16 reported evidence on the effects (both positive and negative) of pharmacological agents on cognition, whereas there was only one chapter on psychological approaches. What is needed for psychological interventions is a 'product champion' and the necessary funding for a substantial program of innovative research. Just in case there is any response to this advert, Table 17.3 gives a few suggestions for this next phase. It includes a recommendation for a set of studies on the interactions between remediation and pharmacotherapy which may prove to be additive, multiplicative or just complementary. If remediation researchers are going to succeed in this next phase, they must improve their thinking dispositions so that they take cognisance of the alternative evidence which is available (and highly replicated) in the educational and cognitive psychology fields. To go back to the quotation at the beginning of this chapter—we do have a partly written manual if only we rehabilitation researchers would refer to it.

Table 17.3 Some recommendation for the next phase of remediation studies

---
- To use theoretical approaches to instructional training developed in the educational field e.g. scaffolding (Wood, 1998) to develop training packages
- All evaluations (laboratory and clinical) should adhere to the following:
  to characterize participants comprehensively with a wide range of cognitive, symptomatic and behavioral measures
  to link hypotheses of specific remediation to specific outcomes, i.e. cognitive flexibility training should improve tasks of cognitive flexibility but have little impact on planning
  to evaluate improvements not only on well known neuropsychological tests but also on more ecologically valid tests of everyday performance and also on brain imaging
- To evaluate the interaction between cognitive remediation and pharmacological treatment.

References

Adams, H.E., Malatesta, V.J., Brantley, P.J. and Turkat, I.D. (1981) Modification of cognitive processes: a case study of schizophrenia. *Journal of Consulting and Clinical Psychology*, **49**, 460–464.

Amabile, T.M., Hennessey, B.A. and Grossman, B.S. (1986) Social influences on creativity: the effects of contracted-for reward. *Journal of Personality and Social Psychology*, **50**, 14–23.

Baddeley, A. and Wilson, B.A. (1994) When implicit learning fails: amnesia and the problem of error elimination. *Neuropsychologia*, **32**, 53–68.

Baron, J. (1985) *Rationality and Intelligence*. Cambridge University Press, Cambridge.

Baron, J. (1994) *Thinking and Deciding*. 2nd edn Cambridge University Press, Cambridge.

Bellack, A.S., Blanchard, J.J., Murphy, P. and Podell, K. (1996) Generalization effects of training on the Wisconsin Card Sorting Test for schizophrenia patients. *Schizophrenia Research*, **19**, 189–194.

Bellack, A.S., Mueser, K.T., Morrison, R.L., Tierney, A. and Podell, K. (1990) Remediation of cognitive deficits in schizophrenia. *American Journal of Psychiatry*, **147**, 1650–1655.

Benedict R.H. and Harris A.E. (1989) Remediation of attention deficits in chronic schizophrenia patients: a preliminary study. *British Journal of Clinical Psychology*, **28**, 187–188.

Benedict, R.H.B., Harris, A.E., Markow, T., McCormick, J.A., Nuechterlein, K.H. and Asarnow, R.F. (1994) Effects of attention training on information processing in schizophrenia. *Schizophrenia Bulletin*, **20**, 537–546.

Brenner, H.D., Roder, V., Hodel, B., Kienzle, N., Reed, D. and Liberman, R.P. (1994) *Integrated Psychological Therapy for Schizophrenic Patients (IPT)*. Hogrefe and Huber Publishers, Göttingen, Germany.

Brown A.L., Campione J.C. and Barclay C.R. (1979) Training self checking routines for estimating test readiness: generalization from list learning to prose recall. *Child Development*, **50**, 501–512.

Brown, C., Harwood, K., Hays, C., Heckman, J. and Short, J. E. (1993) Effectiveness of cognitive rehabilitation for improving attention in patients with schizophrenia. *Occupational Therapy Journal of Research*, **3**, 71–86.

Bryson, G., Bell, M. and Lysaker, P. (1997) Affect recognition in schizophrenia: a function of global impairment or a specific cognitive deficit. *Psychiatry Research*, **71**, 105–113.

Delahunty, A. and Morice, R. (1993) *A Training Programme for the Remediation of Cognitive Deficits in Schizophrenia*. Department of Health, Albury, NSW.

Delahunty, A., Morice, R. and Frost, B. (1993) Specific cognitive flexibility rehabilitation in schizophrenia. *Psychological Medicine*, **23**, 221–227.

Della Sala, S. and Logie, R.H. (1997) Impairments of methodology and theory in cognitive neuropsychology: a case for rehabilitation? *Neuropsychological Rehabilitation*, **7**, 367–385.

Ericsson, K.A., Chase W.G. and Faloon S. (1980) Acquisition of memory skill. *Science*, **208**, 1181–1182.

Evans, J.J., Chua, S.E., McKenna, P.J. and Wilson, B.A. (1997) Assessment of the dysexecutive syndrome in schizophrenia. *Psychological Medicine*, **27**, 635–646.

Field, C.D., Galletly, C., Anderson, D. and Walker, P. (1997) Computer-aided cognitive rehabilitation: possible application to the attentional deficit of schizophrenia, a report of negative results. *Perceptual and Motor Skills*, **85**, 995–1002.

Frith, C.D. (1992) *The Cognitive Neuropsychology of Schizophrenia*. Lawrence Erlbaum Associates, Inc., Hove, UK.

Goldberg T.E. and Weinberger, D.R. (1994) Schizophrenia, training paradigms, and the Wisconsin Card Sorting Test redux. *Schizophrenia Research*, **11**, 291–296.

Goldberg, T.E., Weinberger, D.R., Berman, K.F., Pliskin, N.H. and Podd, M.H. (1987) Further evidence for dementia of the prefrontal type in schizophrenia? A controlled study of teaching the Wisconsin Card Sorting Test. *Archives of General Psychiatry*, **44**, 1008–1014.

Goldman, R.S., Axelrod, B.N. and Tompkins, L.M. (1992) Effect of instructional cues on schizophrenia patients' performance on the Wisconsin Card Sorting Test. *American Journal of Psychiatry*, **149**, 1718–1722.

Green, M.F. (1993) Cognitive remediation in schizophrenia: is it time yet? *American Journal of Psychiatry*, **150**, 178–187.

Green M.F. (1996) What are the functional consequences of neurocognitive deficits in schizophrenia. *American Journal of Psychiatry*, **153**, 321–330.

Green, M.F. (1998) *Schizophrenia From a Neurocognitive Perspective: Probing the Impenetrable Darkness*. Allyn & Bacon, Needhan Heights, MA.

Green, M.F., Satz, P., Ganzell, S. and Vaclav, J.F. (1992) Wisconsin Card Sorting Test performance in schizophrenia: remediation of a stubborn deficit. *American Journal of Psychiatry*, **149**, 62–67.

Hermanutz, M. and Gestrich, J. (1991) Computer-assisted attention training in schizophrenics. A comparative study. *European Archives of Psychiatry and Clinical Neurosciences*, **240**, 282–287.

Hodel, B. and Brenner, H.D. (1994) Cognitive therapy with schizophrenic patients: conceptual basis, present state, future directions. *Acta Psychiatrica Scandinavica Supplement*, **90**, 108–115.

Hunkin, N. Squires, E.J., Parkin, A.J. and Tidy, J.A. (1998) Are the benefits of errorless learning dependent on implicit memory? *Neuropsychologia*, **36**, 25–36.

Jaeger, J. and Douglas, E. (1992) Neuropsychiatric rehabilitation for persistent mental illness. *Psychiatric Quarterly*, **63**, 71–94.

Keefe, R.S.E. (1995) The contribution of neuropsychology to psychiatry. *American Journal of Psychiatry*, **152**, 6–15.

Kern, R.S., Wallace, C.J., Hellman, S.G., Womack, L.M. and Green, M.F. (1996) A training procedure for remediating WCST deficits in chronic psychotic patients: an adaptation of errorless learning principles. *Journal of Psychiatry Research*, **30**, 283–294.

Koh, S.D. and Peterson, R.A. (1978) Encoding orientation and the remembering of schizophrenic young adults. *Journal of Abnormal Psychology*, **87**, 303–313.

Kuipers E., Garety P., Fowler D., Dunn G., Bebbington P., Freeman D. and Hadley, C. (1997) London–East Anglia randomised control trial of cognitive behavioural therapy for psychosis. I. Effects of treatment phase. *British Journal of Psychiatry*, **171**, 319–327.

Laws, K.R., McKenna, P.J., Kondel, T.K. (1998) On the distinction between access and store disorders in schizophrenia: A question of deficit severity? *Neuropsychologia*, **36**, 313–321.

Lepper, M.R. and Greene, D. (eds) (1978) *The Hidden Costs of Reward*. Erlbaum, Hillsdale, NJ.

Lysaker, P. and Bell, M. (1995) Work rehabilitation and improvements in insight in schizophrenia. *Journal of Nervous and Mental Disease*, **183**, 103–106.

Machado, L.A. (1980) *The Right to be Intelligent*. Pergamon Press, Oxford.

Medalia, A., Aluma, M., Tryon, W. and Merriam, A.E. (1998) Effectiveness of attention training in schizophrenia. *Schizophrenia Bulletin*, **24**, 147–152.

Meichenbaum, D. and Cameron, R. (1973) Training schizophrenics to talk to themselves: a means of developing attentional controls. *Behavior Therapy*, **4**, 515–534.

Metz, J.T., Johnson, M.D., Pliskin, N.H. and Luchins, D.J. (1994) Maintenance of training effects on the Wisconsin Card Sorting Test by patients with schizophrenia or affective disorders. *American Journal of Psychiatry*, **151**, 120–122.

Morice, R. and Delahunty, A. (1996) Frontal/executive impairments in schizophrenia. *Schizophrenia Bulletin*, **22**, 125–137.

Morris, R.G., Rushe, T., Woodruffe, P.W.R. and Murray, R.M. (1995) Problem solving in schizophrenia: a specific deficit in planning ability. *Schizophrenia Research*, **14**, 235–246.

Mueser, K.T., Bellack, A., Douglas, M.S. and Wade, J. (1991) Prediction of social skill acquisition in schizophrenic and major affective disorder patients from memory and symptomatology. *Psychiatry Research*, **37**, 281–296

Nuechterlein, K.H. and Dawson, M.E. (1984) A heuristic vulnerability/stress model of schizophrenic episodes. *Schizophrenia Bulletin*, **18**, 387–425.

Nuechterlein, K.H., Dawson, M.E., Green, M.F. (1994) Information processing abnormalities as neuropsychological vulnerability indicators for schizophrenia. *Acta Psychiatrica Scandinavica*, **90(384)**, 71–79.

Nuechterlein, K.H. and Subotnik, K. (1998) The cognitive origins of schizophrenia and prospects for intervention. In: Wykes, T., Tarrier, N. and Lewis, S. (eds), *Outcome and Innovation in Psychological Treatment of Schizophrenia*. Wiley, Chichester, UK, pp. 17–42.

O'Carroll, R.E., Russell, H.H., Lawrie, S.M. and Johnstone, E.C. (1999) Errorless learning and the cognitive rehabilitation of memory impaired schizophrenic patients. *Psychological Medicine*, **29(1)**, 105–112.

Olbrich, R. and Mussgay, L. (1990) Reduction of schizophrenic deficits by cognitive training: an evaluative study. *European Archives of Psychiatry and Clinical Neurosciences*, **239**, 366–369.

Penn, D.L., Spaulding, W., Reed, D. and Sullivan, M. (1996) The relationship of social cognition to ward behavior in chronic schizophrenia. *Schizophrenia Research*, **20**, 327–335.

Rossell, S.L. and David, A.S. (1997) Improving performance on the WCST: variations on the original procedure. *Schizophrenia Research*, **28**, 63–76.

Shallice T. W. (1988) *From Neuropsychology to Mental Structure*. Cambridge University Press, Cambridge.

Shallice, T., Burgess, P. and Frith, C. (1991) Can the neuropsychological case-study approach be applied to schizophrenia. *Psychological Medicine*, **21**, 661–673.

Spaulding, W., Reed, D., Storzbach, D., Sullivan, M., Weiler, M. and Richardson, C. (1998) The effects of remediational approach to cognitive therapy for schizophrenia. In: Wykes, T., Tarrier, N. and Lewis, S. (eds), *Outcome and Innovation in Psychological Treatment of Schizophrenia*. Wiley, Chichester, UK, pp. 145–160.

Spaulding, W., Fleming, S.K., Reed, D., Sullivan, M., Storzback, D., Lam, M. (1999) Cognitive functioning in schizophrenia: Implications for psychiatric rehabilitation. *Schizophrenia Bulletin*, **25**, 275–290.

Startup, M. (1996) Insight and cognitive deficits in schizophrenia: evidence for a curvilinear relationship. *Psychological Medicine*, **26**, 1277–1281.

Steffy, R.A. and Galbraith, K. J. (1980) Relation between latency and redundancy-associated deficit in schizophrenic reaction time performance. *Journal of Abnormal Psychology*, **89**, 419–427.

Stratta, P., Mancini, F., Mattei, P., Casacchia, M. and Rossi, A. (1994) Information processing strategy to remediate Wisconsin Card Sorting Test performance in schizophrenia: a pilot study. *American Journal of Psychiatry*, **151**, 915–918.

Summerfelt, A.T., Alphs, L.D., Wagman, A.M.I., Funderburk, F.R., Hierholzer, R.M. and Strauss, M.E. (1991) Reduction of perseverative errors in patients with schizophrenia using monetary feedback. *Journal of Abnormal Psychology*, **100**, 613–616.

Terrace, H.S. (1963) Discrimination learning with and without errors. *Journal of Experimental Analysis of Behavior*, **6**, 1–27.

Thorndike, E.L. and Woodworth, R.R. (1901) The influence of improvement in one mental function upon the efficiency of other functions. *Psychological Review*, **8**, 247–261

Van der Gaag, M. (1992) *The Results of Cognitive Training in Schizophrenia Patients.* Eburon, Delft, The Netherlands.

Vollema, M.G., Geurtsen, G.J. and van Voorst, A.J.P. (1995) Durable improvements in Wisconsin Card Sorting Test performance in schizophrenic patients. *Schizophrenia Research*, **16**, 209–215.

Vygotsky, L.S. (1962) *Thought and Language.* Wiley, NY.

Wexler, B.E., Hawkins, K.A., Rounsaville, B., Anderson, M., Sernyak, M.J. and Green, M.F. (1997) Normal neurocognitive performance after extended practice in patients with schizophrenia. *Schizophrenia-Research*, **26**, 173–180.

Wood, D. (1998) *How Children Think and Learn: The Social Contexts of Cognitive Development.* 2nd edn. Blackwell Publishers, Inc., Oxford.

Wykes, T. (1994) Predicting symptomatic and behavioural outcomes of community care. *British Journal of Psychiatry*, **165**, 486–492.

Wykes, T. (1998) What are we changing with neurocognitive rehabilitation? Illustrations from two single cases of changes in neuropsychological performance and brain systems as measured by SPECT *Schizophrenia Research*, **34**, 77–86.

Wykes, T. and Dunn. G. (1992) Cognitive deficit and the prediction of rehabilitation success in a chronic psychiatric group. *Psychological Medicine*, **22**, 389–398.

Wykes, T., Tarrier, N. and Lewis, S. (eds) (1998) *Outcome and Innovation in Psychological Treatment of Schizophrenia.* Wiley, Chichester, UK.

Wykes, T., Reeder, C., Corner, J., Williams, C. and Everitt, B. (1999) The effects of neurocognitive remediation on executive processing in patients with schizophrenia. *Schizophrenia Bulletin*, **25**, 291–308.

Young, D.A. and Freyslinger, M.G. (1995) Scaffolded instruction and the remediation of Wisconsin Card Sorting Test deficits in chronic schizophrenia. *Schizophrenia Research*, **16**, 199–207.

Conclusions

Cognitive impairment is now recognized as an important feature of schizophrenia. It is common for patients with schizophrenia to perform poorly on a wide range of cognitive tests, with this fact recognized for the past 50 years. Patients with more severe cognitive impairments are more likely to have more severe negative symptoms and deficits in adaptive functioning. Overall outcome is also correlated with cognitive impairments, with patients with a chronic course of illness more likely to perform poorly on cognitive tests than patients with more episodic illnesses. This relationship is also present on a longitudinal, predictive basis, in that more severe cognitive impairment early in the course of illness predicts a more adverse outcome over time.

Impairments in cognitive functioning commonly are believed to be a consequence of other aspects of the illness, including severe hallucinations or delusions, poor motivation or iatrogenic effects of treatment. These factors are actually of considerably less importance in terms of cognitive functioning than would be expected at first glance. The potential causal role of positive symptoms is undermined by the finding that cognitive impairments are found to be unchanged in severity after the remission of positive symptoms following an acute episode. Thus, the severity of positive symptoms is uncorrelated with the severity of cognitive impairments within individual patients. Since positive symptom severity repeatedly has been found to be uncorrelated with the severity of most cognitive impairments in large samples of patients with schizophrenia, hallucinations and delusions are uncorrelated with most common neuropsychological measures of cognitive functioning within, as well as across, patients.

Poor motivation is not a good explanation for cognitive impairments in schizophrenia, because of the well-known finding that different aspects of cognitive functioning in schizophrenia vary in their average level of impairment. If cognitive impairments were being produced by a global factor such as poor motivation, there is no explanation for why some cognitive tests are performed at levels consistent with the patient's level of premorbid functioning and other are performed 3–5 standard deviations more poorly. The very notion of identification of differential deficits, known for years to be a desirable methodological goal, would be implausible if poor motivation caused all cognitive impairment. Finally, somatic treatments in schizophrenia cannot be the main cause of cognitive deficits. First, cognitive deficits were noted historically before somatic treatments for schizophrenia were developed. Second, cognitive impairment is common and can be severe in neuroleptic-naive patients. Third, typical neuroleptic medication has been demonstrated repeatedly to have no effects on the majority of aspects of cognitive functioning in schizophrenia, other than improving a limited set of attentional functions. Anticholinergic medications co-administered with typical neuroleptics have been shown in the past to worsen various aspects of memory functioning, but patients who are not treated with anticholinergics also have memory deficits Thus, cognitive functioning is an intrinsic part of schizophrenia, endogenous to the illness, and is not completely accounted for by correlates of schizophrenia or its treatment.

Despite the ease with which these statements are made, the typical clinician working with patients with schizophrenia does not know these facts. In addition, much of the academic community studying schizophrenia is often unconcerned about or unaware of new advances in the treatment of this illness and how it can impact on cognition. As a result, the current book fills a critical need.

This book is divided into three sections. The first section provides high level but readable background information on the important aspects of cognitive functioning in schizophrenia. The second section provides information on the correlates of cognitive functioning, in the domains of correlations with classical symptoms of the illness as well as with social and adaptive functional deficits. The final section provides information on the treatment of cognitive functioning in schizophrenia, from the older less effective treatments with conventional antipsychotics, to current results with novel antipsychotics, to developing treatment strategies using experimental compounds and off-label uses for the medications.

Each of the chapters is written by individuals who are acknowledged to be at the forefront of the area. The coverage is also wide and comprehensive, but is also focused within each chapter. The result is a comprehensive set of relatively brief and readable chapters that avoid the broad-brush coverage typical of wide-ranging review articles that attempt to cover all aspects of the field and are often written by individuals whose expertise in some of the areas is limited.

Index

A77636 305
N-acetyl-aspartate:creatine ratio 83
N-acetyl-aspartyl-glutamate 138
acetylcholine 313–15
  drugs increasing cholinergic transmission
    314–15
  drugs stimulating M1/M4 muscarinic receptors
    315
  implications for schizophrenia 314
  role in cognition 313–14
acute schizophrenia 211
α_2-adrenergic receptor
  in prefrontal cortex, drugs stimulating 311–12
  role in cognition 309
β-adrenergic receptors, drugs stimulating 312
affective flattening 194
affect perception 183, 185–6
age of onset 11
Age Scaled Scores 11
alogia 162
alternating semantic categories test 17
Alzheimer's disease 79, 141, 184, 269, 311,
  313
Alzheimer's Disease Assessment Scale 315
amantidine, and psychosis 131
α-amino-3-hydroxy-5-methyl-4-
  isoxazoleproprionate (AMPA) 126, 316
  receptor 316–17
amisulpride and cognitive enhancement 292
AMPA *see* α-amino-3-hydroxy-5-methyl-4-
  isoxazoleproprionate
ampakines 317, 318
amphetamine 309, 312
  attention 132
  ketamine psychosis 132
  prefrontal cortex 306–7
anhedonia 194
anticholinergics, abuse of 277
antipsychotics 241–65, 274–6
  atypical 275–6
    cognitive enhancement 291–5

executive dysfunction 62–3
typical 274
see also individual drugs
aphasia 107
arecoline, and working memory 271
aripipazole
  cognitive enhancement 293, 294
  prefrontal cortex dopamine 307
articulatory loop 18
articulatory suppression 19
aspartate, altered binding of 138
atropine 313
  and short-term memory 270
attention
  drugs affecting
    amphetamine 132
    clozapine 132
    haloperidol 132, 133
    ketamine 132
    lorazepam 132, 133
  selective 56
  supervisory attentional system 21–2, 25–8,
    132
  sustained 179–80
  and working memory 132–3
  see also information processing
attention deficit hyperactivity disorder 311
Auditory Consonant Trigrams Test 26
Auditory Continuous Performance Test 17
auditory verbal hallucinations 93, 213
autonoetic agnosia 36
avolition 194

backward masking 165
basolateral amygdala 312
benztropine 274, 275
  receptor binding 276
  and working memory 42, 273
bias
  response 117
  self-serving 218